Elizabeth Bradshaw.

UNDER THE INFLUENCE

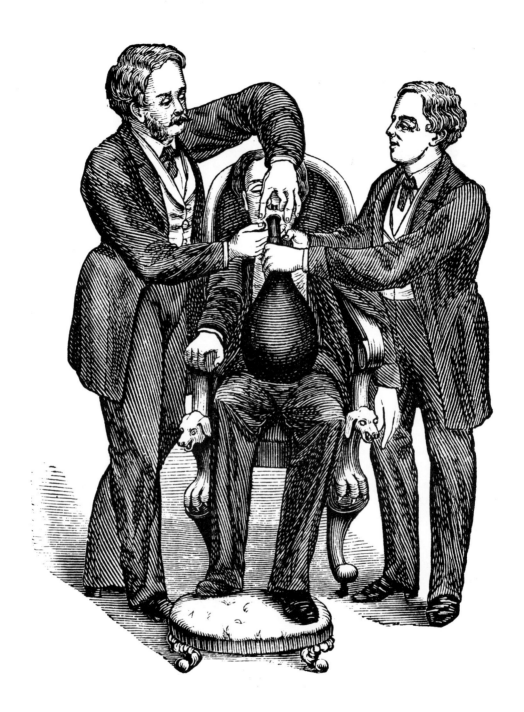

The patient is seated as represented. All the teeth to be extracted, it is presumed, have been examined. A napkin or rubber apron is then placed before him . . . to prevent soiling the clothing with blood. The prop is then placed between the teeth, on the side opposite to that from which the teeth are to be removed. The patient is then instructed to make a long exhalation, in order to empty the lungs as far as possible of atmospheric air. Immediately upon completion of this effort, the assistant should place the tube in the mouth, and the operator proceed to close the nostrils and the lips, as represented in the cut. Then request the patient to inhale and exhale freely through the tube. As soon as this is performed regularly, his mind should be diverted as much as possible from the operation by encouraging and cheerful conversation. Snoring or heavy breathing will be perceived after a few inhalations, followed by a change of colour and twitching of the muscles. When three or four inhalations have occurred subsequent to the appearance of these symptoms, it is time to withdraw the tube. The assistant should remain by the side of the patient, so that, should restlessness occur, he may without delay render all necessary aid . . . . At the close of the operation, the patient's head should be inclined forward and the prop removed from between the teeth. The assistant should be prepared with a small spittoon for the use of the patient, until he has recovered sufficiently to resume control of his actions . . . .

In the one or two cases reported, it was subsequently proved that death was caused by debility, and might reasonably have been expected at any moment . . . .

The circumstances under which experience taught me to use extreme caution in its administration are as follows:

To persons of habitual intemperance.

In disease of the heart.

Pulmonary disease.

Excessive plethoric habit.

Debilitated dyspeptics.

Very aged people.

Children under seven years of age.

I feel confident that, if such cases are avoided, no one of ordinary skill need apprehend difficulty from nitrous oxide.

(Thomas, 1870)

By courtesy of the Wellcome Trustees

For

Ru, Adrian and Lucy

UNDER THE INFLUENCE

A History of Nitrous Oxide and Oxygen Anaesthesia

> Dr. Wells – who sat next to him – noticed the circumstance, and as the audience was retiring, asked me why a man could not have a tooth extracted without pain while under the influence of the gas . . . (Colton, 1886).

W. D. A. SMITH

First published 1982 by
Scientific and Medical Division
MACMILLAN PUBLISHERS LTD
London and Basingstoke
Companies and representatives throughout the
world

Printed in Great Britain by
Unwin Brothers Limited
The Gresham Press, Old Woking, Surrey

ISBN 0 333 31681 9

CONTENTS*

*Textual cross references between chapters quote the part numbers of the original series of articles published in the *British Journal of Anaesthesia*. The following parts about Henry Hill Hickman are not reproduced in this book:

Part IV: *Brit. J. Anaesth.* (1966), **38,** 58
Part IVA: *Brit. J. Anaesth.* (1970), **42,** 347
Part IVB: *Brit. J. Anaesth.* (1970), **42,** 445
Part IVC: *Brit. J. Anaesth.* (1978), **50,** 519
Part IVD: *Brit. J. Anaesth.* (1978), **50,** 623
Part IVE: *Brit. J. Anaesth.* (1978), **50,** 853

PREFACE

I know less about my ancestors than about some of the characters in this book, but a brief family history may help illustrate the significance of the discovery and practice of anaesthesia. My mother (1888 – 1951) was a freelance journalist whose several pseudonyms derived from an old family tree. She was twice anaesthetised for surgical operations although in her lifetime there was nothing remarkable about that. I never met her parents. Thomas Forster Brown, her father, was a mining engineer and my great great great uncle, Westgarth Forster (1772 – 1835), was a mining engineer and pioneer geologist (Forster, 1809; Nall, 1883): but otherwise her genealogy means little more to me than a pattern of names and dates. Her mother was said to regard dentists as socially inferior.

My father (A.W., 1884 – 1964) was a dental surgeon. He put up his plate in Bentinck Street, London, and then moved to Wimpole Street. In his later years he teased me that he was still entitled to administer dental anaesthetics and he thought that they were best given without oxygen. Dr Trewby (1883 – 1956) (fig. 0.1 and Chapter 13, fig. 9) usually anaesthetised his patients and sometimes my father would take over so that Trewby could do the extraction. There were four occasions when my father had reason to be grateful for general anaesthesia. The last of these was when, in his seventies, his remaining teeth were extracted. I have no doubt that he received plenty of oxygen.

My paternal grandfather (J.W., 1850 – 1930) was sent out into the world with a 'bob'[1] in his pocket at the age of sixteen. He cleaned the windows of a chemist shop, served behind the counter and eventually had his own pharmacy. Then he studied in the evenings to become a dentist and in due course set up practice in Bayswater, London. He died following an appendicectomy while on holiday in Hastings, but at least he had the benefit of general anaesthesia for

1 Slang for a shilling (5p).

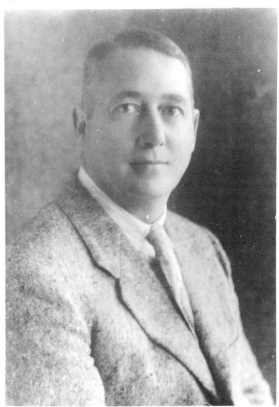

FIG. 0.1

Dr Joseph Frederick Trewby (1883 – 1956) with kind permission of his daughter, Mrs. A. B. Messum.

the operation. By a narrow margin his mother could have received chloroform for his birth; but I doubt that she did.

As a small boy my father was taken to see his ninety-five year old maternal grandmother whose memory reached back to the Napoleonic wars – certainly no obstetric anaesthesia for her.

Before 1846 surgical operations were brief and horrific although attitudes to pain were probably different from those of today and some surgeons even believed that pain contributed a desirable stimulus to recovery.[2] General anaesthesia was unknown. That the inhalation of ether could relieve much of this suffering was demonstrated on 16 October that year at the Massachusetts General Hospital, Boston, by William Thomas Green Morton. News of this crossed the Atlantic and spread world-wide. The way was set for anaesthesia and surgery as we know them today.

Horace Wells, however, had already demonstrated to his own satisfaction that pain relief during dental extraction could be achieved using nitrous oxide. In December 1844, he had one of his own teeth extracted, without any sensation of pain, after inhaling nitrous oxide and his immediate response was to exclaim, 'A new era in tooth pulling!' He repeated the experiment successfully on several patients in his home town of Hartford, and then, in 1845, he went to Boston to demonstrate his new method before a medical class: but his audience was unimpressed. Morton, who had been his pupil and for about four weeks his partner, had helped make the arrangements and was present.

Although there is record of Wells having used nitrous oxide during the removal of a testicle in August 1847, and then for an amputation and for removal of a fatty tumour in January 1848 (Archer, 1944), the greater potencies of ether and chloroform ensured their continued use during surgical operations in preference to nitrous oxide. Dental patients had to wait nearly twenty years for Gardner Quincey Colton (1814–1898), an itinerant lecturer, to introduce the 'new era in tooth pulling' using nitrous oxide (for accounts of itinerant lecturers see Gibbs, 1960 and Miles, 1968).[3] He set up branches of the Colton Dental Association throughout the United States for the extraction of teeth. Nitrous oxide returned to stay.

From that time nitrous oxide played an increasing part in general anaesthesia and analgesia. Today it is one of the most frequently used inhalation anaesthetics, although anaesthetists usually supplement it with other agents, either in order to reinforce its limited potency or to provide muscle relaxation, unless they are just using 50 per cent nitrous oxide in order to relieve pain without loss of consciousness (for an early pioneer of nitrous oxide analgesia see Richards et al., 1976).

AIRS, LAUGHING GAS AND ANAESTHESIA

The history of nitrous oxide begins with its discovery by Joseph Priestley in 1773 (Chapter 1). He called it dephlogisticated nitrous air. Shortly afterwards he identified dephlogisticated air – now called oxygen – and he urged physicians to explore the use of this and other gases in the treatment of their patients. Dr Thomas Beddoes took up the challenge and founded the Medical Pneumatic Institution in Bristol (Levere, 1977), equipping it with apparatus designed and supplied by James Watt of steam engine fame. Through James Watt's son, Gregory, Beddoes came to know young Humphry Davy and upon Mr Davies Giddy's recommendation Davy was employed as medical superintendent (Cartwright, 1952). Davy then made his mark with diverse experiments on nitrous oxide. His classic book describing these researches (Davy, 1800) led to his appointment at the Royal Institution (fig. 0.2). Having demonstrated that nitrous oxide was respirable, Davy found that the effects of breathing it could be hilarious. Furthermore he discovered that it could relieve toothache, so he suggested its use during surgical operations although neither he nor anyone else followed this up at the time. What Priestley had called dephlogisticated nitrous air was soon nicknamed 'laughing gas' and it was after seeing a demonstration of its inebriating effects at a popular lecture by Colton in 1844 that Wells tried the crucial experiment upon himself.[4]

When anaesthesia was fifty years old, Colton gave this account of its beginnings (Colton, 1886):

Dr Crawford W. Long performed a surgical operation while the patient was under the influence of Sulphuric Ether in 1842. But there is no evidence that he ever performed any other operation with it, or that he made any publication

---

2 For descriptions by patients of surgical operations see Riding (1963); Moore (1978); Wilson (1860); and Robinson (1946). For matter-of-fact descriptions of surgical operations in the 1830s by a trainee surgeon (son of John Collins Warren who permitted the first demonstrations of anaesthesia in Boston by Wells and Morton) see Jones (1978). A description of pre-anaesthetic surgery is given also in Cartwright (1952) and Irwin (1955). For early attitudes to anaesthesia see Farr (1977 and 1980).

3 For a delightful description of popular lectures given in Bristol in 1836 see Weller (1981).

4 Nitrous oxide 'trips' have been recorded in the twentieth century. Shedlin et al. (1973) give directions for getting 'high' – see also Dillon (1967); Daily Telegraph (1969); Smith (1971).

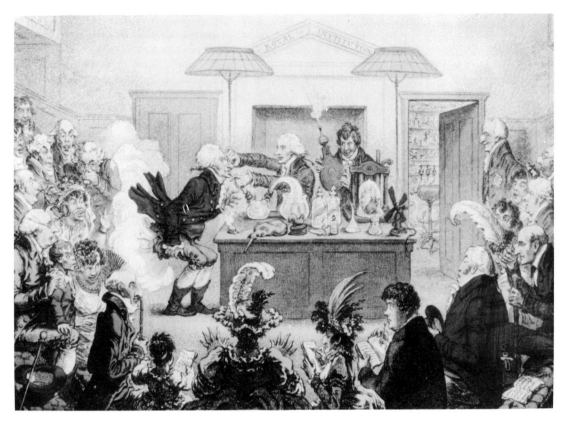

FIG. 0.2

Gillray's famous cartoon of 1802 showing Davy holding a pair of bellows at the Royal Institution. For further details see George (1947).

of it. Evidently he did not consider or claim that he had made a discovery . . . .

On the evening of 10th December, 1844, I gave an exhibition of the effects of laughing gas in the city of Hartford, Conn. Among those who inhaled it was a young man by the name of Cooley, who while under its influence, in jumping about, ran against some wooden benches or settees on the stage, bruising his legs badly . . . he was astonished to find his legs bloody; and said he did not know he had run against a bench, and felt no pain after the effects of the gas had passed off. Dr Wells – who sat next to him – noticed the circumstance, and as the audience was retiring, asked me why a man could not have a tooth extracted without pain while under the influence of the gas. I replied that I did not know, as the idea had never occurred to me. Dr Wells then said he . . . would try it upon himself if I would bring a bag of gas to his dental office . . . . The next morning . . . I . . . administered it to Wells,

and Dr Riggs extracted a molar tooth for him . . . . This was the *first* operation performed in modern anaesthesia, and it was a forerunner of all other anaesthetics . . . .

At the request of Dr Wells, I instructed him how to make the gas, and then went off on my exhibition business. Dr Wells got up the apparatus, made and tested the effects of the gas, and then went to Boston to make his discovery known. He called upon Dr Morton, his former pupil in dentistry, also on many other dentists and physicians, stating what he had discovered and done. They all treated him as a visionary enthusiast. He obtained permission of the elder Dr Warren to address a class in surgery at Cambridge College. At the close of his remarks, he administered the gas to a boy and extracted a tooth. The boy screamed out, though he said he didn't know when the tooth was drawn. The students, however, hissed, and pronounced the pretended discovery a humbug . . . . Wells returned to Hartford . . . . He used the gas during all the year 1845 . . . . During this year . . . no one claims that any dentist or surgeon used the gas, or any other anaesthetic, save Wells alone . . . .

During the month of September, 1846, Dr Morton went to Jackson, a chemist of Boston, to learn how to make the Nitrous Oxide or laughing gas, as he wished to test the truth of Wells's pretended discovery. Dr Jackson advised him to try Sulphuric Ether, and said, 'That gas exhilarates, makes people laugh, dance, etc. If that will destroy pain, Suphuric Ether will do the same', but he advised him not to incur the expense of the apparatus to make the gas. Upon this suggestion, Dr Morton purchased some ether and tried it on a boy named Eben Frost. This first experiment with Ether took place on 30th September, 1846 – almost two years after Wells had used the gas – and was suggested by Wells's experiment! Dr Morton reported the success of his operation to Dr Jackson, which they followed up by a series of experiments between them, with Ether. They applied jointly for a patent . . . . Morton, in order to mystify the public, called it 'Letheon' and began to sell the rights . . . . Dr Morton deserves great credit for his perseverance in pushing it into use and demonstration in the Massachusetts General Hospital . . . .

At the suggestion of Dr Marcy . . . Dr Wells tried Ether on one occasion . . . . But he did not like the symptoms and the odour was bad . . . .

When in New Haven in June, 1863, I was preparing to give an exhibition of the amusing effects of the gas, and invited a number of gentlemen to attend a private preliminary entertainment at which I gave a history of the discovery of anaesthesia, and detailed the experiments of Wells; stating also that I had never been able to induce a dentist to try the gas. Dr J. H. Smith, a distinguished dentist of New Haven said he would try the gas, provided I would administer it. I replied that I would be very glad to do it, as I wished to demonstrate what could be done with it . . . . The first patient who came in was a wealthy old lady, for whom we extracted seven teeth with the gas. On recovery she was so pleased with the result, that she said I might mention her name to my audience, and state that she had seven teeth extracted without pain, and without any ill or unpleasant effects from the gas. I

did so. In three weeks and two days, we extracted a little over three thousand teeth!

Whatever credit I deserve in connection with this matter is derived from the fact that I *revived* the use of the gas after it had been condemned, dead and forgotten as an anaesthetic from 1848 to 1863 . . . . That poor Wells failed to convince the world of its value does not mitigate in the slightest degree against the honour he deserves as the discoverer of anaesthesia. He did all that a man could do under the circumstances.[5]

Contemporary and later accounts differ in detail, emphasis and elaboration, according to personal involvement or to the favoured 'discoverer'. Many authors have taken sides (e.g. McQuitty, 1969) or dispensed orders of merit (e.g. Sykes, 1960). Cartwright (1952) on the other hand, took the view that no one person should be singled out as 'the discoverer' because all the early experimenters were interdependent. The rivalries between Morton, Jackson and Wells in particular were charged with bitterness and their lives ended unhappily. Wells committed suicide in 1848. Morton and Jackson battled on. Morton died of a stroke at the age of forty-eight when visiting New York to uphold his claim. Jackson became an alcoholic, then spent the last seven years of his life in an asylum, dying in 1880 at the age of seventy-five.

In Chapter 6 I have played down the question of who 'discovered' anaesthesia, for the reason stated therein and because the answer must depend upon the precise definition of a discovery. I may also be suspect of partiality. It is certainly because my main theme is nitrous oxide and not any other anaesthetic that I have chosen Colton to quote at length. In so doing I have selected someone who was actively involved from the beginning without staking any claims to the 'discovery' for himself, who lived long enough to see anaesthesia in perspective, who was respected on both sides of the Atlantic and who

5 Other contemporary accounts well worth reading are those of H. J. Bigelow (1846) which includes good examples of amnalgesia, Crawford Long (1849) and J. Marion Sims (1877). These have been reprinted by the Wood Library-Museum in Chicago. See also Bigelow (1876). Colton (1873) also gave an earlier account which described three administrations for dental extractions at New Britain, Conn., in 1862. The dentist involved then used the gas successfully in over 600 patients during the following year. In 1863 he joined forces with Dr J. H. Smith and Colton in New Haven for three weeks. Colton (1888) neglected to mention the episode of 1862 in his later account.

remained sane. When he was 74 years old, Colton gave this insight into his early upbringing:

> When I was a boy in the country, my good orthodox minister thought it very sinful to read a play of Shakespeare. Probably he never read a play himself, and never dreamed that the same lessons he taught from the pulpit were reproduced in these plays, in which vice and virtue receive their proper reward (Colton, 1888).

ON READING, WRITING AND PUBLISHING

Although there is plenty of interest in the history of anaesthesia, I gave it scant attention during my early years in the specialty, except that I looked up its main characters in J. Alfred Lee's *Synopsis of Anaesthesia* before sitting examinations. The subject came to life for me when I read Barbara Duncum's *The Development of Inhalation Anaesthesia*. By then I had a better idea what anaesthesia was all about. Duncum allowed her characters to speak for themselves through generous quotations and her work was thoroughly researched, well documented and very much more than a compilation of summarised dated events. In these respects I have tried to follow her example.

In 1964, a thesis I was preparing on *Outpatient Anaesthesia with particular reference to Nitrous Oxide* (for the degree of M.D. in the University of London) required an introductory chapter. I was obliged to attend to the history of nitrous oxide and this soon became an absorbing subject for research in its own right. Five months set aside for writing up the main work at home were devoted wholly to its historical background. Four years later the thesis was presented with a supplementary volume containing reprints of a ten-part series of historical articles which had been published in the *British Journal of Anaesthesia*. Further contributions have been added.

In 1971, the British Oxygen Company kindly offered to publish the original ten parts in book form, to mark the bicentenary of the discovery of nitrous oxide. I declined (I hope not ungraciously) because this would not have provided opportunity for taking a fresh look at the material, for re-writing and expanding it where appropriate, or for relating the history of nitrous oxide anaesthesia more to its general historical setting. Further parts were in mind and to have agreed might have compromised the production of a more satisfactory book at a later date.

In the present economic climate the cost of extensive alterations would be prohibitive for the anticipated circulation of a book on this subject, so I have acquiesced to the idea of republishing the collected articles. New material which has accumulated since their original publication is included in this preface.

Articles on Henry Hill Hickman, however, have been omitted. Hickman practised near the borders of Shropshire, Worcestershire and Herefordshire early in the nineteenth century. In the light of animal experiments he suggested the induction of suspended animation by 'the introduction of certain gases into the lungs' as a means of relieving the suffering of surgery. That was twenty years before Wells tried the crucial experiment upon himself using nitrous oxide. But there is no firm evidence that Hickman adminstered nitrous oxide to his animals or that he considered its administration to patients. So far as we can tell his story is of marginal relevance to nitrous oxide. Active research into this pioneer of anaesthesia continues. At least one further article is planned and rewriting of some of the earlier work would now be required, so the half dozen instalments which have been published about him so far are being saved for another day.

PRIESTLEY, AIRS AND ELECTRICITY

To understand why Priestley called nitrous oxide 'dephlogisticated nitrous air', and oxygen 'dephlogisticated air', requires knowledge of the phlogiston theory to which he clung long after others had abandoned it (see McKie, 1959). A key to his chemical terminology is provided in a footnote on the first page of Chapter 2 (see also Austin, 1972).

Whilst grappling with Priestley's chemistry I became aware of the breadth of his other interests, and attracted by the modern ring about his ideas on education. I welcomed an excuse to delve deeper into his works when, in 1969, the late Dr K. Bryn Thomas, then President elect of the Section for the History of Medicine of the Royal Society of Medicine, invited me to contribute a bicentenary lecture on Joseph Priestley in 1972, to commemorate his discovery of nitrous oxide.

The advance notice was appropriate to the magnitude of the task. It also provided opportunity for arranging a practical illustration of Priestley's early scientific and medical interests and of the level of contemporary knowledge. Mr Kahl Horner of the University of Leeds' Department of Anaesthesia built a reproduction of Priestley's second electrical machine, using Priestley's illustration of it as a guide

(Chapter 1, fig. 2). This was demonstrated at the end of the lecture. Sparks crackled up to an inch long; pith balls swung from silken strands; electric bells tinkled; a whirligig whirled and paper figures danced. One of the original machines was used for therapy at the Leeds General Infirmary in Priestley's time.

Another version of this lecture was given at the University of Leeds in 1974, to commemorate the discovery of oxygen. For this occasion some of Priestley's vividly described experiments with carbon dioxide were repeated and filmed over one of the old vats at Theakston's Brewery, Masham. The lecture was published in the *University of Leeds Review* and with kind permission is reproduced here as Chapter 1.

While working up the first bicentenary lecture I concluded that Priestley discovered nitrous oxide in 1773 and not in 1772. This was mentioned in the lecture but a more detailed re-appraisal of the discoveries of nitrous oxide and of oxygen was published in 1972 as Part IA of the series. This made minor correction to and supplemented Part I which was published in 1965. The narrative requires that Part IA be presented first so this has become Chapter 2 and Part I has become Chapter 3. The slight overlap of these chapters may be regretted but it is the price to be paid for collecting reprints rather than writing a book. (For a recent appraisal of Priestley as 'Aerial Philosopher' and of contemporary knowledge see McEvoy, 1978 and 1979.)

PRACTICAL HISTORY AND AUTO-EXPERIMENTATION

In 1968, the Fourth World Congress of Anaesthesiologists was held at the Royal Festival Hall in London. For the first time there were sessions on the history of anaesthesia. They were organised by Bryn Thomas who invited me to contribute something on nitrous oxide. Half an hour was allocated and plenty of notice was given. At the time Dr Klaus Siebold and I were planning a series of experiments to measure the uptake and elimination of nitrous oxide in ourselves in the context of short anaesthetics. We designed our experiments to match stages in the development of nitrous oxide anaesthesia. Dr Michael Hargreaves (fig. 0.3) joined us to administer the anaesthetics and Mr Albert Pegg (fig.0.4) filmed the experiment. We also used film to bring to life some of the experimental work of Humphry Davy and a comic song called *Laughing Gas* (see below). I was thus able to enliven the lecture with a series of brief colour films (Smith *et al.*, 1969). Bryn Thomas referred to this experimental approach

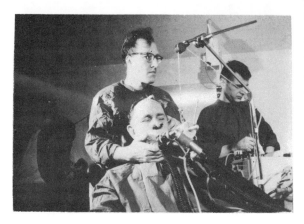

FIG. 0.3

An experiment in the hyperbaric chamber, the Western Infirmary, Glasgow. Front, from left to right, Michael Hargreaves, the author and Klaus Siebold. Back view of Geoffrey Clarke.

as 'Practical History', as did Clarke and Bearn (1971), who described the author as an auto-experimenter.

Experiments representing the trials of Wells and Colton, in which nitrous oxide was rebreathed from bladder or bag and also non-rebreathed through valves (Chapter 6), were filmed in Leeds. We turned horribly blue and overbreathed but the anaesthetics were not pursued to the stage of incipient convulsions.

We then used the hyperbaric chamber at the Western Infirmary, University of Glasgow, to repeat and to film anaesthetics administered at raised ambient pressures (Chapter 11). We began with the administration of 50 per cent nitrous oxide with oxygen at two atmospheres absolute (although Paul Bert used 50 per cent nitrous oxide with air in his

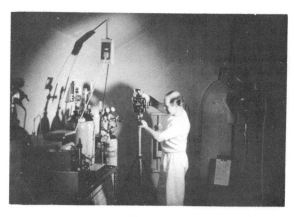

FIG. 0.4

Albert Pegg setting up in the hyperbaric chamber.

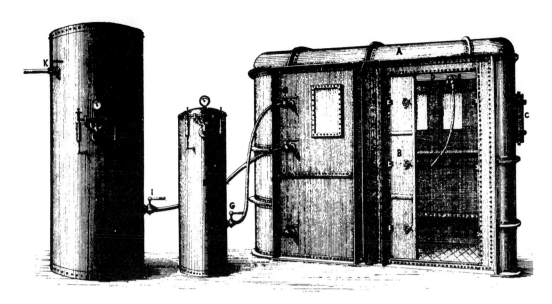

FIG. 0.5

In 1882, after 15 years' experience giving 10 000 conventional nitrous oxide anaesthetics, Claude Martin followed the example of Paul Bert and his disciples (Deroubaix, Guillermin, Blanchard) and administered hyperbaric anaesthetics for dental extractions and a few other operations, using this '*cloche*' or '*chambre metallique*' (2.2 × 1.6 × 2.2 m). The chamber was entered through the sliding door B (shown open—sealed against rubber when closed). Suspended from the ceiling at D was a concertina bag for nitrous oxide and oxygen mixtures. This could be replenished during an operation from a pre-pressurised reservoir F through taps G. Tank H allowed air from the compressor to cool before being supplied to the chamber, the pressure of which was adjusted by manipulation of taps I and J. Occupants were able to receive anything they required, without interference with the chamber pressure, by alternate opening and closing of the two doors of hatch C. Martin (1883) detailed his observations during the first 46 of about 150 hyperbaric anaesthetics administered to patients ranging in age from 10 to 66 years, using various ambient pressures up to 1.6 atmospheres. At first, using 85 per cent nitrous oxide at ambient pressures between 1.2 and 1.4 atmospheres, Martin found 'un sommeil inquiet presque pas anesthésique', but increasing the pressure to 1.6 atmospheres 'le sommeil était plus profond'. He also tried giving 88 per cent nitrous oxide at 1.25 atmospheres. In practice he manipulated the pressure to suit circumstances. The excitement stage seemed to him more marked than hitherto and there was a higher incidence of post-anaesthetic nausea and vomiting although this soon cleared. Dental extractions, of course, were carried out after removal of the mask. Some patients developed earache requiring temporary adjustment of the pressure and he made an occasional note of facial sweating (compare Winter *et al.*, 1972).

original hyperbaric anaesthetic for animals). We followed this by a series of anaesthetics using 85 per cent nitrous oxide; first at 1.2 atmospheres to represent Preterre's first human hyperbaric anaesthetic for a surgical operation by M. Labbé at the suggestion of Paul Bert; then at 1.4 and 1.6 atmospheres to represent the anaesthetics of Claude Martin (fig. 0.5); and finally at 2 atmospheres.

Upon return to Leeds, to complete the series, we filmed experiments in which we non-rebreathed nitrous oxide at atmospheric pressure with 12.5 per cent oxygen (Hewitt's first successful nitrous oxide and oxygen mixture – Chapters 11 and 13), with 8 per cent oxygen (more representative of Hewitt's later clinical practice) and with 20 per cent oxygen.

Time to loss of consciousness was measured in all these experiments and the uptake and elimination of nitrous oxide were measured in the non-rebreathing experiments (Smith *et al.*, 1974; Mapleson *et al.*,

1974). Dr Geoffrey Clarke acted as liaison officer for the hyperbaric experiments in Glasgow and he recorded our encephalograms. The whole hyperbaric venture was not unlike a military exercise in its detailed planning. One weekend two heavily laden cars transported the team and all the apparatus from Leeds to Glasgow. All the hyperbaric experiments were carried out in a single five-day week and everything was driven back to Leeds the following weekend.

DAVY'S BREATHING BOX AND WATT'S BREATHING CLOSET

Chapter 3 includes a description of how Davy was 'enclosed in an air-tight breathing box, of the capacity nine cubic feet and a half' – a very small box in which to enclose any man. But Davy also stated that 20 quarts of nitrous oxide thrown into the box mingled with 32 times this bulk of air, indicating a capacity of about 26 cubic feet – still small but practicable. A letter from James Watt to Davy (Davy, 1858) proposed a breathing closet of eight or nine feet cube and this may have been the source of the confusion (Smith *et al.*, 1969). Figure 0.6 (drawn specially for the World Congress lecture by Miss R. Bailey, University of Leeds Department of Medical Illustration) shows a sketch of James Watt's breathing closet from his description of it. The feather was for mixing the gases.

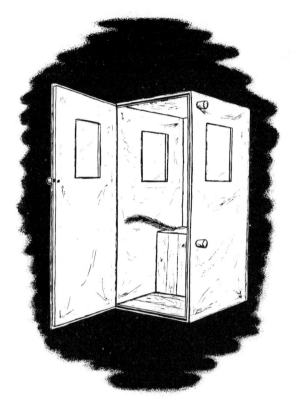

FIG. 0.6

An artist's impression of James Watt's 'breathing closet', from his description of it in a letter to Humphry Davy – by Miss R. Bailey. The feather was for mixing the gases.

MERCURIAL AIRHOLDER AND BREATHING MACHINE

Also described in Chapter 3 is how Davy used a Mercurial Airholder and Breathing Machine to demonstrate the uptake of nitrous oxide in himself and to measure his own lung volume. The apparatus (fig. 0.7) was designed by Clayfield (1800) and illustrated in Davy's '*Researches . . .* ' (1800). It was a very early spirometer (see Spriggs, 1977 and 1978; Gandeira, 1977; Bishop, 1977). It appears

transparent in the figure because it was made of glass. It was called mercurial because mercury was used to seal the receiver, or bell, instead of water. A weight at 'I' (the actual weight is not shown) forced the receiver down into the mercury. To compensate for the variation in upthrust with immersion of the receiver the counterpoise weight was suspended from a spiral pulley. A reconstruction of this apparatus was made for the World Congress (fig. 0.8). (Using glass 3 mm thick, the weight 'I' required was 5 kg so perhaps thinner glass was used in the original apparatus.) Reconstruction both of this airholder and of Priestley's electrical machine gave all concerned respect for contemporary craftmanship.

A COMIC SONG

Chapter 4 enters the era of laughter and missed opportunities that followed Davy's '*Researches . . .* '. M. Henry entertained audiences with laughing gas at the Adelphi Theatre in 1824 (Chapter 4, fig. 2) and three years later another playbill of the Theatre Royal, Haymarket, shows that he was again in London.

The Laughing Gas!! having been received every evening with re-iterated plaudits and peals of laughter will be continued Three Nights More. On Monday, March 19th, Wednesday, 21st and Friday 23rd, 1827. M. Henry will have the honour of Repeating his splendid and Magnificent Spectacle . . . . After which he will administer the Nitrous Oxide or Laughing Gas!! to any of the Audience disposed to inhale it, The wonderful Effects of which must be seen to be believed! (Stone Collection, Victoria and Albert Museum, London).

While those so disposed continued to inhale the laughing gas, others began to sing about it, and from the time that I lit upon the illustrated song sheet (c.1830) *Laughing Gas, a New Comic Song, sung with unbounded Applause by Mr W. Smith of the Royal Surrey Theatre* (Chapter 4, fig. 4), I wanted to bring it to life. The World Congress provided an excuse. I was warned that nothing could fall flatter than a failed musical joke but my aim was to revive a colourful quantum of history. The resurrection was made possible by the combined efforts of Peter Honri who sang it (see Honri, 1973); John Huntley and Bruce Beresford (British Film Institute); Albert Pegg (University of Leeds); Mrs C. P. Dalton who came, and induced others to come, in period dress (she also

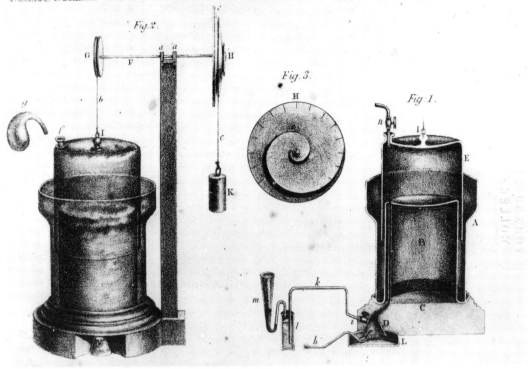

FIG. 0.7

Clayfield's Mercurial Airholder and Breathing Machine, used by Davy and illustrated in his '*Researches* . . .' (1800) (see also Clayfield, 1800). Clayfield got the idea from 'an inspection of Mr Watt's machine for containing factitious airs'. The bell was made of 'strong glass' and it had a capacity of 200 cubic inches (3.3.1). This was sealed over mercury, which necessitated a spiral pulley for achieving counterpoise, regardless of the position of the bell. (For an earlier version made partly of Lignum Vitae see Clayfield (1795).)

provided suitable apparel for volunteer members of the University Department of Anaesthesia); the Leeds City Varieties Theatre; and Radio Leeds which was responsible for attracting the main body of the audience. The complete film was shot between the end of the Radio Leeds morning sing-song and the beginning of the City Varieties Saturday matinee, exactly one month before it was due to be shown. Its reception at the lecture was gratifying. The master film is held by the British Film Institute.

DR SYNTAX, NITROUS GAS AND ELECTRICITY

The analgesic properties of nitrous oxide were put to rhyme as early as 1820. The anonymous doggerel of *Dr Syntax in Paris* (Chapter 5) described a visit to a dentist called Le Charlatan. Le Charlatan prescribed inhalation of 'nitrous gas, to assuage the torments of the face' after twisting out the offending tooth. He also used 'Galvanism' to confirm which was the bad

tooth. This remarkable verse seemed to anticipate the first recognised clinical use of nitrous oxide by twenty-five years and the use of electrical diagnosis in dentistry by half a century.

In 1819, Giovanni Aldini (1762 – 1834), nephew of Galvani, published a book giving *General Views on the Application of Galvanism to Medical Purposes, principally in cases of suspended animation*. In this he wrote:

. . . powerful proof of the very delicate impression produced by galvanic influence on the touch, is the method already communicated to me by Mr Fowler, an eminent dentist in London, for ascertaining the state of the teeth. When caries is concealed from sight, Mr Fowler employs the following method to discover the affected tooth. He first insulates the patient, and places his hand upon the electric chain; he then applies a small

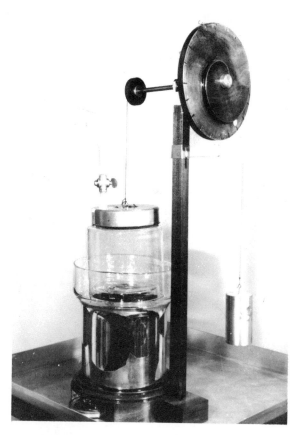

FIG. 0.8

A reproduction of Clayfield's Mercurial Airholder and Breathing Machine, made in the University of Leeds by the Departments of Chemistry and Anaesthesia, donated to the Wellcome Institute for the History of Medicine and now held at the Science Museum, South Kensington. Note the size of the lead weight on top of the receiver (see text). This apparatus required 1300 ml of mercury.

piece of wire to the dens sapientiae, and draws it gradually over the surface of the tooth; he then applies it to the next tooth in the same manner, and proceeds in the like method with the rest, until he comes to the diseased tooth, which is discovered by violent pain being produced, and an involuntary commotion in the body. It has always been remarked, when the tooth is extracted, that it exhibited a carious part, which, in its proper situation, was not visible. This method, therefore, is of great importance, as it frequently happens in such cases, that the dentist, not being able to distinguish the diseased from the healthy tooth, is obliged to draw some that are sound before he can discover it.

xviii

The details of this account match those in the doggerel about Le Charlatan so precisely that it seems very likely to have been the source used by the author of *Dr Syntax in Paris*.

Fowler got the idea from John Robison 26 years earlier (Fowler, 1793). Robison wrote to him:

> I made a piece of zinc having a sharp point, projecting laterally from its end. I applied this point to a hole in a tooth, which sometimes ached a little, and applied the silver in an extensive surface to the inside of the cheek. When the metals were brought into contact, I felt a very smart and painful twitch in the tooth, perfectly resembling a twitch of the toothach.

The likely source of Le Charlatan's knowledge of electrical diagnosis having come to light raised hope of finding a contemporary account of the inhalation of nitrous oxide after dental extraction. This has not been fulfilled. However, there may be more than coincidence in the 'fudge' quoted from *Dr Syntax in Paris* at the head of Chapter 5 and *The Fudge Family in Paris* published by Thomas Moore under the pseudonym 'Thomas Brown the Younger', in 1818. This went into eight editions in the same year.[6]

A PATIENT PROVIDES HIS OWN NITROUS OXIDE

When Colton re-introduced nitrous oxide anaesthesia to America in 1862 (Chapter 6), it was not generally known that this was foreshadowed in England at or near Burton-upon-Trent (Chapter 7). Mr Turton, an engineer, asked William Lloyd Poundall, a dentist, to extract one of his teeth while he was under the influence of laughing gas. The patient provided his own nitrous oxide and he had with him Mr Hallam, a druggist. The gas was breathed from a bottle rather than from a bag which argues against Turton having witnessed one of Colton's demonstrations, although there is a suggestion that he had been to America. The first written account of this episode appeared in a letter from Poundall to the editor or the *British Journal of Dental Science* in 1870 (Cohen, 1941). Corroboration of his claim entailed an exercise in amateur detection which culminated in 1964 by my telephoning a descendant, the late

6 Other accounts of Paris which have been searched include Anon (1815); Jouy (1815); Jerdan (1817); Croly (1818); and Anon (1819). For an excellent biography of William Combe, author of the original Dr Syntax books, of which *Dr Syntax in London* and *Dr Syntax in Paris* are imitations, see Hamilton (1969).

Mr A. B. Poundall, who immediately read out another account from a booklet prepared by W. L. Poundall for his patients in 1881. It was as if I had been given a direct line into the past.

I cannot say what gave Turton the idea of using nitrous oxide but I can add very tentative clues. It is mentioned in Chapter 7 that there were two brothers Hallam and that the daughter of the elder married a Mr Mee who was an architect and also organist at Barton-under-Needwood Church. Barton-under-Needwood is five miles from Burton-upon-Trent and less than thirty miles from Himley where Henry Hill Hickman's mother-in-law was baptised. She was also a Mee. The wife of the younger Hallam, Jane, was born in Ohio (personal communication, Mrs T. Randall, archivist, Staffordshire Record Office).

The next British anaesthetist known to have administered nitrous oxide for dental extractions was Samuel Lee Rymer. He tried to emulate Colton but reported in 1864 '. . . that the *uniform* success claimed by Dr Colton is a matter of perplexity' (Chapter 6 – see also Cohen et al., 1979).

THE PARIS EXHIBITION, AN AMERICAN DENTIST AND DEMONSTRATIONS IN LONDON

Colton visited Paris for the Universal Exhibition in 1867 and the following year nitrous oxide anaesthesia took root in Great Britain. If Le Charlatan (Chapter 5) ever existed in Paris he would probably have been dead and buried by then, but another dentist, Thomas Wiltberger Evans, an American with a lucrative and high-class practice, was very much alive. He became an enthusiastic disciple of Colton. In 1868, at his own expense, Evans journeyed from Paris to London where he devoted one week to demonstrating the new anaesthetic technique, having first set up apparatus for manufacturing the gas in the Langham Hotel (fig. 0.9). Chapter 8 contains one account of this turning point and Chapter 9 gives

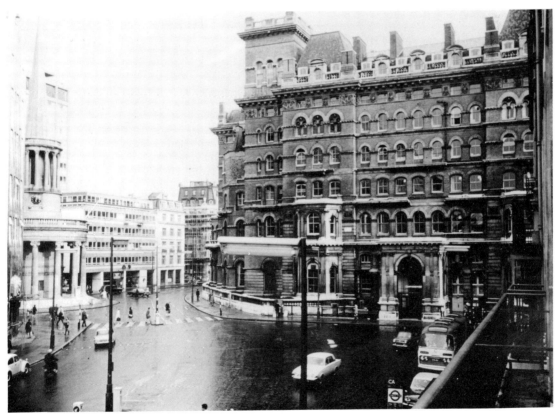

FIG. 0.9

The large building on the right was the Langham Hotel where T. W. Evans set up apparatus for making nitrous oxide. It now belongs to the British Broadcasting Corporation.

another. The former was part of the original series. The latter (reproduced here by kind permission of the *British Dental Journal*) was a centenary lecture to the Lindsay Club, given at the British Dental Association in 1968. The second supplements the first and produces experimental evidence to support one explanation for the failure of Horace Wells and of Samuel Lee Rymer (Chapter 6) and for the successes of Colton and his followers. This agrees with Bigelow's explanation of 1876:

> Wells's want of success can now be satisfactorily explained. He had, through Colton, in following Davy's instructions, made use of the traditional exhilirating gas bag and of Davy's exhilirating dose. This volume of gas is inadequate to produce anaesthesia with any certainty; and Wells failed to suggest a larger dose. This small omission closed his chances . . . .

Some overlap between these two chapters is inevitable, but their treatments are different.

TWENTY YEARS OF NITROUS OXIDE ANAESTHESIA (CHAPTER 10)

The first few years following the visit of Evans to London saw developments in which some of today's practices had their origins, for example: Clover and Fox used nitrous oxide and air, a first step towards using oxygen; Cattlin introduced the reservoir bag; Coleman's economising apparatus used lime to absorb exhaled carbon dioxide; Clover tackled problems of flow resistance and gas leaks by using a 'supplemental' bag; Clover and Coleman combined the use of nitrous oxide with ether, and so on. However, some of the initial enthusiasm may soon have subsided because by 1884 Buxton complained,

> Of one thing there is no uncertainty – that our present methods are clumsy and unscientific; that in their adoption we risk the welfare of our patient, and by shutting our eyes to their imperfections we close the door to useful research . . . .

Four years later Buxton, Hewitt and Silk each published an anaesthetic text book.

HALLAM AGAIN

In the Odontological Museum at the Royal College of Surgeons of England there are some very early examples of nitrous oxide anaesthetic apparatus, such as valved stopcock, noseclip, etc. (J.80.1, 11, 21, 22 and 23 in the museum catalogue). They match advertisements by Samuel S. White of America (Thomas, 1870) of which an example is given in fig. 0.10. These items were donated by S. Hallam. Further specimens were given later by John Hallam of Broadgreen Hospital, Liverpool. John Weymss Hallam (1910–64) was Director of the Maxillo–Facial Unit at Broad Green. I am indebted to his wife for writing to me in 1971:

> His father was Samuel Hallam, L.D.S., R.C.S., qualified at the Royal Dental Hospital in 1904, died in 1957, and was in private practice in Rodney Street, Liverpool for over 50 years. I know that he gave some early equipment to the Royal College and, I think, John gave the remainder on his father's death. The old man was very proud of his collection but, alas, I do not know where it came from . . . . His father . . . was a business man in Leeds. My mother-in-law (née Marianne Stuart Wemyss, daughter of Thomas Wemyss of Harehills Lane, Leeds) married Sam on June 19th 1907 . . . . There was some talk of Burton-on-Trent and early nitrous oxide anaesthesia but it is all so long ago – before the war – that I cannot recall any details.

(The marriage certificate of 1907 records Samuel Hallam's father as 'Samuel Hallam (deceased) Hotel Proprietor'. According to Leeds Directories he was proprietor of the Midland Hotel at 4, Wellington Street in 1882, although resident at Fulstow House, Fulstow, Louth. He moved to the Northern Hotel at 30 and 32 Wellington Street which, by 1907, was known as Hallam's Hotel.)

OXYGEN (CHAPTER 11)

While Evans was demonstrating nitrous oxide anaesthesia in London and while London dentists were beginning to use it, Edmund Andrews in Chicago was exploring the use of nitrous oxide and oxygen mixtures. For brief operations he thought that nitrous oxide by itself was the safest anaesthetic known. He was impressed by its speed of action and by its freedom from the unpleasant side effects of ether and chloroform. He hoped that adding oxygen would enable him to use it for general surgery (his prime interest was urology – see Kiefer, 1974) but he was thwarted by the dilution of nitrous oxide with impurities generated in its manufacture, such as nitrogen.

I have seen no evidence to suggest that Andrews'

HARD-RUBBER INHALER.

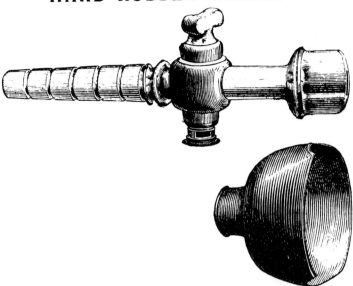

With two flexible Rubber Valves in Stop-cock (one opening inward to allow the gas to pass in at inspiration, which closes by the force of the expiration). Silver-plated Cap at end of Stop-cock with orifice, as shown in cut, to allow the escape of the expirations.

Price $4 00
Inhaler without Valve, price 2 00
Flexible Rubber Hood, to cover mouth and nostrils, price . 1 00

SAMUEL S. WHITE.

NOSE COMPRESS.
INTRODUCED BY DR. S. S. NONES.

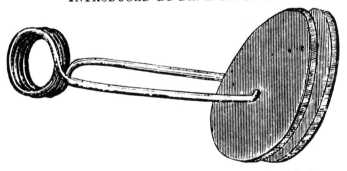

Convenient for the administering of Gas, where the Inhaler used is without a Face-piece.

Price . . . . 50 cents.

SAMUEL S. WHITE.

FIG. 0.10
Advertisement from Thomas (1870), by courtesy of the Wellcome Trustees.

trial of nitrous oxide and oxygen anaesthesia influenced subsequent events. It was another ten years before Paul Bert introduced hyperbaric nitrous oxide and oxygen anaesthesia, and twenty years before Hewitt produced practical clinical apparatus for administering reasonably controlled mixtures of nitrous oxide and oxygen – his 'regulating stopcock' (figs. 0.11 and 0.12).[7]

Economy and convenience rather than the potential hazards of withholding oxygen were what motivated Hewitt's 'enquiry into several methods of adminstering nitrous oxide gas' of 1886. He thought Coleman's economizing apparatus cumbrous and not very successful. He settled for administering nitrous oxide through non-rebreathing valves until it had effect, and then making the patient rebreathe nitrous

oxide from a 1¼ gallon bag. The rebreathing reduced wastage of gas to the atmosphere, but because it also conserved some of the oxygen remaining in the lungs it permitted a slightly extended administration. The patient absorbed more nitrous oxide and on average the time available for dental extraction after removal of the face mask was increased from about 39 seconds to 56 seconds. He devised prototype apparatus for the

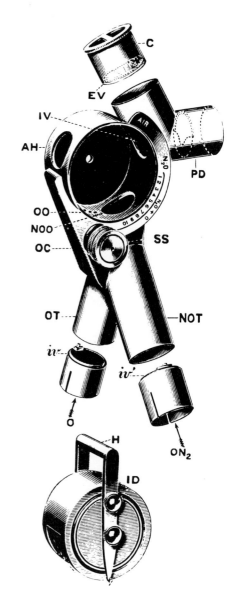

FIG. 0.11
A popular version of Hewitt's Regulating Stop Cock for administering nitrous oxide and oxygen made by George Barth.

7 I have tested three early examples of Hewitt's apparatus in the laboratory, from collections at Oxford (by courtesy Mr R. H. Salt), St. Thomas's Hospital (by courtesy Dr W. D. Wylie) and Liverpool (by courtesy of Professor Cecil Gray). The most generous proportions of oxygen that they would deliver were 8.8 per cent, 11.8 per cent and 10 per cent respectively. Regrettably plans to carry out further performance tests on historical apparatus were never realised.

FIG. 0.12
An exploded diagram of George Barth's version of Hewitt's Regulating Stop Cock.

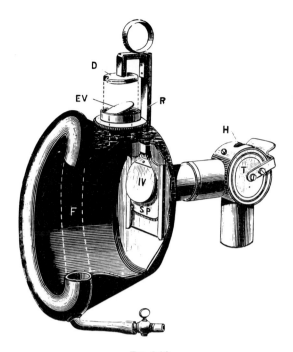

purpose (fig. 0.13) which was superseded by a more convenient system of valves and taps (fig. 0.14).

At that time the effects of hypoxia were regarded merely as a nuisance. To quote from Hewitt (1889):

> We have . . . in nitrous oxide an agent which quickly produced anaesthesia with certain incidental symptoms due to the want of oxygen: . . . it is the manifestation of these . . . which constitutes the main objection to the gas . . . experience has taught us that the phenomena are practically unattended by risk to the patient; yet they have their objectionable aspect, not only from the point of view of the administrator, but also from that of the operator, to whom jactitation is highly inconvenient.

In his text book of 1893, Hewitt had progressed to claiming that there was no anaesthetic more devoid of danger than nitrous oxide administered with sufficient oxygen to prevent asphyxial complications,

FIG. 0.13

Hewitt's prototype apparatus for allowing either non-rebreathing or rebreathing of nitrous oxide (Hewitt, 1885). The sliding plate (R) in its upper position allows the patient to breathe through the inspiratory (IV) and expiratory (EV) valves. Depression of (R) closes (EV) and removes (IV) from the inspiratory port, thus permitting rebreathing into a bag attached to the two-way stop-cock (T).

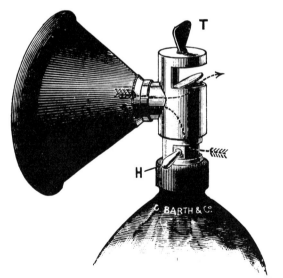

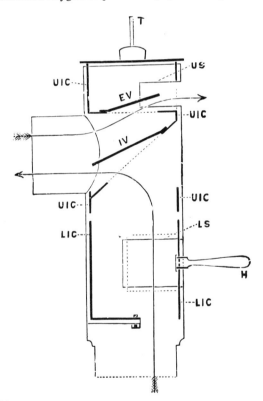

FIG. 0.14

Hewitt's later valved stop-cock. The inspiratory and expiratory valves (IV) and (EV) are mounted within the upper vertical cylinder (drawn with heavy line). Rotating this cylinder by means of tap (T) throws the valves in or out of operation. The lower vertical cylinder is rotated by means of the lever (H) so that either nitrous oxide is admitted from the bag, or the port in the base of this cylinder is closed off and air is admitted through the lateral slot (Hewitt, 1893).

and he advocated this for 'persons with feeble and dilated hearts' and for those 'who . . . might evince symptoms of embarrassed breathing at the acme of nitrous oxide anaesthesia.' But he added: 'Seeing, however, that nitrous oxide when administered free from oxygen is a practically safe anaesthetic in moderately healthy subjects, it is unnecessary here to emphasise the advantage of this mixture.' By 1897, Hewitt was recommending the general adoption of nitrous oxide and oxygen anaesthesia for dental operations.

MANUFACTURE AND IMPURITIES

Although Chapter 12 discusses the early manufacture, storage and purity of nitrous oxide, it relates directly to the more recent past. The original article was published in an issue of the *British Journal of Anaesthesia* devoted to higher oxides of nitrogen as impurities in nitrous oxide. There had been a catastrophe. With hindsight it can be seen that there had been both warnings and recommendations. Martin (1883) had echoed and re-inforced Davy when he wrote: '*C'est une remarque déjà ancienne . . . . Il est urgent qu'il se passe au moins vingt-quatre heures entre sa fabrication et son emploi; de plus, il est bon qu'il soit pendant ce temps en contact avec l'eau*'.

So far as is known the firm supplying the apparatus in figure 9 of Chapter 12 (Messrs Crapper & Co.) was not directly related to the inventor of the water closet (see Reyburn, 1969). A gas holder of that period survives in Sheffield (fig. 0.15).

Chapter 12 draws attention to the transient appearance of the Medical Pneumatic Apparatus Company in 1856, and to its use of wrought iron bottles for the storage of compressed oxygen. The method of manufacture and the purity of the oxygen were not mentioned but production would have been on a small scale. In 1849, Stephen White had set up a process using nitrate of soda or potash but this did not survive. In 1851 Boussingault set up a process using barium oxide. There were practical difficulties in its commercial development but these were partly resolved by the Brin brothers and in 1886 'Brin's Oxygen Company Limited' was formed. Towards the end of the century their produce was expected to contain a minimum of 91 per cent oxygen.[8] Between 1895 and 1902 Hampson in this country and Linde in Munich applied for various patents concerned with the liquefaction and fractionation of oxygen. By 1906 the Brin Company had taken over both the Hampson

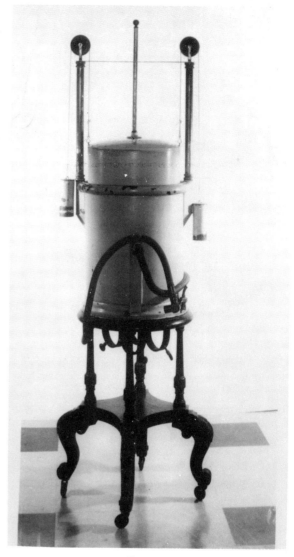

FIG. 0.15

An early gas holder now in the University Department of Anaesthetics, University of Sheffield, by courtesy Professor Andrew Thornton.

and the Linde patent rights and in that year it changed its name to the British Oxygen Company Limited which was able to market oxygen of about 97 per cent purity. The Brin Company relied largely upon the market created by the limelight. Fortunately with the advent of the electric light came the development of the oxy-acetylene blowpipe which made a major contribution to the expansion of the British Oxygen Company. The greatest demand for oxygen did not come from the medical profession.

8 Around this time Hewitt (1886) reported a sample of nitrous oxide to contain 6 per cent nitrogen and 1.5 per cent oxygen.

The medical section of the British Oxygen Company was not established until 1937 (B.O.C. – Archives).

DR STEPHEN COFFIN

Chapter 13 enlarges upon the use of Hewitt's 'mixture' and upon the development of the nasal inhalation of anaesthetics. Chapter 14 covers the two decades between World Wars and I am indebted to Dr Stephen Coffin for the following intimate peep into this period:

You say you are coming to the period when Dr Bellamy Gardner was most active. Let us assume, therefore, omitting the time before and during the war when I didn't know him, the opening date to be immediately after the first war, say 1919. From 1919 onward the anaesthetists in private dental anaesthetic practice using nasal nitrous oxide and oxygen anaesthesia were (as I remember them and I may omit some):

1 Immediately after the war: Dr Bellamy Gardner . . . Dr Ramsay Phillips . . . Dr Trewby . . . Dr Stephen Coffin . . . .
2 Dr Robert Macintosh commenced a few years later, until he went to Oxford.
3 Dr Macintosh later started the firm (popularly known as the 'Mayfair Gas Co') comprising himself, Dr McConnell, Dr Bernard Johnson and later Dr Roche and another whose name I cannot remember. He asked me to join him in practice, but being associated with Dr Bellamy Gardner I had to refuse.
4 A few years after the war many others came along and competition became fierce!

Dr Coffin went on to describe the version of Hewitt's regulating stop cock made by George Barth (fig. 0.11) the lever of which controlled the oxygen concentration from 1 per cent to 10 per cent. An additional knob marked 'Extra O₂' gave an extra 10 per cent oxygen at one turn and a further 10 per cent oxygen at a second turn which he described as 'quick and reliable'.

For nasal $N_2O.O_2$ the above apparatus was adapted thus: the expiratory valve was removed and into the valve chimney a wide bore metal tube (with suitable holes to allow flow to the face or nose piece) was inserted with a right angle turn at the upper end. Onto the free end of this was attached a tube (same bore as present day corrugated hose) carrying at the further end the mouthpiece. This had a valve, spring loaded off, which could be turned on by thumb pressure when required. Instead of the face piece a fitting carrying two tubes to the nose piece was attached. My own nose piece had no expiratory valve and had a narrow flange rubber edge giving a very accurate yet comfortable fitting if required. It was seldom held tight to the nose. The rubber bags were not side by side but the O_2 was within the N_2O (separate, with no mixing of gases – the Levy bag)[9] so that when N_2O was used under pressure, both N_2O and O_2 pressures were equal. My bag was quite large – about $14'' - 16''$, I would say, from top to bottom. This was bigger than usual, but much the same, I think, as Dr B.G.'s.

My personal practice for chair anaesthetics was to induce nasally with an open, propped, mouth at about 10 per cent O_2 with a very loosely applied (really not touching) nose piece and fast flow. Induction was comfortable and rapid and the mouth piece seldom required. Throat pack was by tangerine sized good quality honey comb sponges which were nice and resilient. My cylinder stand had two 50 gallon cylinders and had a large bore silencer filled with spun glass and it gave a very quiet flow. I used two stands in parallel with a switch over cock, giving 200 gallons for a long anaesthetic when required. My technique was not economical of gas. There were no fancy adjuvants to reinforce the N_2O in difficult cases.

I would like to mention what a beautiful nasal gas Dr B.G. used to give. Good colour, quiet, it all looked so simple. 'True art is to conceal art'. I tried to emulate him.

It might interest and amuse you to know that at one time. B.G. had an idea that 'gas' was a term that would scare and put off patients and he wanted to persuade people to call it 'aeris'; but luckily it never caught on! (see Gardner, 1931).

Immediately after the 1914/18 war the only supplier of $N_2O.O_2$ and apparatus was George Barth of Poland Street (so far as I can remember). This was run by two brothers, named Poole. The one I always dealt with was a very pessimistic old chap – I wonder what he would have thought of things now! Coxeter bought up Barth & Co, and then came Charles King. Now BOC has swallowed the lot . . . !

I always found that in a nasal $N_2O.O_2$ so many *small* things counted. I always stood on the patient's left side, not behind him . . . .

9 See Hovell *et al.* (1972) and Chapter 13.

I am of the generation who, as you might say, was not taught anything. After leaving the army, one went into practice with experience during the war (I gave quite a number of anaesthetics during that time) and one learnt as one went, by discussion with one's friends, reading, at medical meetings, and bitter trial and error! Today's high-powered teaching, with periods as anaesthetic registrar under consultants, was unknown!

Your photograph of B.G. is excellent. The very sensitive sketch of Trewby is nice. I knew him well. A nice person . . . .

OXYGEN LACK (HYPOXIA)

Interactions between the disciplines of anaesthesia, pharmacology, physiology, physics and chemistry during the last quarter century have facilitated the introduction of new inhalation and intravenous anaesthetics and new muscle relaxants: and they have increased understanding of drug action and of the body's uptake, distribution and elimination of nitrous oxide and other agents, old and new. Association between anaesthesia and applied respiratory physiology has sharpened attention to blood gases in general and to oxygenation in particular. Chapter 14 stresses the hazards of not administering enough oxygen.

Soon after the Second World War I was taught to induce anaesthesia in outpatients using 100 per cent nitrous oxide until the onset of 'regular respiration' and then to use a mixture of nitrous oxide and oxygen. The emphasis was more upon the maintenance of anaesthesia using nitrous oxide than upon the maintenance of adequate oxygenation. But when I came to anaesthetise patients in Jamaica I found cyanosis difficult to assess through pigmented skin, and patients with anaemia (especially sickle cell anaemia) are put at particular risk by hypoxia. My awareness of the problem was accentuated one day when a patient sang beneath the mask during the induction of anaesthesia *'Pretend you're happy when you're blue'*!

This stimulated me to question previous teaching and, in 1960, to publish a modest contribution to the anaesthetic literature which initiated the sequence of events leading up to the publication of this book. Although it was never intended as an historical article it is reprinted here as Chapter 15 for the insight it gives into the use of nitrous oxide for outpatient anaesthesia at the time. The preceding article in the

same journal (Green and Jolly, 1960) discussed the use of intravenous methohexitone prior to the inhalation of nitrous oxide and oxygen and this too paid attention to the avoidance of hypoxia. Attitudes were changing. Even so, in the month of August, 1961, at a reputable dental hospital, of 410 patients anaesthetised in the dental chair, 301 received 100 per cent nitrous oxide for an average of 45 seconds[10] during the induction of anaesthesia, nineteen were seen to jactitate and many more were obviously hypoxic (Smith, 1964). This state of affairs soon changed and before long all patients at that hospital were administered not less than 20 per cent oxygen throughout anaesthesia (Gould, 1965).

Also published in 1960 was J. G. Bourne's *Nitrous Oxide in Dentistry: its dangers and alternatives* in which he commented: 'Today, the facilities for giving anaesthesia to ambulatory dental patients and the method almost universally used are Victorian. From time to time a new gas machine is introduced. This may give a semblance of progress: what is needed is an altogether fresh approach.' One can imagine Buxton stirring in his grave.

REFERENCES

Anon (1815). *Journal of a Trip to Paris during the summer of 1815.* London: Bewsley.

Anon (1819). *The Englishman in Paris: a satyrical novel. With sketches of the most remarkable characters that have recently visited that celebrated capital.* London: Sherwood, Neely & Jones.

Aldini, J. (1819). *General Views on the Application of Galvanism to Medical Purposes, principally in cases of suspended animation.* London: Callow and Burgess and Hill.

Archer, W. H. (1944). 'Life and letters of Horace Wells discoverer of anaesthesia chronologically arranged'. *J.Am.Coll.Dentists,* **11**, 83.

Austin, A. T. (1972). Glossary in Davy, H. *Researches Chemical and Philosophical; chiefly concerning Nitrous Oxide. A Facsimile reproduction.* London: Butterworth.

Bigelow, H. J. (1846). 'Insensibility during surgical operations'. *Boston Med. & Surg. J.,* **35**, 309.

Bigelow, H. J. (1876). 'A history of the discovery of modern anaesthesia'. *Am. J. Med. Sci.,* **71**, 164.

Bishop, P. J. (1977). 'A bibliography of John Hutchinson'. *Medical History,* **21**, 384.

Bourne, J. G. (1960). *Nitrous Oxide in Dentistry: its Dangers and Alternatives.* London: Lloyd Luke (Medical Books).

Buxton, D. W. (1884). 'The experimental study of the action of anaesthetics: IV'. *Brit. J. dent. Sci.,* **27**, 147.

Cartwright, F. F. (1952). *The English Pioneers of Anaesthesia (Beddoes: Davy; Hickman).* Bristol: Wright.

Clarke, E. and Bearn, J. G. (1971). 'Practical History. The role of experimentation in medical history'. In: Clarke, E. ed. *Modern Methods in the History of Medicine.* London: The Athlone Press of the University of London.

Clayfield, W. (1795). 'Description of a mercurial apparatus' in Beddoes, T. and Watt, J. (1795): *Considerations on the Medicinal Use and Production of Factitious Airs.* Bristol: Bulgin and Rosser.

Clayfield, W. (1800). 'Description of a mercurial airholder suggested by an inspection of Mr Watt's machine for containing factitious airs'. *Phil. Mag.,* **7**, 148.

10 Hewitt (1893) administered nitrous oxide for an average time of 51 seconds before removing the mask.

Cohen, R. A. (1941). 'Some historical notes on dental anaesthesia with special reference to nitrous oxide'. *Dental Gazette*, **8,** 56.

Cohen, R. A., Donaldson, J. A., McAuley, J. E., Messer, F. W., Poynter, F. N. L., Spencer, E. M., and Vinski, I. (1979). *The Advance of the Dental Profession: A Centenary History 1880–1980,* p.244. London: British Dental Association.

Colton, G. Q. (1873). 'Nitrous oxide'. *Mon. Rev. dent. Surg.,* **2,** 26.

Colton, G. Q. (1886). *Anaesthesia, who made and developed this great discovery. A statement 'delivered upon the mellowing of occasion'.* New York: A. G. Sherwood & Co.

Colton, G. Q. (1888). *Shakespeare and the Bible. Parallel passages and passages suggested by the Bible with the Religious Sentiments of Shakespeare.* New York: Thomas R. Knox.

Croly, G. (1818). *Paris in 1815, a poem.* 2nd ed. dedicated to J. W. Croker. London: John Murray.

Daily Telegraph (3 June 1969). 'Laughing-gas party teenagers die in car'. London.

Davy, H. (1800). *Researches, Chemical and Philosophical: chiefly concerning nitrous oxide, or dephlogisticated nitrous air, and its respiration.* London: J. Johnson.

Davy, J. (1858). *Fragmentary Remains, Literary and Scientific.* London: Churchill.

Dillon, J. (1967). 'Nitrous oxide inhalation as a fad'. *Calif. Med.,* **106,** 444.

Duncum, B. M. (1947). *The Development of Inhalation Anaesthesia: with special reference to the years 1846–1900.* London: Oxford University Press.

Farr, A. D. (1977). Thesis. 'Medical Developments and Religious Belief with special reference to Europe in the 18th and 19th Centuries—a Study of the History of Science and Technology'. Submitted for the degree of Doctor of Philosophy at the Open University.

Farr, A. D. (1980). 'Early oppostion to obstetric anaesthesia'. *Anaesthesia,* **35,** 896.

Forster, W. (1809). *A Treatise on a Section of the Strata commencing near Newcastle upon Tyne and concluding on the West side of the Mountain of Cross Fell.* Newcastle: Preston and Heaton.

Fowler, R. (1793). *Experiments and Observations relative to the influence lately discovered by M. Galvani, and commonly called animal electricity.* London: J. Johnson.

Gardner, H. B. (1931). '"Aeris", new name for laughing gas'. *Lancet,* **i,** 1161.

Gandeira, B. (1977). 'John Hutchinson in Australia and Fiji'. *Medical History,* **21,** 365.

George, M. D. (1947). *Catalogue of Political and Personal Satires.* vol. VIII: 1901–1910, p.112. British Museum.

Gibbs, F. W. (1960). 'Itinerant Lecturers in Natural Philosophy'. *Ambix,* **8,** 111.

Gould, R. B. (1965). 'Anaesthesia at the Royal Dental Hospital'. *Brit. J. Anaesth.,* **37,** 212.

Green, R. A., and Jolly, C. (1960). 'Methohexital in dental anaesthesia'. *Brit. J. Anaesth.,* **32,** 393.

Hamilton, H. W. (1969). *Dr Syntax: a silhouette of William Combe.* London: Chatto & Windus.

Hewitt, F. W. (1885). 'A new method of administering and economising nitrous oxide gas'. *Lancet,* **i,** 840.

Hewitt, F. W. (1886). 'An enquiry into several methods of administering nitrous oxide gas'. *J. Brit. dent. Assoc.,* **7,** 86.

Hewitt, F. W. (1889). 'On the anaesthesia produced by the administration of mixtures of nitrous oxide and oxygen. Preliminary notice'. *Lancet,* **i,** 832.

Hewitt, F. W. (1892). 'On the effects of nitrous oxide when administered with oxygen at ordinary atmospheric pressures with remarks on 800 cases'. *Trans. Odont. Soc., G.B.,* **24,** NS, 194.

Hewitt, F. W. (1893). *Anaesthetics and their administration. A manual for medical and dental practitioners and students.* London: Charles Griffin.

Hewitt, F. W. (1897). *The Administration of Nitrous Oxide and Oxygen for Dental Operations.* London: Claudius Ash.

Hewitt, F. W. (1898). 'Administrations of anaesthetics conducted at the London Hospital during the year 1897'. *Lancet,* **i,** 843.

Honri, P. (1973). *Working the Halls.* Farnborough: D. C. Heath Ltd.

Hovell, B. C., Masson, A. H. B., and Wilson, J. (1972). Alfred Goodman Levy (1866–1954): A Biography. *Brit. J. Anaesth.,* **44,** 115.

Irwin, R. A. (1955). *Letters of Charles Waterton of Walton Hall, near Wakefield: naturalist, taxidermist and author of 'Wanderings in South America' and 'Essays on Natural History'.* pp. 81–4. London, Rockliff.

Jerdan, W. (1817). *Six weeks in Paris, or a cure for Gallomania.* 3 vols. London: J. Johnson.

Jones, R. M. (1978). *The Parisian Education of an American Surgeon. Letters of Jonathan Mason Warren (1832–1835).* Philadelphia: The American Philosophical Society.

Jouy, E. de (1815). The Paris Spectator; or *L'Hermite de la Chaussée d'Antin* containing observations upon Parisian manners and customs at the commencement of the nineteenth century. 3 vols. London: Longman, Hurst, Rees, Orme and Brown. (From *Gazette de France*). Translated by W. Jerdan.

Kiefer, J. H. (1974). 'Edmund Andrews: the Forgotten Pioneer of Chicago Urology'. *Illinois Med. J.,* **146,** No. 3.

Lee, J. A. (1953). *A Synopsis of Anaesthesia,* 3rd ed. Bristol: John Wright.

Levere, T. H. (1977). 'Dr Thomas Beddoes and the Establishment of his Pneumatic Institution: a tale of three presidents'. *Notes and Records of the Royal Society of London,* **32,** 41.

Long, C. W. (1849). 'An account of the first use of Sulphuric Ether by Inhalation as an anaesthetic in surgical operations'. *Southern Med. & Surg. J.,* **5,** 705.

McEvoy, J. G. (1978). 'Joseph Priestley, 'Aerial Philosopher': Metaphysics and Methodology in Priestley's Chemical Thoughts'. *Ambix,* **25,** Part I, p.1; Part II, p.93; Part III, p.153 and Part IV (1979), **26,** 16.

McEvoy, J. G. (1979). 'Electricity, knowledge, and the nature of progress in Priestley's thought'. *Brit. J. Hist. Sci.,* **12,** 40.

McKie, D. (1959). 'The Phlogiston theory'. *Endeavour,* **18,** 144.

MacQuitty, B. (1969). *The Battle for Oblivion.* London: Harrap.

Martin, M. C. (1883). *De l'anesthésia par le protoxyde d'azote avec ou sans tension, suivie d'une note sur la germination en presence du protoxyde d'azote sous pression. Mémoire lu à la Société de Médecine de Lyon.* Paris: Delahaye & Lecrosnier.

Mapleson, W. W., Smith, W. D. A., Siebold, K., Hargreaves, M. D., and Clarke, G. M. (1974). 'Nitrous oxide anaesthesia induced at atmospheric and hyperbaric pressures, Part II: Comparison of measured and pharmacokinetic data'. *Brit. J. Anaesth.,* **46,** 13.

Miles, W. D. (1968). 'Public lectures on chemistry in the United States'. *Ambix,* **15,** 129.

Moore, A. R. (1978). 'Pre-anaesthetic mastectomy: a patient's experience'. *Surgery,* **83,** 200.

Moore, T. (1818). *The Fudge Family in Paris.* London: Longman, Hurst, Rees, Orme and Brown.

Nall, W. (1883). 'A Memoir of the Author's Life'. In: Forster, W. *A Treatise on a Section of the Strata from Newcastle upon Tyne to Cross Fell.* 3rd ed. Newcastle upon Tyne: Andrew Reid.

Reyburn, W. (1969). *Flushed with Pride: The Story of Thomas Crapper.* London: MacDonald.

Richards, W., Parbrook, G. D., and Wilson, J. (1976). 'Stanislaw Klikovich (1853–1910). Pioneer of nitrous oxide and oxygen analgesia'. *Anaesthesia,* **31,** 933.

Riding, J. E. (1963). 'Under Chloroform' and preceding reprint from the Cornhill Magazine, vol. I, p.499, 1860. *Brit. J. Anaesth.,* **35,** 334.

Robinson, V. (1946). *Victory over pain,* p.209. New York: Henry Schuman.

Shedlin, M., Wallichensky, D., and Salyer, S. (1973). *Laughing Gas.* Berkeley: And/or Press.

Sims, J. M. (1877). 'The discovery of anaesthesia'. *Virginia Med. Monthly,* **4,** 81.

Smith, W. D. A. (1964). 'A study of 410 dental anaesthetics. Part

I: Introduction, methods, material and anaesthetic techniques'. *Brit. J. Anaesth.*, **36,** 620.

—— (1969). Thesis: *Outpatient Anaesthesia with particular reference to Nitrous Oxide.* University of London.

—— (1971). 'Pharmacology of nitrous oxide'. In: *Pharmacological Topics in Anaesthesia,* ed. Millar, R. A., p.108. Boston: Little, Brown & Co.

——, Siebold, K., Hargreaves, M. D., and Pegg, A. (1969). 'The development of nitrous oxide anaesthesia and a comparison of anaesthetic techniques'. *Proc. 4th Wld. Cong. Anaesth.,* p.208. Amsterdam: Excerpta Medica.

——, Mapleson, W. W., Siebold, K., Hargreaves, M. D., and Clarke, G. M. (1974). 'Nitrous oxide anaesthesia induced at atmospheric and hyperbaric pressures. Part I: Measured, pharmacokinetic and EEG data'. *Brit. J. Anaesth.,* **46,** 3.

Spriggs, E. A. (1977). 'John Hutchinson, the inventor of the spirometer – his north country background, life in London, and scientific achievements'. *Medical History,* **2,** 357.

—— (1978). 'The history of spirometry'. *Brit. J. Dis. Chest.,* **72,** 165.

Sykes, W. S. (1960). *Essays on the First Hundred Years of Anaesthesia,* vol. I. Edinburgh: Livingstone.

Thomas, F. R. (1870). *Manual of the discovery of nitrous oxide or laughing gas and its manufacture.* Philadelphia: S. S. White.

Weller, R. M. (1981). 'Chemistry for the ladies'. *Anaesthesia,* in press.

Wilson, J. E. (1860). *Memoir of George Wilson, M.D., F.R.S.E.,* Regius Professor of Technology in the University of Edinburgh and Director of the Industrial Museum of Scotland, by his sister, p.293. Edinburgh: Edmonston & Douglas.

Winter, P. M., Hornbein, T. F., Smith, G., Sullivan, D., and Smith, K. H. (1972). 'Hyperbaric nitrous oxide anaesthesia in man: determination of anaesthetic potency (MAC) and cardiorespiratory effects'. *Proc. A.S.A. Annual Meeting, Boston.*

ACKNOWLEDGEMENTS

Grateful acknowledgement is extended to the British Oxygen Company for generous support of the publication of this book. (The Company Secretary, Mr C. A. B. Leslie, made available a draft history of the firm and has been most helpful in other ways.) The Editorial Board of the *British Journal of Anaesthesia* and the Council of the Association of Anaesthetists of Great Britain and Ireland have also given kind and active encouragement as has the Board of Directors of the Wood Library-Museum. Detailed acknowledgements are made in the text, in legends and at the end of each chapter. The earlier articles of the original series were typed by Miss Ann Wright and special thanks are due to Mrs Sheila Barlow for undertaking the greater part of the typing and associated secretarial work. Apart from coping with family and job, my wife contributed criticisms, suggestions, guarded approval and spontaneous but timely yawns.

1

JOSEPH PRIESTLEY, FRS, LLD (1733–1804), AND THE 'DISCOVERY' OF OXYGEN*

Nearly two hundred years ago, after breathing what we call *oxygen*, Joseph Priestley (Plate 1) wrote: 'I fancied that my breast felt peculiarly light and easy for some time afterwards. Who can tell that in time, this pure air may become a fashionable article in luxury. Hitherto only two mice and myself have had the privilege of breathing it.' Priestley called it *dephlogisticated air*. The name *oxygène* was coined later by Lavoisier, who was quicker than Priestley to perceive the significance of some of its properties, and to quantify them. Unknown to either of them at the time, oxygen was also isolated by Scheele, and Mayow had already recognized that only part of atmospheric air supported combustion. But although the bicentenary of the 'discovery' of oxygen is the occasion for this lecture, it is not the main subject of it. Rather will we catch, reflected in the life and work of Joseph Priestley, a glimpse of the period in our history around the time of some seven or eight generations ago.

Priestley was born in Owler Lane, Fieldhead near Birstall, six miles from Leeds. After boyhood in Yorkshire he attended the dissenting academy at Daventry. His first post was as assistant minister at Needham Market. Then he moved to a congregation at Nantwich where he ran a school. At the age of twenty-eight he became tutor at the Warrington Academy where he married Mary Wilkinson, daughter of an iron-founder, and they had a daughter. He was ordained, granted an honorary Doctor of Laws, and elected a Fellow of the Royal Society. At thirty-four Priestley came to Leeds where he took charge of the Mill Hill Chapel, and had two sons. At forty he went into the employ of a future Prime Minister, the Earl of Shelburne, at Calne, nominally as librarian but more as a friend. There he had a third son. At forty-seven he moved to Birmingham, took charge of the New Meeting House, and began to

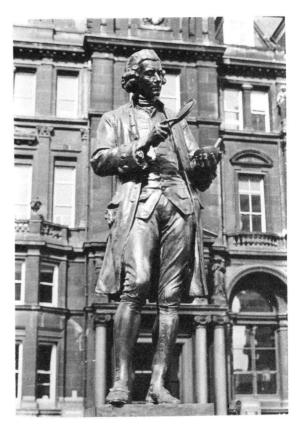

PLATE 1

The statue of Joseph Priestley by Alfred Drury, RA, in City Square, Leeds, facing the present Mill Hill Chapel. (The statues of City Square were formally handed over to the City in September, 1903.) Corry described Priestley thus: 'Dr Priestley was about middle stature, or five feet eight inches high. He was slender and well proportioned; his complexion was fair, his eyes grey and sparkling with intelligence . . . He often smiled but seldom laughed . . . His common dress was a black coat without cape, a fine linen or cambric stock, a cocked hat, a powdered wig, shoes and buckles . . . When engaged in making philosophical experiments he commonly wore a white apron, and canvas covers drawn over his sleeves . . .'

(Photograph by Dr M. D. Hargreaves, Department of Anaesthesia)

*A lecture delivered at the University of Leeds on 3 October 1974. The lecture was published in the *University of Leeds Review* and with kind permission is reproduced here as Chapter 1.

write his Memoirs. (Birmingham, like Leeds, was then a market town without parliamentary representation.) Priestley was happy in Birmingham, particularly with his industrial and medical friends who formed the Lunar Society (it met near full moon); but his eleven years there ended sadly. Having discomforted the theologically orthodox, and urged repeal of the Test Acts (which discriminated against dissenters) at a time when controversy was coloured by revolutionary trends in America and France, he fell victim to misunderstanding and misrepresentation, and finally to the Church and King Riots, with the destruction of his Meeting House, his home, his unique library and 'elaboratory', and a wealth of manuscripts. He found haven in the New College at Hackney, but in 1794, aged 61, he emigrated to America, settling in Northumberland, Pennsylvania. Two years later his wife died and he survived her by eight years.

Those are the bare bones of Priestley's life. His bibliography hints at his animation. Apart from periodicals and multiple editions Crook (1966) listed 128 titles under his authorship, grouping 70 as theological and religious, 19 as political and social, 18 as scientific, 8 as educational and psychological, 7 as historical and 6 as philosophical and metaphysical. Corry, a contemporary biographer, wrote: 'A critical analysis of the multifarious production of Dr. Joseph Priestley would require a combination of talents of which few human beings are in possession.' I can offer only an introductory sketch. I will not attempt analysis of his theology or of his politics, and I will not explore his career beyond his employment with the Earl of Shelburne, when he isolated oxygen and began to appreciate its biological significance.

Joseph Priestley was born in 1733. He was the eldest son of a dresser of woollen cloth. His mother had children in quick succession and Joseph was soon committed to the care of her father, a farmer near Shafton. When he was nearly seven the Great Frost of 1739–40 caused much hardship, and that winter his mother died after childbirth. Priestley came home and went to school locally, but when nine he was adopted by an aunt, Mrs Keighley.

My excellent Aunt, Priestley wrote, was truly Calvinistic . . . left in good circumstances, her home (Heckmondwike Hall) was the resort of all the dissenting ministers in the neighbourhood . . . the most obnoxious on account of their heresy were almost as welcome to her if she thought them honest and good men, as any others . . . brought up with the sentiments of piety, but without bigotry . . . I was . . . confirmed in Calvinism . . . The weakness of my constitution, which often led me to think that I should not be long lived, contributed to give my mind a still more serious turn; and having read many books of *experiences*, and in

consequence believing that a *new birth*, produced by the immediate agency of the Spirit of God, was necessary to salvation, and not being able to satisfy myself that I had experienced anything of the kind, I felt occasionally such distress of mind as it is not in my power to describe, and which I still look back on with horror . . . the remembrance of what I sometimes felt in that state of ignorance and darkness gives me a peculiar sense of the value of rational principles of religion.

Furthermore, the elders would not admit Priestley a communicant because, he explained: '. . when they interrogated me upon the sin of Adam, I appeared to be not quite orthodox, not thinking that all the human race (supposing them not to have any other sin of their own) were liable to the Wrath of God, and the pains of Hell for ever, on account of that sin only . . . .'

Priestley went to Batley Grammar School, learning Latin and Greek, and in the holidays Hebrew. But he left owing to illness and abandoned plans to enter the Ministry. Instead he considered trade—for which he studied languages—and perhaps physic. At home, with help from local ministers, he learned French, Italian and High Dutch; geometry, algebra, and various branches of mathematics. His reading included Gravesande's *Introduction to the Philosophy of Isaac Newton*, Watts' *Logic*, and Locke's *Essay on Human Understanding*. He taught a Baptist minister Hebrew, meanwhile learning Chaldee and Syriac and beginning to read Arabic. He learned Mr Annet's shorthand and suggested improvements. Perhaps he used this on Sundays for he wrote: ' . . . it was my custom to recollect and commit to writing, as much as I could from the sermons . . . until I was able from the heads of the discourse to supply the rest myself. For not troubling to commit to memory much of the amplification, and writing at home almost as much as I had heard I insensibly acquired a habit of composing with great readiness.' When he was about fourteen he contributed a laudatory verse to Annett's second edition. Later Priestley encouraged his pupils to compose verse, believing this to facilitate writing prose.

His health improved and his aunt wanted him to enter the strictly Calvinistic Mile End Academy, but he objected, considering himself then an Arminian—so Dr Doddridge's academy was chosen for its scholarship. Doddridge died that year and the academy moved to Daventry under Dr Ashworth. Priestley was excused all first year studies and much of the second. He wrote:

. . . the academy was peculiarly favourable to the serious pursuit of truth . . . students were about equally divided upon every question of importance, such as Liberty and Necessity, the Sleep of the Soul, and all the articles of theological orthodoxy and heresy . . . these topics were the subject of continual discussion. Our tutors were also of different opinions, Dr. Ashworth taking the orthodox side of every question, and Mr. Clark, the sub-tutor, that of heresy, although always with the greatest modesty . . . Our lectures had the air of friendly conversations . . . we were referred to authors on both sides of every question . . . .

A reference to Dr Hartley's *Observations on Man* engaged Priestley's closest attention, and in his own words: ' . . . produced the greatest effect on my general turn of thinking through life. It established me in the doctrine of necessity; it greatly improved that disposition to piety which I brought to the Academy, and it freed me from that rigour with which it had been tinctured.' Hartley explained memory, the formation of ideas, and of their associations (a concept of particular interest to Priestley) by supposing that particles of the brain retain a disposition to vibrate as they have formerly vibrated. And each human action, Hartley maintained, resulted from the previous circumstanes of body and mind, in the same manner, and with the same certainty as other effects do from their mechanical causes. Years later Priestley re-published parts of Hartley's work, adding introductory essays, and revealing insight. He wrote:

I was educated so strictly and properly that the slightest oath, or irreverent use of the name of God, gives me a sensation that is more than mental. It is next to shuddering . . . whereas other persons . . . of strict virtue and honour in other respects, feel not the least moral impropriety in the greatest possible profaneness of speech. But by a different education I might have been as profane as they, and without remorse. Now no principle conceived to be innate . . . can operate more certainly, or more mechanically, than this which I know to have been acquired with respect to myself . . . without reflection and observation I should have concluded . . . that the *dread of an oath* had been natural and invariable in mankind.

At Daventry Priestley and his room mate, Mr Alexander, rose early to read ten folio pages of Greek, and generally a Greek play in the week besides. Priestley commented, however: 'My attention was always more drawn to mathematical and philosophical studies than his was . . . But all the while I was at the Academy . . . I never lost sight of the great object of my studies, which was the duties of a Christian Minister. Particularly I there composed the first copy of my Institutes of Natural and Revealed Religion.' These were published seventeen years later. His main discouragement at Daventry was an impediment of speech, but he admitted: 'Without such a check I might have been disputatious in company, or . . . seduced by the love of popular applause as a preacher . . . '.

In 1755, Priestley cheerfully agreed to assist a superannuated Minister at Needham Market, in Norfolk. He catechized the children there using the Catechism of Isaac Watts, which was phrased according to the age group of children, then an innovation. Priestley owed something to the editors of Watts' works—Jennings and Doddridge. Jennings's brother John, who founded Kibworth Academy, lectured in the traditional Latin, but he introduced French, geography and science, and he encouraged free enquiry. His pupil, Doddridge, followed suit but lectured in English. Ashworth, who was Doddridge's pupil, carried on the tradition and taught Priestley.

Priestley used the draft of his 'Institutes' for lectures to his congregation on religion, but, he wrote: 'I soon found that I had acted imprudently . . . When I came to treat of the *Unity of God* . . . several of my audience were attentive to nothing but the soundness of my faith in the doctrine of the Trinity . . . It was soon discovered that I was an Arian. From the time of this discovery, my hearers fell off apace.' His speech deteriorated, and although his aunt financed a visit to a London 'curer' of speech defects, after temporary improvement he was worse than ever. Meanwhile to help clarify his ideas, Priestley perused the whole of the Old and New Testaments. He wrote: 'In consequence of much pains and thought (I became) persuaded of the falsity of the doctrine of atonement, of the inspiration of the authors of the books of scriptures as writers, and of all idea of supernatural influence, except for the purpose of miracles . . . But I was still an Arian . . . contenting myself with seeing the absurdity of the Trinitarian system.' Some of his conclusions were published in 1761: the rest years later in the *Theological Repository* which he edited.

Anxious to supplement his meagre salary, which never exceeded £30 per annum although he was promised £40 (£20 per annum went on board), Priestley proposed himself as schoolmaster, but parents would not expose their children to his unorthodoxy. He did, however, give ten lectures on the use of globes, ten hearers paying half a guinea each which enabled him to purchase a pair of globes. (The contemporary price for a pair of 12 in. globes was £3.) Two verdicts on Priestley's character at this time are worth quoting. Mr Spink, who knew him at Needham Market, recalled ' . . . his opponents could not but commend him for the easy access all persons had who came to controvert his opinions, and the calm patience with which he heard them.' And the Reverend Tom exclaimed to a critic: 'My young friend, Dr. Priestley's sentiments are not mine. I hope they will never be yours; and I am sorry they are his; but from my acquaintance with him at Needham Market, I shall always respect him for the openness and honesty of his character.'

In 1758, Priestley was recommended for a tutorship at Warrington Academy 'on account of critical and classical learning, not common in one so young', but Dr Aikin was preferred. The Trustees of the Academy were: 'not without some apprehension of his being thought too young to sustain the character of tutor . . . the subordinates might expect a person more advanced in years . . . more known in the world, and longer experienced in life and manners. They are informed, too, that he has some hesitations and interruptions in his manner of speaking.'

He then received an invitation to serve a congregation at Nantwich, which he gladly accepted. For economy he travelled as far as London by sea, probably embarking at Ipswich. In Nantwich Priestley was boarded with Mr John Eddowes, tobacconist and grocer, who taught him to play a little on the English flute. Ministerial duties being light, and the congregation favourably disposed, he established a school of thirty boys and a dozen young ladies. 'My school', he wrote, 'enabled me to buy a few books and some philosophical instruments, such as a small air pump, and an electrical machine . . . These I taught my scholars in the highest class to keep in order and to make use of, and by entertaining their parents and friends with experiments, in which the scholars were generally the operators, and sometimes the lecturers too, I considerably extended the reputation of my school; though I had no other object originally than gratifying my own taste . . . '. School was from 7 am to 4 pm, with an hour off for lunch and only red letter days as holidays. After school he taught in the family of Mr Tomkinson, attorney, at Dorfold Hall, a mile away, probably walking there, as his son put it: ' . . . very firmly and expeditiously'. He also found time to compose a very successful *Rudiments of English Grammar* which went into several editions. In a later work he dealt with the theory of language, and he applied linguistics to his study of the Bible.

In 1761, Priestley was appointed tutor at the Warrington Academy. This academy was a new venture. There was a choice of subjects and tutors were full time. Priestley was allocated Languages and Belles Lettres, which he interpreted broadly, although he wrote: 'I should have preferred the office of teaching the mathematics and natural philosophy, for which I had at that time a great predilection.'

He composed, and in due course published, lectures on 'The Theory of Language', and on 'Oratory and Criticism', and he introduced lectures on 'History and General Policy', on 'The Laws and Constitution of England', and on 'The History of England'. To recommend these studies he composed an 'Essay on a Course of Liberal Education for Civil and Active Life: with Syllabusus', in which he wrote: 'So awakened are all the States of Europe . . . to . . . their true interests . . . that . . . without superior degrees of wisdom and vigour in political measures, everything we have hitherto gained will be infallibly lost. In this critical posture of affairs more lights and superior industry are required . . . and consequently a different and better furniture of mind is requisite to be brought into the business of life. This is certainly a call upon us to examine the state of education in this country . . . '. And about teaching techniques he wrote: 'Let (the) text be the subject of a regular but familiar discourse, not exceeding an hour . . . Let the lecturer give his pupils . . . encouragement to enter occasionally into conversation, by proposing queries, or making . . . objections or remarks . . . Let time be spent in receiving from the students a minute account . . . of the preceding lecture . . . Upon every subject of importance, let the tutor make reference to the principal authors . . . and if controversial . . . on both sides of the question . . . Let the tutor select questions as exercises . . . to be treated in the form of orations, theses, or dissertations . . . . '. He added: 'A proper mixture of dignity and freedom will prevent or repress all impertinent or unseasonable remarks. A tutor must be conscious of having made very ridiculous pretensions, and of having given himself improper airs, if it give him any pain to tell his class that he will reconsider a subject; or even to acknowledge himself mistaken.' Priestley also mentioned the importance of informal and casual conversation in learning.

In addition to the above he published a 'Chart of Biography', on which prominent lives were plotted by year and by occupation. He followed this with a 'New Chart of History'. His 'Syllabus for the Study of History' included: 'The terms of fortification explained, by the help of a model . . . to enable young gentlemen to understand modern history, the newspapers, and to judge the progress of a siege'. Following the syllabus he wrote: 'I advise that more attention be given to Commercial Geography . . . we are probably strangers to some of the most useful productions of the earth . . . attention excited to the subject by teaching it to youth . . . would be the best provision for extending it . . . A knowledge of chemistry is absolutely necessary to the extension of this useful branch of science.' Dr Turner of Liverpool was invited to lecture on chemistry, and this was Priestley's first direct contact with the subject.

Priestley also taught elocution, logic, Hebrew, and, one year, anatomy (at Daventry he had read the section on anatomy in Chamber's *Cyclopaedia*). 'Finding no public exercises', he wrote, 'I introduced them . . . every Saturday the tutors . . . the students, and often strangers, were assembled to hear English and Latin compositions . . . the delivery of speeches, and the exhibition of scenes in plays.' He had considered the requirements of education and the mechanics of learning. It was in recognition of his educational contributions that he was granted an honorary Doctor of Laws by Edinburgh University. Both Benjamin Franklin and Mr Jefferson acknowledged his worth in this field.

Between 1757 and 1783, Warrington Academy admitted a total of 396 students. Twenty-two entered medicine. The first of these, Dr Percival, supported the recommendation for Priestley's honorary degree. To the son of another, Dr Bostock who attended in Priestley's time, was bequeathed by Dr Robert Cappe of York, whose father was a friend of Priestley's, ' . . . all my electrical apparatus whatever, the machine will be the more acceptable to him when he knows that it is one of the first constructed by Dr Priestley.' That particular machine has been handed down to the Royal Society. We will return to this later.

Almost the last student to be admitted was Malthus. This was after Priestley's time, but just before Priestley died, President Jefferson wrote to him: 'Have you seen the new work of Malthus on population? It is one of the ablest that I have ever seen.' Malthus quoted 'An Essay on the Population of England' by Richard Price, who was a close friend of Priestley and had recommended him for his FRS and to the Earl of Shelburne. Lectures 58 and 59 in Priestley's course on history were about the populousness of Nations, in which he commented: ' . . . it cannot be doubted but that the world is growing more populous than ever . . . The extreme of population is far from desirable.'

Priestley was also aware of the relevant and topical subject of pollution. In 1778 he wrote: 'The confinement and hard labour of working manufacturers, together with the bad air they breathe, are vey destructive.' In 1786, Dr Percival said in a letter to James Watt who, with Priestley, was among the members of the Lunar Society: 'In conversation with Dr Priestley . . . I learned . . . that you have established a method of destroying smoke which issues from . . . furnaces and other works . . . a discovery which promises to be of great importance to the inhabitants of Manchester, who appear peculiarly incident to pulmonic affections, and I am apprehensive will become more so from the rapid increase of the cotton manufacturing'.

Let us now take up the story again back at Warrington. In December 1765, Priestley described a visit to London: ' . . . being introduced to Dr. Price, Mr. Canton, Dr. Watson and Dr. Franklin, I was led to attend to the subject of experimental philosophy . . . I mentioned to Dr. Franklin an idea . . . of writing the history of the discoveries of electricity . . . and that I would willingly undertake it, provided I could be furnished with the books necessary . . . (which) he readily undertook. I set about the work, without having the least idea of doing more than writing a distinct and methodical account of all that had been done by others. Having, however, a pretty good machine . . . ' (according to his brother Timothy it was one of Nairne's) 'I was led to endeavour to ascertain several facts which were in dispute; and this led me by degrees into a large field of original experiments.' Here began Priestley's scientific career, at the age of 32. Symbolic of this, and of contemporary knowledge, is our own electrical machine (Plate 2), made recently by Mr Kahl Horner in the Department of Anaesthesia, to the same design as that bequeathed by Dr Robert Cappe of York.

The preface to Priestley's *History and Present State of Electricity* is noteworthy. He wrote: 'The immediate use of natural science is the power it gives us over nature . . . whereby life is made more comfortable and happy . . . Human happiness depends chiefly upon having some object to pursue, and upon the vigour with which our faculties are exerted in the pursuit.' He discussed the organization of science, the need for specialization reviews, for smaller societies and the organization of transactions, and for funds and encouragements. 'I wish', he wrote, 'all the incorporated philosophical societies in Europe would join the funds . . . to fit out ships for the complete discovery of the face of the earth: and for many capital experiments which can only be made in such extensive voyages.' Perhaps that was partly why Priestley was invited to join Captain Cook's second voyage—although it is said that a later work on *Vision, Light and Colours* was more directly instrumental. Clergymen on the Board of Longitude, however, objected, and the invitation was withdrawn.

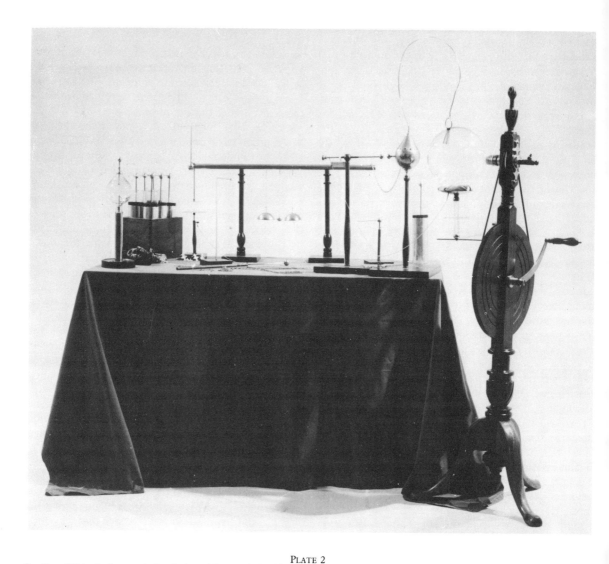

PLATE 2
Replica of Priestley's second electrical machine, made by Mr K. D. Horner, Department of Anaesthesia, from Priestley's published description and drawing, and exhibited at the City of Leeds 'O$_2$' bicentenary exhibition, 10 September – 26 October 1974. (Overall dimensions were checked against the only known surviving, but incomplete, machine, which was that originally owned by Dr Robert Cape of York and handed down to the Royal Society. This has been on display at the Science Museum, South Kensington.) Frictional electricity was generated between the rotating glass globe, and the leather rubber underneath. Electrical connection was made to the globe by suspended needles, and to the rubber by a chain. Such a machine was used for therapy at the General Infirmary at Leeds.

Priestley discussed theories of electricity. He gave practical hints and described his own experiments. He tried to compare the electrical conductivities of metals, and he discovered that charcoal was a conductor. On the penultimate page, following up an experiment suggested by Franklin, he wrote: 'May we not infer . . . that the attraction of electricity is subject to the same laws as that of gravitation, and is therefore according to the squares of the distances . . . '. He electrified animals, and observed: 'I killed a pretty large kitten with the discharge of a battery of thirty-three square feet . . . I endeavoured to bring it back to life by distending the lungs, blowing with a quill into the trachea, but to no purpose.' He described his own electrical machine (the one handed down from Robert

Cappe was of a slightly later design), and he used this to charge a battery of 64 Leyden jars, which he discharged on to metal plates. Then he used a microscope to examine the rings formed on the metal surfaces as a result of the electrical 'explosion'.

The microscope at present on show in the Leeds 'O_2' Exhibition (10 September – 26 October 1974) was purchased by Priestley from Benjamin Martin of Fleet Street in September 1767. That was the year that he came to Leeds and took charge of the Mill Hill Chapel. (Travel between London and Leeds then took two and a half days—if God permitted. For goods the flying wagon took five days.) The following year he published 'A Familiar Introduction to the Study of Electricity', and opposite the title-page he advertised his new electrical machine, which was manufactured mainly by his brother Timothy in Manchester. It was one of these which was owned by Robert Cappe. Leeds Infirmary accounts show that 11s. had already been paid to Mr Miers for electrifying, and later the Infirmary Minutes recorded that: '. . . an electrical machine is very necessary for this house.' Timothy Priestley was duly paid £5. 11s. 6d. for one of the new machines. The enthusiast was William Hey, surgeon to the Infirmary, a Methodist but scientific friend of Priestley. Doubtless Hey was familiar with John Wesley's indications for electrifying.

In order to illustrate his scientific works, Priestley learned perspective, then he used some of these illustrations for his *Familiar Introduction to the Theory and Practice of Perspective* which he published while in Leeds. He dedicated it to Joshua Reynolds. Many of the diagrams were three-dimensional and unfolded from the surface of the page.

But Priestley now had congregational responsibilities again. He resumed his speculative theology, and indulged in theological pamphleteering, for example: 'Considerations on Differences of Opinion Among Christians with a letter to the Reverend Mr Venn in answer to his' was one title advertised in the *Leeds Mercury*. Meanwhile Priestley helped found the Leeds Subscription Library, and he published his 'Essay on the First Principles of Government' in which he maintained that a man in his day, who had been tolerably well educated in an improved Christian country, had greater potential for being, and for making happy, than a person some centuries before; and he expected this trend to continue. He wrote: 'The great instrument in the hand of *Divine Providence* of this process of the species towards perfection, is *Society*, and consequently Government;'

and, ' . . . the good and happiness of the members, that is the majority of the members of any state, is the great standard by which every thing related to that state must be finally determined'. Later, Jeremy Bentham recalled that: 'Priestley was the first who taught my lips to pronounce the sacred truth—that the greatest happiness of the greatest number is the foundation of morals and legislation.' Priestley also extended his interest in the history of science. His purchase of a microscope in 1767 was doubtless in preparation for his *History and Present State of Discoveries Relating to Vision, Light and Colours*, but this left him out of pocket, and he abandoned ambitious schemes for further similar works.

When Priestley came to Leeds in 1767, the Minister's house next door to the Chapel was not ready, so he lodged in Meadow Lane, by Jaques' Brewery, where fermenting liquor supplied him with abundant fixed air (as Joseph Black named it), or carbon dioxide, for him to experiment with, at least until he accidentally contaminated a brew with ether. He found that a red rose held over the vats turned purple, and frogs seemed nearly dead, but recovered. Lighted candles were extinguished, as were lighted chips, but a red hot poker was not sooner cooled. He found that smoke 'united with this kind of air' and floated like clouds which he found very amusing to look upon. Pouring water between two vessels over the vat he sometimes made a glass of exceedingly pleasant sparkling water, so he developed apparatus specially for impregnating water with fixed air (said to be the beginning of the soda water industry). In due course the Royal College of Physicians recommended this apparatus to the Lords of the Admiralty, as likely to be of use in sea scurvy. Details were conveyed to the *Endeavour* for use during Captain Cook's second voyage. Meanwhile Dr Withering administered fixed air for phthisis, and William Hey and Dr Percival gave enemas impregnated with fixed air for putrid disorders. Thus began Priestley's 'Experiments and Observations on Different Kinds of Air' which was published in the *Philsophical Transactions* in 1772. It won him the Royal Society's Copley Medal in November 1773, and focused greater attention upon the specific properties of gases.

Priestley's thinking about 'airs' may have begun when he was eleven years old, when, according to his brother Timothy, he observed the survival of spiders put into air-tight bottles. At Warrington he tried to repair air injured by respiration, by discharging electricity into it. Then on 23 August 1771, he wrote to his great friend Theophilus Lindsay: 'I have of late been very busy about some experiments on air, with respect to respiration and vegetation, and flatter myself that I have discovered what I have long been in quest of . . . that process in nature by which air, rendered noxious by breathing, is returned to its former salubrious condition. Air in which animals have died, and which kills other animals instantly, afterwards is made fit for respiration again by plants living in it, and they thrive amazingly.'

Next Priestley experimented with nitric oxide, which he called nitrous air. Stephen Hales had recorded the red fumes that this produced when exposed to common air, and Priestley, mixing known quantities of nitrous and of common air, over water, found a diminution in volume in proportion to the common air's fitness for respiration. This was the basis of his quantitative test for the 'Goodness' of air—a welcome alternative to the survival time of mice. We may see this as analysis for oxygen, but oxygen was then unknown.

Experimenting further with nitric oxide, Priestley derived nitrous oxide, which he called dephlogisticated nitrous air. This discovery is usually dated 1772, but what Priestley did in 1772 was to expose nitrous air to a paste of iron filings and brimstone, over water. After five to six hours this got hot and effervesced. The gas contracted to one quarter of its initial volume, and it extinguished a candle. He thought that the residual gas was phlogisticated air, that is, nitrogen. He had not discovered a new air. In 1773 or early in 1774, he exposed nitrous air to iron nails over mercury, for two months. This time three-quarters of the initial volume remained. It allowed a candle to burn, sometimes with an enlarged flame, but it killed animals and its ability to support combustion was destroyed by water. These were new properties. He probably made this discovery late in 1773 because he began his next recorded experiment on 18 December (Smith, 1972). He reasoned that because this air supported combustion, it must have been able to take up phlogiston, which was thought to be the imponderable principle of inflammability. Nitrous air, he supposed, was already saturated with phlogiston, and so extinguished a candle—it could not take up any more. The new air supported combustion, and therefore the nitrous air with which he began must have been dephlogisticated. Later he repeated the experiment of 1772, but took serial gas samples. These did support combustion during the last stages of the reaction, but only before the water had time to act. Presumably Priestley did not find nitrous oxide

in 1772 because he lost it into solution.

On 1 August 1774, using a large burning lens, Priestley heated mercuric oxide over mercury, and obtained an air that supported combustion. Because of this property he assumed that it was dephlogisticated nitrous air, although he was at a loss to explain it. His experiments were then interrupted by travels with the Earl of Shelburne in Europe. He met Lavoisier and told him about his new experiment. In November, back in England, Priestley found that this air supported combustion even after agitation with water—therefore it was *not* dephlogisticated nitrous air. In March 1755, a mouse lived twice as long in this air as it would have done in common air, and the remaining air was still at least as good as common air—so Priestley reasoned that the mouse must have been breathing dephlogisticated air. He had in fact prepared the same air as early as 1771 by heating saltpetre, but the significance of this escaped him. The precise date of his 'discovery' of dephlogisticated air or oxygen, depends upon one's definition of a discovery.

Priestley's experiments on different kinds of air stimulated physicians to explore their medical application. Dr Beddoes, for example, founded the Medical Pneumatic Institution in Clifton. The superintendent was young Humphry Davy, who investigated nitrous oxide. Davy discovered that its inhalation relieved toothache, and he actually suggested its use during surgical operations. The immediate fruits of Davy's work, however, were to get him a job at the Royal Institution, and to popularize nitrous oxide as laughing gas, encouraging its inhalation upon the stage, and at public lectures. At such a lecture in America, in 1844, Horace Wells, a dentist, noticed that a participant appeared oblivious of an injury sustained under its influence. Wells then breathed the gas from a bladder, without air or oxygen, immediately before having one of his own teeth pulled by a colleague. The extraction was painless. Today, nitrous oxide, *and* oxygen are the commonest ingredients of anaesthesia, and used also for analgesia. Some anaesthetic machines also carry carbon dioxide, and oxygen is, of course, used for therapy. Hence anaesthetists' curiosity about Joseph Priestley.

By 1773, Priestley had joined the Earl of Shelburne whose seat, Bowood, was in Wiltshire. Priestley lived nearby in Calne, but spent the greater part of winter at his Lordship's London house. Perhaps Priestley exposed nitrous air to iron nails just before leaving for London, and found nitrous oxide when he returned two months later.

An immediate sequel to his discovery of oxygen was his paper 'Observations on Respiration and the Use of Blood', dated 1776. Priestley confirmed the usual colour changes in sheep's blood, noting that the change might occur in the lungs. He found that dark blood turned red more quickly and completely in dephlogisticated air than in common air; and furthermore, that the goodness of air was reduced by repeated exposure to dark blood. On the other hand nitrous air repeatedly exposed to red blood was diminished, and lost some of its power of diminishing common air. Said he: 'As the principal use of blood seems to be its power of receiving and discharging phlogiston' (we could say discharging and receiving oxygen), 'and as the degree in which it possesses this power is easily ascertained by the eye, it might not, perhaps, be unworthy of being particularly attended to by physicians'. Later that year, John Hunter, advocating blowing air into the lungs of the apparently drowned, acknowledged that: 'Perhaps the dephlogisticated air, described by Dr. Priestley, may prove to be more efficacious than common air.'

This is an appropriate point at which to leave Dr Joseph Priestley at Calne, early in 1777, in the company of his servants, his children and his wife, reading a letter just received from Paris in which Benjamin Franklin wrote: 'I rejoice to hear your continual progress in those useful discoveries. I find that you have set all the philosophers of Europe at work upon the *fixed air*; and it is with great pleasure I observe how high you stand in their opinion; for I enjoy my friend's fame as my own.'

In many ways Priestley may have reflected some of the trends of his time, but undoubtedly he contributed vision, light and colour.

REFERENCES

Crook, R. E. *A Bibliography of Joseph Priestley*; Library Association: 1966
Lester, D. N. R. (1962). The History of Batley Free Grammar School, 1612–1972, based on a thesis submitted for the degree of MEd at the University of Leeds.
Smith, W. D. A. (1972). *Brit. J. Anaesth.*, **44**, 297.

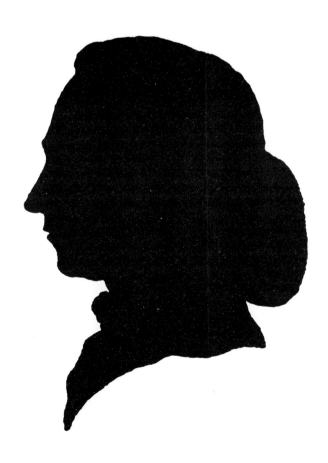

2

THE DISCOVERY OF NITROUS OXIDE AND OF OXYGEN

"It may be asked: Did Priestley 'discover' nitrous oxide?" (Hartog, 1941).

Priestley's "discovery" of nitrous oxide.

If Priestley did "discover" nitrous oxide, it may be asked: When did he discover it? Various dates between 1772 and 1777 have been suggested (table I).

TABLE I. *Dates quoted by various authors for the discovery or the first preparation of nitrous oxide.*

Before 1766	Robison (1803) cited Partington (1962)
1772	Davy (1812); Roscoe and Schorlemmer (1884) cited Hewitt (1893); Buxton (1914); Flagg (1916); Gardner (1916); Gwathmey (1925); Sykes (1939); Goldman (1941); Lundy (1943); King (1946); Parry-Price (1946); Robinson (1946); Clement (1951); Seward and Bryce-Smith (1957); Wylie and Churchill-Davidson (1960); McKie (1961); Keys (1963); Heironimus (1964); Wood-Smith and Stewart (1964); Faulconer and Keys (1965); Smith (1965) by implication; Lee and Atkinson (1968); Paton and Payne (1968); Davison (1971)
1772–3	Cartwright (1952)
1773	Fülöp-Miller (1938), authority not cited; Marston in foreword to Cartwright (1952)
1774	Dallemagne (1948)
About 1774	Robinson (1922), in posthumous edition of Hewitt's *Anaesthetics and their Administration* in which Hewitt had previously given the alternative dates of 1772 or 1776
1776	Watts (1868) cited Hewitt (1893); Braine (1872); Hadfield (1923); Webster (1924); Dogliotti (1935); Collins (1966)
About 1766	Boyle and Hewer (1923)
1777	Lee (1947); Marston (1949)
Date not specified	Blomfield (1922); Duncum (1947); Collins (1952); Gibbs (1965) but he implied that it was not 1772 when he considered nitrogen rather than nitrous oxide to have been prepared

The date quoted most frequently is 1772. This was the date implied in Part I (Smith, 1965), in which Priestley's vivid description of the diminution of nitrous air* by a mixture of iron filings and brimstone

---

*N.B. Nitrous air is nitric oxide.

Dephlogisticated nitrous air is nitrous oxide.

Phlogisticated air is nitrogen.

Dephlogisticated air is oxygen.

Fixed air is carbon dioxide.

Brimstone is sulphur.

Liver of sulphur is potassium polysulphide.

---

made into a paste with water, was quoted as follows:

The diminution of common air by a mixture of nitrous air, is not so extraordinary as the diminution which nitrous air itself is subject to from a mixture of iron filings and brimstone, made into a paste with water. This mixture, as I have already observed, diminishes common air between one fifth and one fourth . . . but when it is put into a quantity of nitrous air, it diminishes it so much than no more than one fourth of the original quantity be left. The effect of this process is generally perceived in five or six hours, about which time the visible effervescence of the mixture begins; and in a very short time it advances so rapidly, that in about an hour almost the whole effect will have taken place. If it be suffered to stand a day or two longer, the air will still be diminished farther, but only a very little farther, in proportion to the first diminution. The glass jar, in which the air and this mixture have been confined, has generally been so much heated in this process, that I have not been able to touch it.

Following this quotation the statement was made that:

The remaining air supported combustion and it smelled more like common air than like nitrous air. He named it "dephlogisticated nitrous air". In his own words (Priestley, 1786): "Dephlogisticated nitrous air is the term by which I first distinguished this species of air, because it admitted a candle to burn in it." This is now known as nitrous oxide.

Although it could be argued that this statement is not entirely untrue, it would not have been true in 1772 and it is certainly misleading.

In 1772 Priestley undoubtedly exposed nitrous air to a mixture of iron filings and sulphur, with water, which he found led to a considerable reduction in its volume. He also found that the residual gas "has not the peculiar smell of nitrous air, but smells more like common air in which the same mixture has stood". At that time Priestley evidently appreciated that he had begun the experiment with nitrous air in the container and ended it with a smaller quantity of something which was not nitrous air. He did not, however, record that the end product had any specific properties other than those possessed by common air.

Later Priestley (1777), discussing the phenomena attending the diminution of nitrous air by iron filings and brimstone, and also by liver of sulphur, wrote:

The first remarkable diminution that I observed was occasioned by the fermentation of iron filings with brimstone, made into a paste with water. This process is attended with much heat, the diminution of the air is exceedingly rapid, and whenever I examined the air that remained, it always appeared to be simply phlogisticated air, neither affecting common air, not being affected by nitrous air, and always extinguishing a candle.

This makes it quite clear that in 1772 Priestley was not aware that he had discovered a new air by exposing nitrous air to a paste of iron filings and brimstone. It even casts doubt upon whether he had prepared a new air at the time.

Reporting experiments and observations made in the year 1773, and the beginning of the year 1774 (Priestley, 1774), Priestley described an experiment in which he exposed nitrous air to iron over mercury (without any sulphur) for about two months. He wrote:

. . . a most remarkable and unexpected change was made in the nitrous air; and in pursuing the experiment, it was transformed into a species of air, with properties which, at the time of my first publication on this subject, I should not have hesitated to pronounce impossible, *viz.* air in which a candle burns quite naturally and freely, and which is yet in the highest degree noxious to animals, in so much that they die the moment they are put into it; whereas, in general, animals live with little sensible inconvenience in air in which candles have burned out. Such, however, is nitrous air, after it has been long exposed to a large surface of iron.

It is not less extraordinary, that a still longer continuance of nitrous air in these circumstances (but *how long* depends upon too many, and too minute circumstances to be ascertained with exactness) makes it not only to admit a candle to burn in it, but enables it to burn with an *enlarged flame*, by another flame (extending everywhere to an equal distance from that of the candle, and often plainly distinguishable from it) adhering to it. Sometimes I have perceived the flame of the candle, in these circumstances, to be twice as large as it is naturally, and sometimes not less than five or six times larger; and yet without anything like an *explosion*, such as in the firing of the weakest inflammable air.

There we have Priestley's "discovery" of an air with new and specific properties: his "discovery" of nitrous oxide. The instantaneous death of mice put into this new air can probably be attributed as much to the effects of unchanged nitric oxide as to the effects of nitrous oxide and of anoxia. The crucial experiment was most probably carried out towards the end of 1773 because on the following page he wrote: "Lastly, one quantity of nitrous air, which had been exposed to iron and quicksilver from December 18 to January 20 . . .".

Continuing his account of the discovery of this new air, Priestley made the following observation:

Nor is the farther progress in the transmutation of nitrous air, in these circumstances, less remarkable. For when it has been brought to the state last mentioned, the agitation of it in fresh water almost instantly takes off

that peculiar kind of inflammability, so that it extinguishes a candle, retaining its noxious quality . . .

Presumably the explanation of this is that much of the nitrous oxide that he had prepared was dissolved in water. This is most probably why he did not "discover" nitrous oxide in 1772. Confirmation of this point would require critical repetition of his original experiments, using modern methods of gas analysis capable of distinguishing the various oxides of nitrogen.

Priestley's repetition of his experiment of 1772.

Priestley also prepared nitrous oxide by exposing nitrous air to liver of sulphur, and he found that this reaction was quicker than when iron was used. This led him to repeat his previous experiments in which the exposure of nitrous air to a mixture of iron filings and brimstone had produced an air which extinguished a candle. In 1777 he was able to write:

I have since, however, observed that nitrous air diminished by iron filings and brimstone does not really differ from that which is diminished by the other processes; but that this process being made in a large quantity of water, either the superfluous nitrous acid vapour, the superfluous phlogiston, or both, were always absorbed before the experiment was made. This I discovered by repeating the process in the following manner.

Having introduced a pot of iron filings and brimstone into a large jar of nitrous air, I examined the state of the air in all the stages of its diminution, from the time that the fermentation began, till it could be diminished no more by that process. In order to get a small quantity of the air, without moving the jar, or disturbing the apparatus contained in it, I fastened a small phial, or a piece of glass tube, to the end of a stiff wire; and filling it with water, I put it up into the vessel, with its mouth downwards; when, the water running out, it would necessarily be filled with the air of the jar, which I could then with the same ease withdraw, and examine.

Proceeding in this manner, I found that, in the last stage of the diminution of this air, and not before, a candle burned in it with an enlarged flame. This process, therefore, exactly resembles that with iron only or liver of sulphur, only that in this case the air must be examined very soon, before the water can have had an opportunity to act upon it . . .

The first preparation of nitrous oxide by Joseph Black.

From these later experiments it could be argued that Priestley did prepare nitrous oxide in 1772, but did not know it. If this is admitted as significant evidence for the *"discovery"* of nitrous oxide, however, it may have to be conceded that the credit is due not to Joseph Priestley, but to Joseph Black.

Robison (1803, cited Partington, 1962), publishing Black's *Lectures on the Elements of Chemistry* after his death, added the following note to the account of ammonium nitrate:

In a bundle, marked "old notes, excerpts, &c." I find some experiments on this salt, which deserves some notice. Dr Black seems to aim at the best process for preparing it for medical purposes by sublimation. He was aiming at the same thing with the salt called *acetous ammoniac*, and is surprised that he can prepare the latter very easily, but that the nitrous ammoniac could not be condensed, although its ingredients are not nearly so volatile as those of the other.

In one experiment with a dry nitrous ammoniac, which he had prepared himself by mixing colourless nitrous acid with the purest volatile alkali, the vapours were incoercible *in part*, and what did condense was almost pure water, greatly exceeding in quantity what could be supposed necessary for the crystals of the salt. He was obliged to give passage to the incondensible vapours. He tried whether they were inflammable, by presenting a bit of lighted paper to the hole in the luting. It did not take fire, but it made the paper burn with prodigious violence. He thought, from this circumstance, that it was the nitrous acid: But putting alkaline ley into the receiver, he did not find it condense more readily, nor produce a nitre. Putting lime water into the receiver, he found no precipitation, when he used the pure salt prepared by himself; but employing some gotten in the shop of Mr Hill (which I mention, because it shows the date of the experiment to be previous to 1766), he had a precipitate. He attributes this to impure alkali, containing inflammable matter. He says, that although the incoercible fumes filled the laboratory, the effect on his breathing and sensations was *very far from being unpleasant*. He suspects that the acid suffers some decomposition, and again wonders at the quantity of water obtained. With some particular view, he had mixed with the salt thrice its weight of finely powdered glass. In three succeeding trials, the mixture detonated, and burst the vessels, although the heat was not much above that of boiling water.

These experiments tally in many particulars, with those in the judicious analysis of this salt by Mr Davy of the Royal Institution. Dr Black has had some experience of the wonderful effects of the *gaseous oxyd of azote*, or *nitrous oxyd*, which have given so much amusement of late, and from which mighty medical consequences are expected by some physicians. This subject will come before us some time hence. [See Appendix.]

The significance of the above reference to Mr Hill's shop and to the date 1766, is that Mr Ninian Hill, and Co, surgeon, was proprietor of a "dispensary shop Leeche's land, south side Trongate, No. 54" (Jones' Directory of Glasgow, 1787; personal communication Miss E. G. Jack, 1970), and that Joseph Black moved from Glasgow to Edinburgh in 1766. There is evidence, however, that Black was still in communication with Mr Hill as late as 1768 (Robinson and McKie, 1970), so it is possible that he purchased chemicals from him after 1766.

The following caution has also been given by McKie and Kennedy (1960): ". . . the historical value of the content of the printed *Lectures* is not very great, and statements are to be ascribed to Black only when they can be confirmed by independent evidence from other sources". Unfortunately none of Black's MS. notes used by Robison appear to have survived (Smeaton, W. A., 1970, personal

communication), and Black did not publish anything on the subject himself. Manuscript lecture notes made by Thomas Cochrane, when he attended Black's lectures in Chemistry in Edinburgh during the session 1767–68, have survived (edited McKie, 1966). These record:

> *Ammon Nitros:* is the most fusible of the Common Salts; w^n the heat is increased is copiously converted into Vapour; the degree of heat Sufficient for its fusion is that of boiling water if exposed to a sudden heat undergoes a deflagration although no inflammable matter be added to it.

Similar notes made by George Cayley (1786), nearly twenty years later, record:

> *Nitros Ammoniac*, also called nitrum semi volatile, & some times Nitrum Fulminans. It is the most fusible of ye compound salts; it melts in glass vessels, in a heat not greatly exceeding boiling water, it appears perfectly fluid & transparent like oil, & begins to emit vapours if ye heat is increased, & soon entirely evaporates, but if ye heat is applied more suddenly it takes fire, w^c gives a presumption y^t ye volatile alkali contains inflammable matters in its composition, & ye other ammoniacs when thrown into melted nitre shows ye same inflammation & there are many other experiments, w^c show y^t there is some of ye principle of inflammability in ye composition of ye volatile alkali . . .

Cochrane's notes suggest that Black had prepared nitrous oxide by heating ammonium nitrate at least as early as 1767, but Cochrane does not reveal any of the properties of the copious vapour into which the ammonium nitrate was converted. George Cayley tantalizes us with his mention of "many other experiments, w^c show y^t there is some of ye principle of inflammability in ye composition of ye volatile alkali". Although details of the experiments were withheld, this hint does lend some support to Robison's note quoted above.*

Background to Priestley's "discovery" of nitrous oxide.

If Priestley did "discover" nitrous oxide, it may also be asked: Why did he discover it?

An early reference to Priestley's interest in air is contained in his *History and Present State of Electricity, with Original Experiments (1767),* in which he wrote:

> Having read, and finding by my own experiments, that a candle would not burn in air that had passed through a charcoal fire, or through the lungs of animals, or in any of that air which the chymists call mephitic; I was considering what kind of change it underwent, by passing through the fire, or through the lungs &c., and

---

* Another set of manuscript notes, dated 1770, and now at the Royal College of Surgeons, Edinburgh, does not throw any further light on the subject.

whether it was not possible to restore it to its original state, by some operation or mixture. For this purpose I gave great intestinal motion to it; I threw a quantity of electric matter from the point of a conductor into it, and performed various other operations upon it, but without any effect.

When Priestley moved from Warrington to Leeds in 1767 he found an abundant supply of carbon dioxide in the brewery adjacent to his temporary home. This was an added stimulus and he began his experiments on different kinds of air which were enthusiastically received when first published in 1772. He then revealed that his interest in nitrous air arose from reading Stephen Hales' *Vegetable Staticks* (1727):

Ever since I first read Dr Hales's most excellent *Statical Essays*, I was particularly struck with that experiment of his, of which an account is given, Vol. I, p. 224, and Vol. II, p. 280, in which common air and air generated from Walton Pyrites, by spirit of nitre, made a turbid red mixture, and in which part of the common air was absorbed; but I never expected to have the satisfaction of seeing this remarkable appearance, supposing it to be peculiar to that particular mineral. Happening to mention this subject to the Hon. Mr Cavendish, when I was in London, in the spring of the year 1772, he said that he did not imagine but that other kinds of pyrites, or the metals might answer as well, and that probably the red appearance of the mixture depended upon the spirit of nitre only. This encouraged me to attend to the subject; and having no pyrites, I began with the solution of the different metals in the spirit of nitre, and catching the air which was generated in the solution, I presently found what I wanted, and a good deal more.

Beginning with the solution of brass, on the 4th of June, 1772, I first found this remarkable species of air, only one effect of which was casually observed by Dr Hales; and he gave little attention to it, and it has been so unnoticed since his time, that, as far as I know, no name has been given to it, I therefore found myself, contrary to my first resolution, under an absolute necessity of giving a name to this kind of air myself. When I first began to speak and write of it to my friends, I happened to distinguish it by the name *nitrous air*, because I had procured it by means of spirit of nitre only; and though I cannot say that I altogether like the term, neither myself nor any of my friends, to whom I have applied for the purpose, have been able to hit upon a better; so that I am obliged, after all, to content myself with it.

Having obtained nitrous air, Priestley investigated its reaction with common air, and he found that:

The diminution of a mixture of this air and common air is not an equal diminution of both kinds, which is all that Dr Hales could observe, but of about one fifth of the common air, and as much of the nitrous air as is necessary to produce that effect; which, as I have found by many trials, is about one half as much as the original quantity of common air. For if one measure of nitrous air be put to two measures of common air, in a few minutes (by which time the effervescence will be over) there will want about one ninth of the original two measures; and if both the kinds of air be very pure, the diminution will still go on slowly, till in a day or two, the whole will be reduced to about one fifth less than the original quantity of common air . . .

He went on to repeat the experiment over mercury, and noted that there was still a reduction in volume, but not as great as when it was carried out over water.

His next major step was to determine that:

. . . this effervescence and diminution, occasioned by the mixture of nitrous air, is peculiar to common air, or *air fit for respiration*; and as far as I can judge, from a great number of observations, is at least very nearly, if not exactly, in proportion to its fitness for this purpose; so that by this means the goodness of air may be distinguished much more accurately than it can be by putting mice, or any other animals, to breathe in it.

This was a most agreeable discovery to me, as I hope it may be an useful one to the public; especially as, from this time, I had no occasion for so large a stock of mice as I had been used to keep for the purpose of these experiments, using them only in those which required to be very decisive; and in these cases I have seldom failed to know beforehand in what manner they would be affected. . . .

. . . Also the degree of diminution being from nothing at all to more than one third of the whole of the quantity of air, we are by this means, in possession of a prodigiously large *scale*, by which we may distinguish very small degrees of difference in the goodness of air.

Priestley made extensive use of his new test of the goodness of air. Previously he had used mice for his investigation of the power of living plants to restore air which had been injured by the respiration of animals. He used the test, belatedly, when he "discovered" oxygen and its power of supporting respiration. He also applied it to the residual air obtained in the experiment of 1772, in which he exposed nitrous air to a paste of iron filings and brimstone over water. Note his comment, ". . . it always appeared to be simply phlogisticated air, neither affecting common air, *nor being affected by nitrous air*, and always extinguishing a candle".

The idea of exposing common air to iron filings and brimstone also came from his reading of Hales' work. He wrote: "I repeated the experiment and found the diminution greater than I had expected." (The origin of the mixture of iron filings and brimstone made into a paste with water is uncertain. It was used by Lemery as early as 1690 (cited Partington, 1962) to imitate volcanic action, by burying it in the ground.) Having followed Hales' example and tried the effect of the paste of iron filings and brimstone on common air, it is not surprising that he should have tried out its effect on nitrous air.

Priestley's trial of the effect of iron upon nitrous air over mercury, in 1773, was not directly related to his experiment with iron filings and brimstone in 1772. His reasons for carrying out the crucial experiment that led to the "discovery" of nitrous oxide are clearly stated:

As fixed air united to water dissolves iron, I had the curiosity to try whether fixed air alone would do it; and as nitrous air is of an *acid* nature, as well as fixed air, I, at the same time, exposed a large surface of iron to both kinds; first filling two eight ounce phials with nails, and then with quicksilver, and after that displacing the quicksilver in one of the phials by fixed air, and in the other nitrous air; then inverting them, and leaving them with their mouths immersed in basons of quicksilver.

In these circumstances the two phials stood about two months, when no sensible change at all was produced in the fixed air, or in the iron which had been exposed to it, but a most remarkable, and most unexpected change was made in the nitrous air.

Sequel to the "discovery" of nitrous oxide: the "discovery" of oxygen.

Because Priestley had recently "discovered" nitrous oxide he was slow in recognizing that he had "discovered" oxygen. He confused oxygen with nitrous oxide. The story is best told in his own words (Priestley, 1775):

. . . having . . . procured a (burning) lens of twelve inches diameter, and twenty inches focal distance, I proceeded with great alacrity to examine, by the help of it, what kind of air a great variety of substances, natural and factitious, would yield, putting them into vessels . . . which I filled with quicksilver, and kept inverted in a bason of same. . . .

With this apparatus, after a variety of other experiments . . . on the 1st of August, 1774, I endeavoured to extract air from *mercurius calcinatus per se*; and I presently found that, by means of this lens, air was expelled from it very readily. Having got about three or four times as much as the bulk of my materials, I admitted water to it, and found that it was not imbibed by it. But what surprised me more than I can well express, was, that a candle burned in this air with a remarkably vigorous flame, very much like that enlarged flame with which a candle burns in nitrous air, exposed to iron or liver of sulphur; but as I had got nothing like this remarkable appearance from any kind of air besides this particular modification of nitrous air, and I knew no nitrous acid was used in the preparation of mercurius calcinatus, I was utterly at a loss how to account for it.

In this case, also, though I did not give sufficient attention to the circumstance at that time, the flame of the candle, besides, being larger, burned with more splendor and heat than in that species of nitrous air; and a piece of red hot wood sparkled in it, exactly like paper dipped in solution of nitre, and it consumed very fast; an experiment which I had never thought of trying with nitrous air.

At the same time that I made the above mentioned experiment, I extracted a quantity of air, with the very same property from the common *red precipitate*, which being produced by a solution of mercury in spirit of nitre, made me conclude that this peculiar property, being similar to that of the modification of nitrous air above mentioned, depended upon something being communicated to it by the nitrous acid; and the *mercurius calcinatus* is produced by exposing mercury to a certain degree of heat, where common air has access to it, I likewise concluded that this

substance had collected something of nitre, in that state of heat, from the atmosphere.

. . . I entertained some suspicion that the mercurius calcinatus, on which I had made my experiments, being bought at a common apothecary's, might, in fact, be nothing more than red precipitate; though, had I been any thing of a practical chymist, I could not have entertained any such suspicion. However, mentioning this suspicion to Mr Warltire, he furnished me with some that he had kept for a specimen of the preparation, and which, he told me, he could warrant to be genuine. This being treated in the same manner as the former, only by a longer continuance of heat, I extracted much more air from it than from the other.

This experiment might have satisfied any moderate sceptic: but, however, being at Paris in the October following, and knowing that there were several very eminent chymists in that place, I did not omit the opportunity, by means of my friend Mr Magellan, to get an ounce of mercurius calcinatus prepared by Mr Cadet, of the genuineness of which there could not possibly be any suspicion; and at the same time, I frequently mentioned my surprize at the kind of air which I had got from this preparation to Mr Lavoisier, Mr le Roy, and several other philosophers, who honoured me with their notice in that city; and who, I dare say, cannot fail to recollect the circumstance.

At the same time, I had no suspicion that the air which I had got from the mercurius calcinatus was even wholesome, so far was I from knowing what it was that I had really found; taking it for granted, that it was nothing more than such kind of air as I had brought nitrous air to by the processes above mentioned; and in this air I have observed that a candle would burn sometimes quite naturally, and sometimes with a beautiful enlarged flame, and yet remain perfectly noxious.

At the same time that I had got the air above mentioned from mercurius calcinatus and the red precipitate, I had got the same kind from *red lead* or *minium*. In this process, that part of the minium on which the focus of the lens had fallen, turned yellow. One third of the air, in this experiment, was readily absorbed by water, but, in the remainder a candle burned very strongly, and with a crackling noise.

That fixed air is contained in red lead I had observed before; for I had expelled it by the heat of a candle, and found it to be very pure. See Vol. I, p. 192. I imagine it requires more heat than I used to expel any of the other kind of air.

This experiment with *red lead* confirmed me in my suspicion, that *mercurius calcinatus* must get the property of yielding this kind of air from the atmosphere, the process by which that preparation, and this of red lead is made, being similar. As I never make the least secret of any thing that I observe, I mentioned this experiment also, as well as those with the mercurius calcinatus, and the red precipitate, to all my philosophical acquaintance at Paris, and elsewhere; having no idea at that time, to what these remarkable facts would lead.

Presently after my return from abroad, I went to work upon the *mercurius calcinatus*, which I procured from Mr Cadet; and, with a very moderate degree of heat, I got from about one fourth of an ounce of it, an ounce measure of air, which I observed to be not readily imbibed, either by the substance itself from which it had been expelled . . . or by water, in which I suffered this to stand a considerable time before I made any experiment upon it.

In this air, as I had expected, a candle burned with a vivid flame; but what I observed new at this time (Nov. 19), and which surprised me no less than the fact I had discovered before, was, that, whereas a few moments agitation in water will deprive the modified nitrous air of its property of admitting a candle to burn in it; yet, after more than ten times as much agitation as would be sufficient to produce this alteration in the nitrous air, no sensible change was produced in this. A candle still burned in it with a strong flame; and it did not, in the least, diminish common air, which I have observed that nitrous air, in this state, in some measure, does.

Priestley then found that even two days of contact with water did not rob this air of its property of allowing a candle to burn. He continued:

These facts fully convinced me, that there must be a very material difference between the constitution of the air from mercurius calcinatus, and that of phlogisticated nitrous air, notwithstanding their resemblance in some particulars.* But though I did not doubt that the air from *mercurius calcinatus* was fit for respiration, after being agitated in water, as with every other kind of air without exception, on which I had tried the experiment, had been, I still did not suspect that it was respirable in the first instance; so far was I from having any idea of this air being, what it really was, much superior, in this respect, to the air of the atmosphere.

In this ignorance of the real nature of this kind of air, I continued from this time (November) to the 1st of March following; . . . But in the course of this month, I not only ascertained the nature of this kind of air, though very gradually, but was led by it to the complete discovery of the air we breathe.

Till this 1st March, 1775, I had so little suspicion of the air from mercurius calcinatus, &c. being wholesome, that I have not even thought of applying it to the test of nitrous air; but thinking (as my reader must imagine I frequently must have done) on the candle burning in it after long agitation in water, it occurred to me at last to make the experiment; and putting one measure of nitrous air to two measures of this air, I found, not only that it was diminished, but that it was diminished quite as much as common air, and that the redness of the mixture was likewise equal to that of a similar mixture of nitrous and common air.

After this I had no doubt but that the air from mercurius calcinatus was fit for respiration, and that it had all the other properties of genuine common air. But I did not take notice of what I might have observed, if I had not been so fully possessed by the notion of there being no air better than common air, that the redness was really deeper, and the diminution something greater than common air would have admitted.

. . . the next day I was more surprised than ever I had been before, with finding that, after the above mentioned mixture of nitrous air and the air from the mercurius calcinatus, had stood all night, . . . a candle burned in it, and even better than in common air.

I cannot, at this distance of time, recollect what it was that I had in view in making this experiment; but I know I had no expectation of the real issue of it. . . . If, however, I had not happened, for some other purpose, to have had a lighted candle before me, I should probably never have made the trial; and the whole train of my future experiments relating to this kind of air might have been prevented. . . .

On the 8th of this month I procured a mouse, and put it into a glass vessel, containing two ounce-measures of the air from mercurius calcinatus. Had it been common air, a full grown mouse, as this was, would have lived in

it about a quarter of an hour. In this air, however, my mouse lived a full half hour; and although it was taken out seemingly dead,† it appeared to have been only exceedingly chilled; for, upon being held to the fire, it presently revived, and appeared not to have received any harm from the experiment.

By this I was confirmed in my conclusion, that the air extracted from mercurius calcinatus, &c. was, *at least, as good as* common air: but I did not certainly conclude that it was any *better*; because, though one mouse would live only a quarter of an hour in a given quantity of air, I knew that it was not impossible but that another mouse might have lived in it half an hour; so little accuracy is there in this method of ascertaining the goodness of air. . . .

This experiment with the mouse, when I had reflected upon it for some time, gave me so much suspicion that the air into which I had put it was better than common air, that I was induced, the day after, to apply the test of nitrous air to a small part of that very quantity of air which the mouse had breathed so long; so that had it been common air, I was satisfied it must have been very nearly, if not altogether, as noxious as possible, so as not to be affected by nitrous air; when, to my surprise again, I found that though it had been breathed for long, it was still better than common air. . . . Thinking of this extraordinary fact upon my pillow, the next morning I put another measure of nitrous air to the same mixture, and, to my utter astonishment, found that it was farther diminished to almost one half of its original quantity. I then put a third measure to it; but this did not diminish it any farther, but, however, left it one measure less than it was even after the mouse had been taken out of it.

Priestley then tried the effect of the air on another mouse which lived for about three-quarters of an hour, but was unable to revive it afterwards, and he again suspected that the mouse had succumbed to cold. He continued:

Being now fully satisfied of the superior goodness of this kind of air, I proceeded to measure that degree of purity, with as much accuracy as I could, by the test of nitrous air. . . . I conclude that it was between four and five times as good as common air.

His researches into what he later called dephlogisticated air did not end there, but the rest of the tale is not directly relevant to this article.

Conclusion.

Present evidence suggests, therefore, that Joseph Black prepared nitrous oxide by heating ammonium nitrate at least as early as 1767, and possibly as early as 1766. Although he never published this experiment he promulgated it in his lectures. There is also inconclusive evidence that he was aware of its property of supporting combustion. In 1772 Joseph Priestley, by exposing nitric oxide to a paste of iron filings and sulphur over water, would have

---

* Misprint for dephlogisticated nitrous air in Priestley's original work.

†A case of "suspended animation" due to the accumulation of carbon dioxide. Priestley had previously rendered animals comatose by holding them over the vats of fermenting liquor in the brewery next door to his home, and found that they recovered in common air.

prepared nitrous oxide, but he was quite unaware of this at the time, presumably because the nitrous oxide was lost into solution before he was able to observe its properties. He did not pursue the experiment at that time. Later, following a completely different line of thought, he prepared nitrous oxide by exposing nitric oxide to iron over mercury, and on this occasion he observed that it permitted a candle to burn with an enlarged flame. The date of this experiment is almost certainly 1773, probably towards the end of the year. On August 1, 1774, Priestley heated mercuric oxide and obtained a gas which supported combustion, as if, it seemed to him, it was nitrous oxide. This puzzled him and he pursued the matter. It was not until November 19 that he found that the gas supported combustion even after agitation with water and from this time he recognized that it could not be nitrous oxide. On March 1, 1775, he applied his test of "goodness" and found that it was as "good" as common air. On March 8 he found that a mouse could live in this gas for more than twice the time it would have done in common air, and testing the "goodness" of the gas that the mouse had breathed he then concluded that it must be "better" than common air. This he confirmed by trying its effect on another mouse and by very careful and repeated tests of its "goodness", and he concluded that it was four to five times as "good" as common air.

APPENDIX

Despite Robison's conviction that the "vapour" produced by Black was nitrous oxide—which was not contradicted by Partington (1963)—ammonium nitrate can sublime as a white cloud on heating just above its melting point. This could have been the "vapour" referred to, in which case it would have had a slightly ammoniacal smell (Dr A. T. Austin, 1972, personal communication). On raising the temperature further, however, nitrous oxide would have been formed. That the temperature was raised is evident from the following extract from another set of notes taken during Black's lectures by N. Dimsdale, in 1767 (MS. 3534 pp. 4–6, National Library of Scotland).

"Ammon: Nitrosum. . . . The same heat requisite to its Fusion, converts it into a stinking Vapour. If it be exposed to a Degree approaching red Heat, it is liable to undergo a sort of Inflammation; . . ."

The description of the vapour as "stinking" does not accord with Robison's version of Black's own notes, which refers to the effect on the breathing and sensations as being "very far from unpleasant". One can only guess the origin of the stink. There may have been impurities or higher oxides of nitrogen, or someone may have found the smell of subliming ammonium nitrate to be objectionable.

Some time after 1775 Priestley (1777) produced nitrous oxide using nitric acid and zinc, but repeat experiments did not always produce the same results and nitric oxide was always present. He had tried adding zinc to nitric

acid as early as 1772 when he was experimenting with different methods of making nitric oxide. In one of these experiments he would have produced oxygen. Having obtained all the gas that he was able to at room temperature, he then boiled the solution in a sand-heat until all the fluid part was evaporated and there remained a brown fixed substance. A part of this he threw into a small red-hot crucible which he immediately covered with a receiver, standing in water. He wrote:

"I observed that very dense red fumes rose from it, and filled the receiver. This redness lasted about as long as that which is occasioned by a mixture of nitrous and common air; the air is also considerably diminished with the receiver . . .

"It is remarkable, however, that though the air within the receiver was diminished about one-fifth by this process, it was itself affected with a mixture of nitrous air, as common air is, and a candle burned in it very well . . ."

The latter observations indicate that he had obtained more than sufficient oxygen to react with both the nitric oxide which was also evolved, and with the nitric oxide which he then added. Presumably his brown residue was a nitrate. Priestley does not appear to have appreciated the significance of this finding.

ACKNOWLEDGEMENTS

I am indebted to Dr W. A. Smeaton, Reader in History and Philosophy of Science, University College, London, who first suggested to me that Priestley did not discover nitrous oxide in 1772. Among other things, he also drew my attention to the unreliability of Robison's text of Black's lectures. I am most grateful to Dr D. Robertson, hon. librarian, the York Medical Society, who provided every facility for my perusal of George Cayley's manuscript notes of Black's lectures. Mr C. G. Wood, librarian, the Andersonian Library, Glasgow, kindly drew my attention to Thomas Cochrane's manuscript notes, and to the recent edition of these edited by McKie (1966) (Mr R. G. Hoare, Division Chairman, the Imperial Chemical Industries Ltd, courteously provided me with a copy). I also wish to thank: Miss E. G. Jack, reference librarian, the University of Glasgow, who, among other things, provided information on Ninian Hill; Miss D. U. Wardle, librarian, the Royal College of Surgeons, Edinburgh, who provided relevant details of another set of Black's lectures; Mr J. W. Cockburn, City Librarian and Curator, Edinburgh; Dr A. T. Austin, Department of Organic Chemistry, University of Leeds; and Mr P. M. Cadell, assistant keeper, National Library of Scotland.

REFERENCES

Blomfield, J. (1922). Anaesthetics in Practice and Theory. London: Heinemann.
Boyle, H. E. G., and Hewer, C. L. (1923). Practical Anaesthetics, 3rd edn. London: Froude and Hodder & Stoughton.
Braine, F. W. (1872). On the chemistry of nitrous oxide. Trans. Odont. Soc., 4, 178.
Buxton, D. W. (1914). Anaesthetics: their Use and Administration, 5th edn. London: Lewis.
Cartwright, F. F. (1952). The English Pioneers of Anaesthesia (Beddoes: Davy: Hickman). Bristol: Wright.
Cayley, G. (1786). A course of Lectures upon Chemistry by Dr. Black. Vol. III, p. 72. MS. notes in the Library of the York Medical Society.
Clement, F. W. (1951). Nitrous Oxide-Oxygen Anaesthesia, 3rd edn. London: Kimpton.

Collins, V. J. (1952). *Principles and Practice of Anesthesiology*. London: Kimpton.

—— (1966). *Principles of Anesthesiology*. London: Kimpton.

Dallemagne, M. J. (1948). *Aspects actuels de L'Anesthésiologie*. Paris: Masson.

Davison, M. H. A. (1971), in *General Anaesthesia*, 3rd edn. (eds. Gray, T. C., and Nunn, J. F.). London: Butterworth.

Davy, H. (1812). *Elements of Chemical Philosophy*. London: J. Johnson.

Dogliotti, A. M. (1935). *Trattato di Anestesia*. Torino: Unione Tipografico-edetrice Torinese.

Duncum, B. M. (1947). *The Development of Inhalation Anaesthesia: with special reference to the years 1846–1900*. London: Oxford University Press.

Faulconer, A., and Keys, T. E. (1965). *Foundations of Anesthesiology*, Vol. 1. Springfield: Thomas.

Flagg, P. J. (1916). *The Art of Anaesthesia*. Philadelphia: Lippincott.

Fülöp-Miller, R. (1938). *Triumph over Pain*. New York: The Literary Guild of America, Inc.

Gardner, H. B. (1916). *A Manual of Surgical Anaesthesia*, 2nd edn. London: Baillière, Tindall & Cox.

Gibbs, F. W. (1965). *Joseph Priestley: Adventurer in Science and the Champion of Truth*. London: Nelson.

Goldman, V. (1941). *Aids to Anaesthesia*. London: Baillière, Tindall & Cox.

Gwathmey, J. T. (1925). *Anaesthesia*, 2nd edn. London: Churchill.

Hadfield, C. F. (1923). *Practical Anaesthetics*. London: Baillière, Tindall & Cox.

Hales, S. (1727). *Vegetable Staticks: or, an account of some Statical Experiments on the Sap in Vegetables: being an essay towards a Natural History of Vegetation. Also, a specimen of an Attempt to Analyse the Air, by a great variety of Chymio-Statical Experiments*. London: W. & J. Innys and T. Woodward.

Hartog, Sir P. J. (1941). The new views of Priestley and Lavoisier. *Ann. Sci.*, **5**, 1.

Heironimus, T. W. (1964), in *Clinical Anesthesia: Nitrous Oxide* (ed. Eastwood, D. W.). Oxford: Blackwell.

Hewitt, F. W. (1893). *Anaesthetics and their Administration: a manual for medical and dental practitioners and students*. London: Charles Griffin.

Keys, T. E. (1963). *The History of Surgical Anesthesia*. New York: Dover.

King, C. (1946). *The Principles of Gaseous Anaesthetic Apparatus*, 2nd edn. London: Baillière, Tindall & Cox.

Lee, J. A. (1947). *A Synopsis of Anaesthesia*. Bristol: Wright.

—— Atkinson, R. S. (1968). *A Synopsis of Anaesthesia*, 6th edn. Bristol: Wright.

Lundy, J. S. (1943). *Clinical Anesthesia: a Manual of Clinical Anesthesia*. Philadelphia and London: Saunders.

McKie, D. (1961). Joseph Priestley and the Copley Medal. *Ambix*, **9**, 1.

—— (ed.) (1966). *Thomas Cochrane: Notes from Doctor Black's lectures on Chemistry 1767/8*. Wilmslow: Imperial Chemical Industries Ltd.

—— Kennedy, D. (1960). On some letters of Joseph Black and others. *Ann. Sci.*, **16**, 134.

Marston, A. D. (1949), in *Modern Practice of Anaesthesia* (ed. Evans, F. T.). London: Butterworth.

Parry-Price, H. (1946). *A short Handbook of Practical Anaesthetics*. Bristol: Wright.

Partington, J. R. (1962). *A History of Chemistry*, Vol. III. London: Macmillan.

Paton, W. D. M., and Payne, J. P. (1968). *Pharmacological Principles and Practice*. London: Churchill.

Priestley, J. (1767). *The History and Present State of Electricity, with Original Experiments*. London: J. Dodsley, J. Johnson and B. Davenport, and T. Cadell.

—— (1772). Experiments and observations on different kinds of air. *Phil. Trans.*, **62**, 216.

—— (1774). *Experiments and Observations on Different Kinds of Air*, Vol. I. London: J. Johnson.

—— (1775). *Experiments and Observations on Different Kinds of Air*, Vol. II. London: J. Johnson.

—— (1777). *Experiments and Observations on Different Kinds of Air*, Vol. III. London: J. Johnson.

—— (1786). *Experiments and Observations relating to various branches of Natural Philosophy; with a continuation of the observations on air*, Vol. III. Birmingham: Pearson.

Robinson, E., and McKie, D. (1970). *Partners in Science: Letters of James Watt and Joseph Black*. London: Constable.

Robinson, H. (1922). *Anaesthetics and their Administration: a Text Book by the late Sir Fred. W. Hewitt*, 5th edn. London: Froude and Hodder & Stoughton.

Robinson, V. (1946). *Victory over Pain: a History of Anesthesia*. New York: Schuman.

Robison, J. (ed.) (1803). *Lectures on the Elements of Chemistry delivered in the University of Edinburgh by the late Joseph Black, M.D.*, Vol. 1. Edinburgh: Longman & Rees.

Roscoe, Sir H. E., and Schorlemmer, C. (1884). *A Treatise on Chemistry*, Vol. 1. London: Macmillan.

Seward, E. H., and Bryce-Smith, R. (1957). *Inhalation Analgesia in Childbirth*. Oxford: Blackwell.

Smith, W. D. A. (1965). A history of nitrous oxide and oxygen anaesthesia. Part I: Joseph Priestley to Humphry Davy. *Brit. J. Anaesth.*, **37**, 790.

Sykes, W. S. (1939), in Claye, A. M., *The Evolution of Obstetric Analgesia*. London: Oxford University Press.

Watts, H. (1868). *A Dictionary of Chemistry and the Allied Branches of Other Sciences*, Vol. IV. London: Longmans, Green & Co.

Webster, W. (1924). *The Science and Art of Anaesthesia*. London: Kimpton.

Wood-Smith, F. G., and Stewart, H. C. (1964). *Drugs in Anaesthetic Practice*, 2nd edn. London: Butterworth.

Wylie, W. D., and Churchill-Davidson, H. C. (1960). *A Practice of Anaesthesia*. London: Lloyd-Luke.

3

JOSEPH PRIESTLEY TO HUMPHRY DAVY

"An historical review may be useful as offering a kind of a map of the science and of the roads by which it has been explored."

(Humphry Davy 1810;
cited John Davy 1839)

Towards the end of the eighteenth century increasing knowledge of "different kinds of air", and of respiration, led to the inhalation of gases for medicinal purposes. Inhalation anaesthesia emerged from this background of "Pneumatic Medicine", although not quite as soon as it might have done. A long-suffering acceptance of pain, and of the improbability of its relief during surgical operations, probably contributed to the delay.

The first attempts to introduce nitrous oxide as an anaesthetic were short-lived. It was temporarily supplanted by ether and chloroform, even for anaesthesia in the ambulant patient. When it was revived, many of the later improvements in anaesthetic technique were considered, at least in embryonic form, but their development had to await the accumulation of experience and basic knowledge, new discoveries and advances in technology.

The isolation of nitrous oxide and oxygen.

"The word 'discovery' is often ambiguous in Science and leads to misunderstandings." Those words could have been applied appropriately to the "discovery" of anaesthesia, but they were written by Hartog (1941) in relation to the allied subject of the "discovery" of oxygen. He continued: "In dealing with experiments and observations like those of Priestley and Scheele on Oxygen, I prefer to say that they 'isolated and recognised' or 'identified' rather than that they 'discovered' oxygen." Priestley (1733–1804) isolated both nitrous oxide and oxygen during the course of his *Experiments and Observations on different kinds of Air*.

Priestley gave the name "nitrous air" to what is now known as nitric oxide. In 1772 he found that nitrous air contracted when allowed to stand in contact with a paste of iron filings and brimstone. Some of the thrill of this discovery is communicated in his description of it:

> The diminution of common air by a mixture of nitrous air, is not so extraordinary as the diminution which nitrous air itself is subject to from a mixture of iron filings and brimstone, made into a paste with water. This mixture, as I have already observed, diminishes common air between one fifth and one fourth . . . but when it is put into a quantity of nitrous air, it diminishes it so much that no more than one fourth of the original quantity be left. The effect of this process is generally perceived in five or six hours, about which time the visible effervescence of the mixture begins; and in a very short time it advances so rapidly, that in about an hour almost the whole effect will have taken place. If it be suffered to stand a day or two longer, the air will still be diminished farther, but only a very little farther, in proportion to the first diminution. The glass jar, in which the air and this mixture have been confined, has generally been so much heated in this process, that I have not been able to touch it.

The remaining air supported combustion and it smelled more like common air than like nitrous air. He named it "dephlogisticated nitrous air". In his own words (Priestley, 1786): "Dephlogisticated nitrous air is the term by which I first distinguished this species of air, because it admitted a candle to burn in it." This is now known as nitrous oxide.

Although he did not realize it at the time, Priestley first liberated oxygen from saltpetre (potassium nitrate) in 1771 (Hartog, 1933). He obtained it again in 1774 by focusing sunlight on mercurius calcinatas (mercuric oxide), having just procured a lens of 12 inches diameter (Priestley, 1776, p. 33). He discovered that a candle burned in it with a remarkably vigorous flame. He wrote (Priestley, 1776, p. 33):

> But what surprised me more than I can well express, was, that a candle burned in this air with a remarkably vigorous flame, very much like that enlarged flame with which a candle burns in nitrous air exposed to iron or liver of sulphur; but as I had got nothing like this remarkable appearance from any kind of air besides this particular modification of nitrous air, and I knew no nitrous acid was used in the preparation of mercurius calcinatas, I was utterly at a loss how to account for it.

In the following year he found that a mouse would live longer in this new air than in an equal volume of common air (pp 33–34). He concluded that it was better than common air (p. 45) and he called it dephlogisticated air. He breathed it:

> The feeling of it to my lungs was not sensibly different from that of common air; but I fancied that my breast felt peculiarly light and easy for some time afterwards. Who can tell that, in time, this pure air may become a fashionable article in luxury. Hitherto only two mice and myself have had the privilege of breathing it.

Patterson (cited Fulton, 1935) has drawn attention to the fact that as early as 1660 Boyle had already committed himself to Paracelsus' earlier conjecture that there is in the air "a little quintessence . . . which serves to the refreshment and restoration of our vital spirits, for which the grosser and incomparably greater part of the Air being unserviceable, it need not seem strange that an animal stands in need of almost incessantly drawing in fresh air". In the same work Boyle calls attention to the fact that the flame of a lamp is put out by removal of air just as the life of an animal is extinguished (cited Fulton, 1935). Priestley saw that there was a similarity between the processes of combustion and respiration, but his appreciation of the significance of his new gas was hindered by his belief in the phlogiston theory. Phlogiston was thought to be the inflammable part of any body and to escape upon combustion. It was also thought to take part in respiration. Priestley considered that the new gas owed its properties to a capacity for absorbing phlogiston, and therefore that it initially contained less phlogiston than common air—hence "dephlogisticated air".

It was Antoine Laurent Lavoisier (1742–94) who paved the way to a fuller understanding of the nature of dephlogisticated air. He also discredited the Phlogiston Theory. These contributions were based on the systematic use of the balance in checking chemical reactions (Hartog, 1941), and on the application of the principle of the Indestructibility of Matter. By 1773 it had already occurred to Lavoisier that the gain in weight of phosphorus or sulphur on combustion might be due to combination with air, or with an elastic fluid contained in air. Later he repeated and extended Priestley's experiments and concluded that common air consisted of a mixture of two elastic fluids, and that one was necessary for combustion and for

respiration while the other would support neither. The former—dephlogisticated air—he renamed "oxygen". Their proportions he found to be about 25 parts to 75 parts (Duncum, 1947, pp. 56–57).

Humphry Davy's experiments with nitrous oxide.

Twenty-six years after the first isolation of nitrous oxide, Humphry Davy (1778–1829) was appointed Superintendent of the Medical Pneumatic Institution which had been set up by Dr. Beddoes (1760–1808) in Clifton, Bristol. Davy was then 21 years old and his status was approximately equivalent to that of a house surgeon (Cartwright, 1952, p. 100).

Beddoes was one of the leading authorities on pneumatic medicine, which was concerned with the administration of medicinal "airs". He was an enthusiast and he so impressed his friends that they encouraged him to set up the Institution and provided him with the necessary funds. Its purpose was to ascertain the effects of the inhalation of gases in various diseases, and to discover the best means of applying them. Apparatus for producing and receiving the various "airs" had already been designed by James Watt (1736–1819) in collaboration with Beddoes (Beddoes and Watt, 1796, 2, p. 184). Davy thus had an exceptional start to his career.

Nitrous oxide was chosen for particular study, and Davy set about investigating its physical, chemical and biological properties. Within a little over a year he had carried out numerous experiments and written them up in his *Researches, Chemical and Philosophical; chiefly concerning nitrous oxide, or dephlogisticated nitrous air, and its respiration* (Davy, 1800b) from which the quotaions given below have been taken.

Although Davy experimented with the preparation of nitrous oxide from nitrous air (Davy, 1800b, p.196), he soon adopted the more efficient method of heating nitrate of ammoniac, which was introduced by Berthollet in 1785 (Davy, 1800a and 1800b, p. 56; Partington, 1960). The nitrous oxide was collected in a gasometer—then described as hydraulic bellows—and stored in an air-holder which was an enclosed tank filled, initially, with water. As the water was drained from the bottom of the tank, nitrous oxide was aspirated into the top from the "hydraulic bellows", which served as a reservoir. The water from the air–holder was

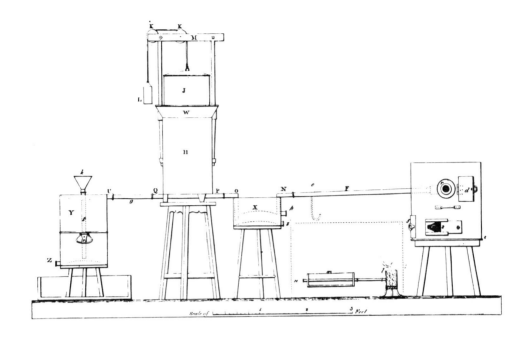

FIG. 1

The apparatus designed by James Watt for Thomas Beddoes and used by Humphrey Davy for
making "Factitious Airs". X—"Refrigeratory". H—"Hydraulic Bellows". Y—"Air Holder". (From
Beddoes and Watt, 1796, plate III, fig. 1, by courtesy of and photographed at the Royal Society of
Medicine. The apparatus was described previously in Beddoes and Watt, 1794.)

allowed to become saturated with the gas and it
was stored in special containers when not in use
(p. 120) (see fig. 1). Clayfield (1800), following the
basic ideas of Watt's hydraulic bellows, designed a
bell-jar-upon-mercury air-holder ("spirometer")
in which counterpoise was achieved by using a
spiral pulley. This was used for quantitative experiments. For qualitative experiments the "airs" were
usually inhaled from oiled-silk bags. A special
mouthpiece with two silk valves was designed, but
this does not seem to have been used to any
extent.

Davy repeated some of Priestley's experiments.
For example, he confirmed that nitrous oxide
supported combustion. He confirmed that water
dissolved about one half of its bulk of nitrous
oxide (Priestley, 1786), but he expressed this more
precisely, i.e. that 100 cubic inches of water
absorbed 54 cubic inches of nitrous oxide at
46°F (p. 236). He tried to measure its solubility in

freshly drawn blood but his results were variable
(pp. 376–378), probably because he had to use
smaller quantities of blood and to contend with its
coagulation. He found that 100 cubic inches of pure
nitrous oxide weighed 50·1 grains at a temperature
of 50°F and an atmospheric pressure of 30·7
(inches of mercury). This great specific gravity
surprised him (p. 95), but a molecular weight of
45 may be derived from his figures which makes a
reasonable comparison with the now known value
of 44.

Before Davy started his experiments with
nitrous oxide, Samuel Latham Mitchill of America
had declared that contact with or inhalation of
nitrous oxide would have dire consequences:
". . . nitrous oxide was the principle of contagion
and capable of producing the most terrible effects
when respired by animals in the minutest quantities
or even when applied to the skin or a muscle
fibre" (cited Davy, 1800b, p. 453). "If full inspira-

tion of the gaseous azote be made there will be sudden extinction of life; and this accordingly accounts for the fact related by Russel (*History of Aleppo*) and confirmed by other observers, of many persons falling down dead suddenly, when struck with the contagion of the plague" (cited Beddoes and Watt, 1796, 5, p. 56). At an early stage, therefore, Davy satisfied himself that "nitrous oxide was respirable, and capable of supporting life for a longer time than any gas, except atmospheric air and oxygene . . ." (p. 335); but he also observed: "Of respirable gases, or those which are capable of being taken into the lungs by voluntary efforts, one only has the power of uniformly supporting life—atmospheric air. Other gases, when respired, sooner or later produce death; but by different modes" (p. 334).

Davy also tested the direct effects of nitrous oxide on exposed tissues:

Having accidentally cut one of my fingers so as to lay bare a little muscle fibre, I introduced it while bleeding into a bottle of nitrous oxide; the blood that trickled from the wound became more purple; but the pain was neither alleviated nor increased. When, however, the finger was taken out of the nitrous oxide and exposed to the atmosphere, the wound smarted more than it had done before. After it had ceased to bleed I inserted it through water into a vessel of nitrous gas; but it did not become more painful than before [p. 386].*

Later, Beddoes repeated Davy's experiment with nitrous oxide and decided that the pain was increased (Davy, 1800b, p. 543).

A wide range of animals was observed during and following the inhalation of nitrous oxide. The majority were warm-blooded, but amphibians, fishes and insects were included (pp. 333–372). The particular lessons he learned were (p. 342):

1st. That nitrous oxide is destructive when respired for a certain time to warm-blooded animals, apparently previously exciting them to some extent.
2nd. That when its operation is stopped before complete exhaustion is brought on, the healthy living action is capable of being gradually reproduced, by enabling the animal to respire atmospheric air.
3rd. That exhaustion and death is produced in the small animals by nitrous oxide sooner than in the larger ones, and in the young animals of the same species in a shorter time than in the old ones, as indeed Dr. Beddoes conjectured a priori would be the case.

---

*Cartwright (1952, p. 200) suggested that this experiment may have been inspired by a previous one of Dr. Ingenhousz (letter of August 4, 1794, cited Beddoes and Watt, 1796, p. 43), in which it was demonstrated that the pain of a blister induced by Cantharides might be relieved by immersion in carbon dioxide. (This observation was subsequently repeated by Thomson, 1839.)

The animal experiments carried out by a Committee of the Odontological Society of Great Britain, sixty-eight years later, added nothing to these conclusions.

He found that animals lived twice as long in nitrous oxide as in hydrogen or water, but that "the external appearance of animals that had been destroyed by nitrous oxide, is very little different from that of those killed by privation of atmospheric air" (p. 347). He did, however, notice differences in the appearances of internal organs (p. 353).

By giving animals mixtures of nitrous oxide and oxygen, or air, to breathe he found that they survived much longer than if they were given nitrous oxide alone:

Into a mixture of one of oxygen and three of nitrous oxide, a small guinea pig was introduced. He immediately began to struggle, and in two minutes reposed on his side, breathing very deeply. He made afterwards no violent muscular motion; but lived quietly for near fourteen minutes; at the end of which time, his legs were much convulsed. He was taken out and recovered [p. 358].

Davy carried out many experiments upon himself. He made his first inspiration of pure nitrous oxide in April 1799: ". . . it passed through the bronchia without stimulating the glottis, and produced no uneasy feeling in the lungs" (Davy, 1799a and 1800b, p. 456). On April 17 (Davy, 1799b) he inhaled the gas in the presence of Dr. Beddoes:

Having previously closed my nostrils and exhausted my lungs, I breathed four quarts of nitrous oxide from and into a silk bag. The first feelings were similar to those produced in the last experiment; but in less than half a minute, the respiration being continued, they diminished gradually, and were succeeded by a sensation analogous to gentle pressure on all muscles, attended by a highly pleasurable thrilling in the chest and extremities. The objects around me became dazzling and my hearing more acute. Towards the last inspirations, the thrilling ceased, the sense of muscular power became greater, and at last an irresistible propensity to action was indulged in; I recollect but indefinitely what followed; I know my motions were various and violent. . . . The next morning the recollections of the effects of the gas were indistinct, and had not remarks written immediately after the experiment recalled them to my mind, I should even have doubted their reality [pp. 457–458].

Davy (1799b) wasted no time in announcing his discovery and he immediately wrote to the editor of *Nicholson's Journal*:

I have this day made a discovery, which, if you please, you may announce in your Physical Journal, namely that the nitrous phosoxyd or gaseous oxyd of azote, is respirable when perfectly freed from nitric phosoxyd (nitrous gas). Dr. Mitchill's theory of contagion is of course completely overturned; the mistake of Priestley and the Dutch chemists probably arose from their having never obtained it pure.

In subsequent experiments Davy found that he "could breathe nine quarts of nitrous oxide for three minutes, and twelve quarts for rather more than four. I could never breathe it in any quantity for more than five minutes" (p. 460). Such long periods of inhalation might be taken to suggest that the nitrous oxide was contaminated with air during its preparation, storage or administration, which probably was the case; but in these experiments he would also have been rebreathing into a bag, and the pure nitrous oxide initially contained in the bag would be diluted by the gases already in the lungs and respiratory deadspace.

Davy then "resolved to breathe the gas for such a time and in such quantities as to produce excitement equal in duration and superior in intensity to that occasioned by high intoxication from opium or alcohol" (p. 484). "On Dec. 26th, I was inclosed in an air-tight breathing box, of the capacity of about nine cubic feet and a half, in the presence of Dr. Kinglake." Even as a small man he cannot have had much room in which to move. His description continues: "After I had taken a situation in which I could, by means of a curved thermometer inserted under the arm, and a stop watch, ascertain the alterations in my pulse and animal heat, twenty quarts of nitrous oxide were thrown into the box" (p. 485). This might have produced a concentration of about 25 per cent nitrous oxide in air. In four minutes, "I began to feel a slight glow in the cheeks, and a generally diffused warmth over my chest, though the temperature in the box was 50°" (p. 486). Twenty quarts were then thrown into the box, followed by a further twenty quarts about thirty minutes later: "My sensations were now pleasant; I had a generally diffused warmth without the slightest moisture of the skin, a sense of exhiliration similar to that produced by a small dose of wine, and a disposition to muscular exertion and merriment." After three-quarters of an hour a further twenty quarts were admitted.

I now had a great disposition to laugh, luminous points seemed frequently to pass before my eyes, my hearing was certainly more acute and I felt a pleasant lightness and power of exertion in my muscles. In a short time the symptoms became stationary; breathing was rather more oppressed, and on account of the great desire of action, I now came out of the box, having been in precisely an hour and a quarter [p. 487].

An appreciable quantity of nitrous oxide must have been taken up and distributed throughout Davy's body by the end of that experiment. It is not surprising that when, having just got out of the box, he tried breathing unmingled nitrous oxide: "A thrilling extending from the chest to the extremities was almost immediately produced."

The description of his subsequent sensations is vivid:

I felt a sense of tangible extension highly pleasurable in every limb; my visible impressions were dazzling and apparently magnified, I heard distinctly every sound in the room and was perfectly aware of my situation. By degrees as the pleasurable sensations increased, I lost all connection with external things; trains of vivid visible images rapidly passed through my mind and were connected with words in such a manner, as to produce perceptions perfectly novel. I existed in a world of newly connected and newly modified ideas. I theorised; I imagined that I made discoveries. When I was awakened from this semi-delirious trance by Dr. Kinglake, who took the bag from my mouth, indignation and pride were the first feelings produced by the sight of persons about me. My emotions were enthusiastic and sublime; and for a minute I walked round the room perfectly regardless of what was said to me. As I recovered my former state of mind, I felt an inclination to communicate the discoveries I had made during the experiment. I endeavoured to recall the ideas, they were feeble and indistinct; one collection of terms, however, presented itself; and with the most intense belief and prophetic manner, I exclaimed to Dr. Kinglake "Nothing exists but thought! The Universe is composed of impressions, ideas, pleasures and pains!" [pp. 488–489].

At one time Davy may even have contemplated breathing nitrous oxide under pressure. In a letter to Mr. Davies Giddy of November 12, 1798, before the researches had got under way, he wrote:

We shall try the gases in every possible way. They may be condensed by pressure and rarefied by heat. Quere— would not a powerful injecting syring, furnished with two valves, one opening into the air holder and the other into the breathing chamber, answer the purpose of compression better than any other apparatus? [Paris, 1831].

During the animal experiments Davy noticed that the water always rose in the jar and that, therefore, some of the nitrous oxide was absorbed by the animal. He had already shown that nitrous oxide was soluble in blood. Later he made a series of experiments to measure the quantity of nitrous oxide absorbed by himself, thus anticipating by more than a century and a half the recent interest in measurements of the uptake of nitrous oxide, which started with those of Severinghaus in 1954.

For these measurements of nitrous oxide uptake, Davy used Clayfield's mercurial air-holder which had a capacity of 200 cubic inches (3·28 litres), and first he practised using it when filled with oxygen or air.

The power of uniformly exhausting the lungs and the fauces to the same extent I did not acquire until after many experiments. At last by preserving exactly the same posture after exhaustion of the lungs before the inspiration of the gas to be experimented upon, and during its compleat expiration, I found that I could always retain nearly the same quantity of gas in the bronchial vessels and fauces; the difference in volume expired at different times never amounting to a cubic inch and a half [pp. 390–391].

But when he came to fill the mercurial air-holder with pure nitrous oxide:

. . . the pleasurable delirium was very rapidly produced, and being obliged to stoop on the cylinder, the determination of blood to my head from the increased arterial action in less than a minute became so great as often to deprive me of voluntary power over muscles of the mouth. Hence I could never rely on the accuracy of any experiment in which the gas had been respired for more than three quarters of a minute [p. 392]. . . . In all the numerous experiments that I made on the respiration of nitrous oxide in this way, a very considerable diminution of gas always took place; and the diminution was generally apparently greater to the eye during the first four or five respirations.

Davy measured the total volume remaining at the end of the experiment, analyzed the remaining gases and calculated the nitrous oxide that they contained. By subtracting this from the initial volume of nitrous oxide in the air-holder he obtained the volume of nitrous oxide absorbed. This value would have included the nitrous oxide retained in the lungs and air passages as well as the nitrous oxide taken up by the pulmonary capillary blood and distributed throughout the body.

The results he obtained during two experiments were equivalent to a rate of uptake of about 2·3 l./min (pp. 394–395), but their assessment is difficult. The purity of the nitrous oxide is not known, the methods of gas analysis were primitive and the effective concentration of nitrous oxide inhaled would have been reduced with each breath as he was rebreathing into an air-holder of about the same volume as his own functional residual capacity.

An indication of the quantity of nitrous oxide taken up by the pulmonary capillary blood may be obtained from the diminution of the contents of the air-holder. The average for the two experiments was equivalent to about 1·3 l./min.

From these experiments [Davy wrote] we learn that nitrous oxide is rapidly absorbed by the venous blood, through the moist coats of the pulmonary veins. But as after compleat voluntary exhaustion of the lungs, much residual air must remain in the bronchial vessels and fauces, as appears from their incapability of completely collapsing, it is evident that the gas expired must be mingled with different quantities of the residual gas of the lungs [p. 396] . . . whilst after a complete expiration, much of the unabsorbed nitrous oxide must remain as residual gas in the lungs. Now when a complete expiration is made after the breathing of atmospheric air, it is evident that the residual gas of the lungs consists of nitrogene . . . mingled with small portions of oxygen and carbonic acid. And these are the only products formed after the respiration of nitrous oxide. To ascertain whether these products were partially produced, during the process of respiration . . . or whether they were wholly the residual gas of the lungs, I found extremely difficult [p. 397] . . . yet I distinctly saw that it was impossible . . . to ascertain . . . unless I could first determine the capacity of my lungs [p. 398].

He then proceeded to measure the capacity of his lungs by repeating the experiments using hydrogen instead of nitrous oxide, having already observed that hydrogen was not absorbed (pp. 399–400). The value obtained was 118 cubic inches (1,935 ml) which was on the low side, but possibly a fair estimate considering his statement that: "This capacity is most probably below the medium, my chest is narrow, measuring in circumference, but 29 inches, and my neck is rather long and slender" (p. 410). The method was later improved by Gréhant (1887) and it anticipated modern closed-circuit methods of measuring the functional residual capacity (Van Slyke and Binger, 1923; Christie, 1932; McMichael, 1939; Meneely and Kaltreider, 1941, 1949; Gilson and Hugh-Jones, 1949).

It would be unfair to say that Davy became a nitrous oxide addict. The evidence does not suggest that his inhalations of nitrous oxide were detrimental to himself or to society, nor that he developed a dependence on the effects of nitrous oxide; but the possibility may have passed through his mind when he wrote: "I ought to observe that a desire to breathe the gas is always awakened in me by the sight of a person breathing, or even by that of an air bag or an air holder" (p. 493). He was not alone in having such a desire: "The desire of some individuals acquainted with the pleasures of nitrous oxide for the gas has been so strong as to induce them to breathe with eagerness, the air remaining in the bags after the respiration of others" (p. 556). It may be significant that it was soon after participating in these experiments that Samuel Taylor Coleridge was noticed to be becoming increasingly under the influence of opium (*Encyclopaedia Britannica*, 1926).

At times Davy must have been severely hypoxic. He recorded experiments in which he breathed hydrogen and nitrogen with feelings of suffocation (p. 466). On one occasion he attempted to inspire nitrous oxide after having made two inspirations of hydrogen:

> . . . but in this experiment the effects of hydrogen were so debilitating, and the consequent stimulation by nitrous oxide was so great, as to deprive me of sense. After the first three inspirations, I lost all power of standing, and fell on my back, carrying in my lips the mouth piece separated from the cylinder, to the great alarm of Mr. Patrick Dwyer, who was noting the periods of inspiration [p. 398].

The most dramatic incident was when he took three inspirations of a gas described as "hydrocarbonate" which was prepared from water and charcoal, having a strong disagreeable smell. It would have contained a high proportion of carbon monoxide.

> The first inspiration brought a sort of numbness and loss of feeling in the chest and about the pectoral muscles. After the second inspiration, I lost all power of perceiving external things, and had no distinct sensation except a terrible oppression of the chest. During the third expiration, this feeling disappeared, I seemed sinking into annihilation and had just power enough to drop the mouth piece from my unclosed lips. A short interval must have passed during which I respired some common air, before the objects around me were distinguishable. On recollecting myself, I faintly articulated "I do not think that I shall die". Putting my finger to my wrist, I found my pulse thread like and beating with excessive quickness.
> In less than a minute I was able to walk, and the painful oppression in the chest directed me to the open air.
> After making a few steps which carried me to the garden, my head became giddy, my knees trembled and I had just sufficient voluntary power to throw myself to the grass. Here the painful feeling in the chest increased with such violence as to threaten suffocation. At this moment I asked for some nitrous oxide. Mr. Dwyer brought me a mixture of oxygen and nitrous oxide. I breathed this for a minute, and believed myself relieved. In five minutes, the painful feelings began gradually to diminish. In an hour they had nearly disappeared, and I felt only excessive weakness and a slight swimming in the head. My voice was very feeble and indistinct. This was at two o'clock in the afternoon.
> I afterwards walked slowly for about half an hour . . . and on my return, was so much stronger and better, as to believe that the effects of the gas had disappeared;

though my pulse was 120 and very feeble. I continued without pain for near three quarters of an hour; when the giddiness returned with such violence as to oblige me to lie on the bed; it was accompanied with nausea, loss of memory, and diminished sensation. In about an hour and a half, the giddiness went off, and was succeeded by an excruciating pain in the forehead and between the eyes, with transient pains in the chest and extremities.

> Towards night these affectations gradually diminished. At ten no disagreeable feeling except weakness remained. I slept sound, and awoke feeling very feeble and hungry. No recurrence of the symptoms took place, and I had nearly recovered my strength by the evening [pp. 468–471].

This alarming tale has no direct bearing on nitrous oxide, except that Davy believed that inhalation of a nitrous oxide-oxygen mixture afforded some relief; but if there had been any truth in Mitchill's warnings, for all that Davy could have known, such a reaction might have resulted from his first inhalation of nitrous oxide. Indeed, during preliminary trial inhalations of impure nitrous oxide, diluted with air, he found that "its effects appeared to be depressing, and I imagined that it produced a tendency to fainting: the pulse was certainly rendered slower under its operation" (p. 455).

Dr. Beddoes took part in some of these experiments and made pertinent notes. On the colour of blood he wrote: "I thought it might be an amusing spectacle to see the different tints of blood flowing from a wound by a leech in the consequence of breathing different airs. The purple from nitrous oxide was very evident. Oxygene, we thought, occasioned a quicker flow and a brighter colour in the blood" (p. 545). Davy had noted that "In all these experiments, after the first minute my cheeks became purple" (p. 488).

Early in his researches Davy had observed the changes in colour of recently withdrawn venous blood when subjected to various gases and gas mixtures in vitro:

> The blood in oxygen and atmospheric air were of a much brighter tinge than that in any of the other gases. On the top the colour was vermilion, but no perceptible absorption had taken place [p. 381].
> The coagulum in nitrous oxide when examined in the mass was dark, and hardly distinguishable in its colour from venous blood. . . . An absorption had taken place in this cylinder, more considerable than in any of the others . . . [p. 382].
> To human blood that had been saturated with nitrous oxide whilst warm and constantly agitated for four or five minutes, to prevent its uniform coagulation, oxygen was introduced; the red purple on the surface of it immediately turned to vermilion, and on agitation this

colour was diffused through it. On comparing the tinge with oxygenated blood, no perceptible difference could be observed [p. 383].

The conclusions that he drew from these in vitro experiments were as follows:

1st. That when nitrous oxide is agitated in fluid venous blood, a certain proportion of the gas is absorbed; whilst the colour of the blood changes from dark red to purple.
2nd. That during the absorption of nitrous oxide by the venous blood, minute proportions of nitrogene and carbonic acid gas are produced, either by evolution from the blood, or from decomposition of part of the nitrous oxide.
3rd. That venous blood impregnated with nitrous oxide is capable of oxygenation and vice versa; that oxygenated blood may be combined with nitrous oxide [p. 387].

A subjective impression clearly expressed by Beddoes was: "Time by my feelings has always appeared longer than by my watch" (p. 547).

Beddoes also found that he could "hold his breath uncommonly long when respiring oxygen gas with nitrous oxide" (p. 546). That the inhalation of nitrous oxide could be made safer by mixing it with oxygen or air was quite evident to Davy:

Modification of the powers of nitrous oxide by mixture of the gas with oxygen or common air, will probably enable the most delicately sensible to respire it without danger, and even with pleasurable effects: heretofore it has been administered to such only in the pure form or mingled with small quantities of atmospheric air, and in its pure form even the most robust are unable to respire it with safety for more than five minutes [p. 553].

Davy's *Researches Chemical and Philosophical*; *chiefly concerning nitrous oxide . . .*, contains a wealth of data based upon planned experimentation, but it is most frequently quoted for a brilliant idea based upon the chance observations that nitrous oxide could relieve headaches and the toothache:

In one instance, when I had a headache from indigestion, it was immediately removed by the effects of a large dose of gas; though it afterwards returned, but with much less violence. In a second instance, a slighter degree of headache was wholly removed by two doses of gas [p. 464].
The power of immediate operation of the gas in removing intense pain, I had very good opportunity of ascertaining.
In cutting one of the unlucky teeth called dentes sapientæ, I experienced an intense inflammation of the gum, accompanied with great pain, which equally destroyed the power of repose and of consistent action.
On the day when the inflammation was most troublesome, I breathed three large doses of nitrous oxide. The pain always diminished after the first four or five

inspirations; the thrilling came on as usual, and uneasiness was for a few minutes swallowed up in pleasure. As the former state of mind, however, returned, the state of the organ returned with it; and I once imagined that the pain was more severe after the experiment than before [p. 465].

As a result of these experiences Davy wrote: "As nitrous oxide in its extensive operation appears capable of destroying physical pain, it may probably be used with advantage during surgical operations in which no great effusion of blood takes place" (p. 556). If Davy had put this idea to the test of experiment before writing up his researches, it is possible that there would now be a very different tale to tell.

ACKNOWLEDGMENTS

This study started with Duncum (1947) and frequent reference was made to this source. Background reading included Cartwright (1952)—particularly relevant to this instalment—Robinson (1946), Sykes (1960 and 1961), Leake (1947) and Keys (1945). Research was carried out in a number of libraries, often with the help and encouragement of their librarians.

REFERENCES

(Page numbers are given in the text when more than one reference is made to a given source)

Beddoes, T., and Watt, J. (1794). *Considerations on the Medicinal use of Factitious Airs, and on the manner of obtaining them in large quantities*, 1st ed., Part II. Bristol: Bulgin and Rosser.
—— (1796). *Considerations on the Medicinal Use and on the Production of Factitious Airs*, 3rd ed. London: J. Johnson.
Cartwright, F. F. (1952). *The English pioneers of anaesthesia: Beddoes, Davy and Hickman*. Bristol: John Wright.
Christie, R. V. (1932). Lung volume and its subdivisions. *J. clin. Invest.*, **11**, 1099.
Clayfield, W. (1800). Description of a mercurial airholder, suggested by an inspection of Mr. Watt's machine for containing factitious airs. *Tilloch's Philosophical Magazine*, **7**, 148.
Davy, H. (1799a). Letter from Mr. H. Davy, introductory to the experiments contained in the subsequent article, and on other subjects relative to the progress of science. *Nicholson's Journal*, **3**, 55.
—— (1799b). Extract of a letter from Mr. H. Davy. *Nicholson's Journal*, **3**, 93.
—— (1800a). A letter from Mr. Davy, Superintendent of the Pneumatic Institution, to Mr. Nicholson, on the Nitrous Oxide, or gaseous oxide of azote, on certain factors relating to heat and light, and on the discovery of the decomposition of the carbonate and sulphite of ammoniac. *Nicholson's Journal*, **3**, 515.
—— (1800b). *Researches, Chemical and Philosophical*; *chiefly concerning nitrous oxide, or dephlogisticated nitrous air, and its respiration*. London: J. Johnson.
Davy, J. (1839). *Memoirs of the life of Sir Humphry Davy*. London: Smith, Elder & Co.
Duncum, B. M. (1947). *The Development of Inhalation Anaesthesia: with special reference to the years 1846–1900*. London: Oxford University Press.

Encyclopaedia Britannica (1926). Coleridge, Samuel Taylor. 13th ed., vol. 5, p. 679. London.

Fulton, J. F. (1935). *A bibliography of two Oxford physiologists, Richard Lower 1631–1691 and John Mayow 1643–1679*. Oxford: Oxford University Press.

Gilson, J. G., and Hugh-Jones, P. (1949). Measurement of total lung volume and breathing capacity. *Clin. Sci.*, **7**, 185.

Gréhant, N. (1864). Recherches physiques sur la respiration de l'homme. *J. Anat. Physiol. (Paris)*, **1**, 523.

—— (1887). Perfectionnement du procédé de mesure du volume des poumons par l'hydrogène. *C.R. Soc. Biol. (Paris)*, **4**, 242.

Hartog, P. J. (1933). Date and place of Priestley's discovery of oxygen. *Nature*, **132**, 25.

—— (1941). The newer views of Priestley and Lavoisier. *Ann. Sci.*, **5**, 1.

Keys, T. E. (1945). *The History of Surgical Anesthesia*. New York: Schuman.

Leake, C. D. (1947). *Letheon: the cadenced story of anesthesia*. Austin: University of Texas Press.

McMichael, J. (1939). A rapid method for determining lung capacity. *Clin. Sci.*, **4**, 167.

Meneely, G. R., and Kaltreider, N. L. (1949). Volume of the lung determined by helium dilution. *J. clin. Invest.*, **28**, 129.

Paris, J. A. (1831). *The life of Sir Humphry Davy*, p. 45. London: Colburn and Bently.

Partington, J. R. (1960). *A Textbook of Inorganic Chemistry*, 3rd ed. (revised), p. 573. London: Macmillan.

Priestley, J. (1772). Observations on different kinds of air. *Phil. Trans.*, **62**, 147.

—— (1776). *Experiments and observations on different kinds of air*, 2nd ed. London: J. Johnson.

—— (1786). *Experiments and Observations relating to various branches of Natural Philosophy; with a continuation of the observations on air*, Vol. III, p. 324. Birmingham: Pearson.

Robinson, V. (1946). *Victory over pain*. New York: Henry Schuman.

Severinghaus, J. W. (1954). The rate of uptake of nitrous oxide in man. *J. clin. Invest.*, **33**, 1183.

Sykes, W. S. (1960). *Essays on the first hundred years of Anaesthesia*, Vol. I. Edinburgh: Livingstone.

—— (1961). *Essays on the first hundred years of Anaesthesia*, Vol. II. Edinburgh: Livingstone.

Thomson, A. T. (1839). Debate on poisoning by charcoal fumes. *Lancet*, **2**, 94.

Van Slyke, D. D., and Binger, C. A. L. (1923). The determination of lung volume without forced breathing. *J. exp. Med.*, **37**, 457.

4

DAVY'S RESEARCHES IN RELATION TO INHALATION ANAESTHESIA

The exceptional merit of Davy's work on nitrous oxide and its relevance to inhalation anaesthesia are self-evident. Its influence on the development of inhalation anaesthesia is less obvious and a variety of opinions has been expressed.

Davy's suggestion that nitrous oxide may probably be used with advantage during surgical operations, for example, received the following comment from Macintosh and Pratt (1940):

These few words, lifted from the unimportant position assigned to them by Davy among a mass of his other deductions, not all of them accurate, have been given much prominence in the history of anaesthesia and it is often implied that Davy was suggesting that nitrous oxide should be used as a general anaesthetic. It is probable, however, that no such idea occurred to him, even though he knew that prolonged inhalation of the gas would produce stupor. If indeed he had conceived the idea of producing surgical anaesthesia by means of nitrous oxide, he would deserve blame rather than praise, in that he, fresh from apprenticeship to a surgeon, made no attempt to follow up this important idea himself or to encourage others to do so. It should, however, be realized . . . that his dominant enthusiasm was chemistry rather than medicine, as was shown by the fact that a year later he resigned his post at the Pneumatic Institution in order to take charge of the chemical laboratory of the newly formed Royal Institution in London. This early promotion resulted in the discontinuance of Davy's experiments with nitrous oxide. Had he remained in Bristol and taken his medical degree as originally intended, it is more than possible that his genius would have led him to utilize nitrous oxide as a means of producing surgical anaesthesia.

Those views were echoed by Duncum (1947, p. 73). Sykes (1960) was more generous to Davy:

Having made the suggestion, he dropped the matter and took no further steps to follow it up. From one point of view, why should he? It is not fair to expect it from a pure chemist. What is surprising is that his suggestion was completely ignored by the very people whom it should have interested most; that surgeons should have continued, for nearly fifty years longer, to operate upon screaming, struggling patients in full consciousness. Surely a lasting testimonial to their thickheadedness.

Cartwright (1952, p. 213) was so enthusiastic about Davy's work on the inhalation of nitrous oxide that he wrote: "It is not too much to say that this part of Davy's book should be read in the original by every anaesthetist." He implied that more notice might have been taken of Davy's results if Beddoes' politics had been more acceptable:

. . . it would be going too far to say that, had he been more Tory in his outlook, he and Davy would have introduced anaesthesia in 1800; but there can be no doubt that every opinion and report that was produced by him and anyone concerned with him was suspect, the wild-cat scheming of a radical enthusiast [p. 77].

Cartwright (1952, p. 312) was probably near the mark when he wrote:

But, when we study the facts, it becomes no longer remarkable that Davy's suggestion of anaesthesia fell on deaf ears. A number of factors conspired together to make the adoption of this idea not only improbable but almost impossible. Of these factors the two most important are, firstly, the outlook of the ordinary eighteenth-century man upon the subject of pain, and secondly the fact that Davy's idea would have been an entirely new and unheard of thing.

The pain associated with operations was one of the limiting factors in the advance of surgery, as pointed out by Duncum (1947, p. 9) when writing about Astley Cooper:

. . . during the first quarter of the nineteenth century [he] laid the foundations of experimental surgery, but because of the uncontrollable factor of pain, much of the knowledge which he gained from his constant dissections of the cadaver could not be applied in operating on the living body . . . .

In 1800, however, Astley Cooper inhaled a possible solution at a meeting of the Askesian Society.*

* The Askesian Society was formed at Plough Court by some young men desirous of improving themselves by philosophical exercises. Its objects were to elucidate, by experiment, either facts generally understood, or to examine and repeat any novel discoveries (Chapman-Houston and Cripps, 1954). Plough Court Pharmacy, later to become Allen and Hanburys, was owned by William Allen who was later a lecturer in Chemistry at Guy's Hospital and a Fellow of the Royal Society.

In either February (Chapman-Houston and Cripps, 1954) or March (Wilks and Bettany, 1892) 1800, William Allen entered in his diary:

Present Astley Cooper, Bradley, Fox and others. We all breathed gaseous oxide of azote. It took a surprising effect upon me, abolishing completely, at first, all sensation: then I had the idea of being carried violently upward in a dark cavern with only a few glimmering lights. The company said that my eyes were fixed, face purple, veins in the forehead very large, apoplectic stertor, etc. They were all much alarmed, but I suffered no pain and in a short time came to myself. [See also Fayle, 1884.]

The immediate stimulus for Allen's experiment probably came from Davy's third communication on nitrous oxide to *Nicholson's Journal* (Davy, 1800a), in which he gave an account of how he prepared the gas for respiration. At that time Astley Cooper would not have read Davy's suggestion that nitrous oxide might be used with advantage during surgical operations*: but even if he had been aware of it, he should be forgiven if the alarming appearance of Allen discouraged him from trying the experiment.

Of particular interest is a contemporary review of Davy's "*Researches . . . concerning nitrous oxide . . .* which was published in a reputable medical periodical (*Annals of Medicine*, 1800):

Of the many singular and highly interesting particulars contained in the volume now before us, no proper analysis could be given within the limits of our periodical publication. For most of these, therefore, we must refer the chemical reader to the original work, which demonstrates, in a remarkable degree, the industry and genius of the author, whose enthusiasm for the discovery of truth, has led him, with a perseverance almost without example, to undergo very great sufferings, and even to run the risk, on many occasions, of immediate death. And we have no doubt, that the intelligent reader, after careful perusal of his experiments, will give him due credit for his meritorious exertions.

We shall content ourselves with merely mentioning, in a general way, the subjects considered in his first three researches; and we shall give a particular account of the fourth, as being more immediately connected with the practice of medicine.

There can be no doubt about the impact of Davy's *Researches* upon this reviewer, who recognized the calibre of the work. The greater part of

the thirty-one pages of the review was devoted to a generous description of Davy's experiments on the respiration of nitrous oxide, including a full account of his observations on the relief of headaches and of toothache. The review ended:

In short, Mr. Davy's experiments, in place of exhausting the subject, have pointed out a new and most extensive field for future investigation. And while he has unquestionably very great merit in having paved the way for succeeding enquiries, we would fain hope that he will not himself desert a pursuit which he has already prosecuted with so much success and so much honour.

It is hard to believe that the readers of this account were not impressed. If they did not read the original work, however, they would not have known about Davy's thought on relieving physical pain during surgical operations. This was not mentioned.

Neither relief of headache or toothache, nor the possible use of nitrous oxide during surgical operations, was mentioned in another very favourable contemporary review which ran to twenty-four pages (*Medical and Chirurgical Reviews*, 1800-1801). This reviewer mentioned that Dr. Beddoes' previous "Notice" had ". . . rendered it a subject of much curiosity, and one that promised important results in its investigation". In his opening comments on Davy's *Researches* he had this to say:

The experiments detailed here are entitled to the more attention, as the ingenious author seems to have been aware of, and to have cautiously guarded against, every circumstance, however minute, which tended in any way to influence the result.

There was a further favourable account in the *Monthly Review* (1801), but this failed to give any hint of the anaesthetic potentialities of nitrous oxide.

It was not long before nitrous oxide was included in the syllabus of chemical lectures for medical students, at least at Guy's and St. Thomas's Hospitals where Babington and Allen's (1802) printed syllabus was used. The relevant paragraph and some manuscript notes made in an interleaved copy in 1806 are reproduced in figure 1. These notes were written by a George Hickman, but he was not a near relative of Henry Hill Hickman (for articles on Hickman see p. vii). The sketch of the apparatus used in the preparation of nitrous oxide suggests that George Hickman saw this demonstrated. A similar printed syllabus does

---

* The introduction to Davy's *Researches . . . concerning nitrous oxide* was dated June 25, 1800, and the publication of this work was noted in Nicholson's (monthly) *Philosophical Journal* of August 1800 (4,240). Its purchase by the Physical Society, Guy's Hospital, in which Astley Cooper was one of the leading figures, was noted in the Minutes on December 6, 1800 (Wills Library, Guy's Hospital Medical School).

Of Nitrous Oxyd Gas.

Procured from the decompofition of *Nitrate of Ammonia* with a gentle heat. Confifts of *Oxygen* and *Azote* in intimate union. In fome of its properties refembles *Acids.*

100 cubical inches at a middle temperature and preffure, weigh about 50 grains—Is decompofed by combuftible fubftances at a very high temperature—Soluble in double its volume of *Water*, to which it communicates a fweetifh tafte.

Remarkable for the intoxicating effects which it produces in refpiration.

Gafeous

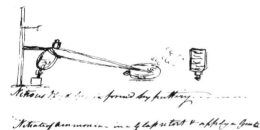

FIG. 1

The section on nitrous oxide in Babington and Allen's *Syllabus of a course of chemical lectures read at Guy's Hospital* (1802), and interleaved manuscript notes made by George Hickman in 1806.

"Soluble in twice its bulk of water and communicates a sweet taste to it. It is soluble in half its bulk of any of the inflammable substance.

"A taper burns in it with an enlarged flame tho: it contains only 16 per cent: oxygen.

"This gas had been thought to be irrespirable but Davy has proved that it may: when respired it produces the most curious sensation.

"It should not be exhibited to hysterical persons it has been known to produce ill effects—tho in the common number of persons it produces only temporary effects.

"Nitrous oxide gas is formed by . . . putting nitrate of ammoniac in a glass retort and applying gentle heat." (By courtesy of The Wills Library, Guy's Hospital Medical School.)

not appear to have been used in Edinburgh at that time, but nitrous oxide was mentioned in a chemistry lecture given by T. C. Hope as early as 1800, as evidenced by notes made by John Lee:

. . . the gaseous oxide of azote—It consists of azotic and oxygen gas—Dr. Mitchell supposes this gas to be the contagion of all diseases—Mr. Davy has discovered its very singular properties—When inhaled it gives highly pleasurable sensations of the most extatic kind —The account given by Dr. Beddoes Jan 18th is perhaps exaggerated . . .*

Following the publication of the reviews of Davy's *Researches, Chemical and Philosophical; chiefly concerning nitrous oxide,* references to nitrous oxide in two of the popular philosophical journals of the day† were infrequent. There is no definite evidence that it was ever used during surgical operations before 1844, but nitrous oxide was mentioned from time to time in the medical literature. There were six references to nitrous oxide in the *Lancet* between October 1823—when it was first published—and 1844. It was also brought to the notice of the public by scientific demonstrations at the Royal Institution (*Tilloch's Magazine*, 1801), at private and public entertainments, and in non-medical literature.

A short course of lectures on pneumatic chemistry was delivered by Davy soon after his arrival at the Royal Institution (*Tilloch's Magazine*, 1801). The concluding lecture, on June 20, was on respiration, and after the lecture:

. . . an opportunity was given to such as wished it, to breathe some of nitrous oxide . . . Mr. Grosvenor Bedford, Mr. Stodart, and Mr. Underwood, breathed the gas; and the effects it produced, especially on the last, were truly wonderful. He experienced so much pleasure from breathing it, that he lost all sense to everything else, and the breathing bag could only be taken from him at last by force.

The note went on say that: "On 23rd June a select party met at the Institution to try the effects of the gaseous oxide."

* Hope was Professor of Chemistry from 1795 to 1844, and he was also Davy's primary sponsor when he was recommended to Count Romford for employment at the Royal Institution (Kendall, 1954). Lee later became Principal of Edinburgh University (Simpson, 1964, Edinburgh University Library, personal communication; see also Cartwright, 1952, p. 117).

† *Nicholson's Journal of Natural Philosophy, Chemistry and the Arts*; and *Tilloch's Philosophical Magazine*, comprehending the various branches of science, the liberal and fine arts and commerce.

James Stodart (1802) subsequently described his experiences of nitrous oxide inhalation in a letter to *Nicholson's Journal*. He apparently inhaled it on June 23 as well as on June 20, and then he ". . . prepared and breathed the gas at different times, and the effects were always pleasurable".

One circumstance [he continued] I wish to notice. A pain in the right side of my face and head, which for some weeks had been very troublesome, was certainly at first increased, after breathing four quarts of the gas. The pain, however, gradually lessened, and in about an hour was quite gone, nor had I any return of it either during the remainder of the day or following night. From this I began to suspect that the gas had been instrumental in some manner in removing the pain. Some symptoms of its return during the following day induced me to give this agent a further trial. With this view I prepared six quarts of the gas, and an hour before my bed time I breathed it . . . (I) slept well during the night, and awoke free from pain in the face. I have felt very little of it ever since. Whether the nitrous oxide was the removing cause or not, I shall not take upon me to determine. I used no other means; nor do I know whether any other person has breathed the gas under similar circumstances. A better acquaintance with this most extraordinary agent would probably lead to important and useful discoveries.

In this instance the relief of pain may not have been due to the inhalation of nitrous oxide, but the possibility was presented plainly enough to readers of *Nicholson's Journal*. If anyone had noticed that this appeared to support Davy's observations on the relief of pain by nitrous oxide, he might have been dissuaded from investigating the matter further by Stodart's description of his subsequent experiences.

The letter continued:

Since writing the above, I have again breathed the nitrous oxide in a very pure state at the Royal Institution, and was as usual lost in pleasure. On recovering, I signified a wish to know the state of my pulse, and was told it was above 140. This was on Saturday the 13th, about three o'clock. I continued under the strong influence of the gas as to muscular action, etc., during the remainder of the day; but awoke next morning with feelings very different to those I had formerly experienced. I felt a tremor, soon became faint, and this faintness increased so much, that for a short space of time I was as if sinking into nothing. I was certainly under considerable alarm. . . . For some hours afterwards I remained in a very low state, during which I am certain that I repeatedly tasted the gas. But my mind was now perfectly tranquil, and at times I had feelings analogous to those I have sometimes experienced during the time of breathing the gas itself. . . . I remain much at a loss to account for the effects produced by the last dose, so contrary to all my former experience; more especially as Mr. Davy does not think the dose was at all extra-

ordinary in quantity, and the gas was not different from that usually prepared. It has stood over water for a day, and was breathed at the same time by Mr. Davy and another gentleman with no unusual consequence.

As Stodart evidently discussed this matter with Davy, he may have mentioned the relief of the pain in the side of his face and head. If he did, Davy may by then have been too taken up with his new interests, such as galvanism and lecturing, to pay much attention; or he may have had his own reasons for being unimpressed by Stodart's story.

Evidence that the inhalation of nitrous oxide was not confined to those in the vicinity of Bristol or London is contained in an editorial note by Robison at the end of Black's *Lectures on the Elements of Chemistry*. Black referred to the experiments of Priestley and of the philosophical chemists in Amsterdam on nitrous oxide and Robison commented (Black, 1803): "Its effects, when breathed for some time, are very wonderful, and were first discovered, I believe, by Mr. Davy. To those who are not hurt by the sight of folly, they are also very amusing."

Bostock (1804), in his essay on respiration, mentioned that Priestley thought that nitrous oxide "was in the highest degree noxious to animals", and that the Society of Dutch Chemists later came to the same conclusion. He continued:

The experiment was, however, repeated by Mr. Davy, and he discovered not only that this gas may be respired for a short time without inconvenience, but that the employment of it is succeeded by a singular excitement of the nervous system, which differs from that produced by alcohol and opium, in not inducing a subsequent state of exhaustion. Mr. Davy also proved, that it is absorbed by the blood in considerable quantity.

He gave a detailed account of Davy's measurements of nitrous oxide absorption and of lung volumes, but he was critical of some of Davy's conclusions.

Ashurst (1897), writing in America about surgery in the days before anaesthesia, commented: ". . . it was the custom of some of our medical schools—at the University of Pennsylvania, for one—for students to breathe 'laughing gas', as it was then called, for a diversion." Fulton and Stanton (1946) drew attention to a thesis written in Philadelphia (Barton, 1808) which may have stimulated this interest in the gas.

In the preface of his *Dissertation on the*

Chymical Properties and Exhilarating Effects of Nitrous Oxide, Barton wrote:

But the account which he (Davy) gave of its operation was generally derided as extravagant and imaginary. Few believed it. The description was supposed to have proceeded from a warmed and highly excited mind [Barton, 1808, p. xiii]. In the United States the chymists partook of the prevalent skepticism as to the alleged properties of the gas [p. xiv].

This is more in keeping with Cartwright's (1952, p. 77) comment on the influence of Beddoes' politics on the aceptance of Davy's work, than with the reviews of his *Researches, Chemical and Philosophical . . .* quoted above.

Having inhaled nitrous oxide following a blow on the head ". . . by accidentally striking it against the sharp edge of a door", Barton (1808, p. 74) observed: "I am decidedly of opinion with Mr. Davy, that this gas has the power of removing intense physical pain". But he made no reference to the possible application of this property.

Barton expressed a strong desire to direct the attention of physicians to nitrous oxide, but its entertainment value remained the main interest in the gas, and Read (1947) cites evidence of its popularity in England at this time:

Judging from the contemporary writer Fiévée, the inhalation of "exhilarating" or "laughing" gas became a vogue . . . for in his *Lettres sur l'Angleterre* he condemned the practice as a national vice of the English!

The effects of respiring nitrous oxide were also recorded in British textbooks on chemistry (Thomson, 1804; Henry, 1815; Ure, 1823). Henry (1815, p. 380) explained its safety thus: ". . . it does not prove fatal because, when received into the lungs, it is mixed and diluted with the atmospherical air present in that organ". Under the heading "Nitrate of Ammonia", Henry (1815, p. 391) also went into the economics of the production of nitrous oxide: "One pound of the compact kind gives, by careful decomposition, nearly five cubic feet of gas, or rather more than 34 doses, so that the expense, estimating the salt at 5*s.* 10*d.* per pound, is about 2*d.* for each dose". Further indication of the general interest in the inhalation of nitrous oxide, implied by these writings, is provided by two contributions to the *Journal of the Science and Arts.* An anonymous contribution in 1818 drew attention to the similarity of the effects of inhaling nitrous oxide and the vapour of sulphuric ether, and Faraday (1819)

advised on the precautions to be taken to avoid the inhalation of impurities so that ". . . it may always be breathed with safety, except by the few who experience effects apparently anomalous to those which belong to the gas".

A decade later, Professor Silliman, writing in the *American Journal of Science* (cited *Tilloch's Magazine*, 1819) again suggested that more attention should be paid to the possible uses of gases in medicine, with particular reference to oxygen and nitrous oxide. He wrote:

Should the revival of the experiments on the respiration of oxygen gas appear to be desired, it would not be difficult to simplify the apparatus and operations so as to bring them within the reach of an intelligent person, even although ignorant of chemistry.

This interesting class of experiments ought to be resumed, not with the spirit of quackery nor of extravagant expectation, but with the sobriety of philosophical research; and it is more than probable that the nitrous oxide, which is now little more than the subject of merriment and wonder, if properly diluted and discreetly applied, would be productive of valuable effects.

Shaw (1889, 1893) suggested that nitrous oxide might have been associated with tooth-drawing, for the relief of pain following extraction, in either London or Paris as early as 1820. He based this on a passage in *Doctor Syntax in Search of the Grotesque* which was published around that time (see Chapter 5). Shaw quoted the following lines:

Dolly cries, "My jaws do burn,
I've caught the toothache from the damp,
So to the doctor let us tramp."
"Here lives, my dear, a skilful man,"
Said Syntax, "called Le Charlatan."
Le Charlatan, with knowing grin,
Welcomed his patient, heard her case,
Received his fee, and took his place.
Our dentist quickly twisted out
The offending tooth, and Dolly rose.
Le Charlatan observed, "Suppose,
Madam, you sniff some nitrous gas
To assuage the torments of your face."

In another "Doctor Syntax" book (1820b, *The Tour of Doctor Syntax through London*), there is a description of a visit to the London Institution during which nitrous oxide was demonstrated. The relevant lines are:

Then he'd varieties of gasses
Which no philosopher surpasses;
Some that produced most strange effects
Upon the nerves of either sex,
One that if you but take a dose*
A sweet delirium bestows;
To dullest alderman gives wit
And to despair a laughing fit. . . .

    * Nitrous Oxyd, or laughing gas.

Animal experiments with nitrous oxide had at least been considered by Brodie in the Royal College of Surgeons at this time. In 1821 he investigated the effects of sulphuric ether on a guineapig, by enclosing the animal under a bell glass and conveying ether vapour to it from a retort. He attributed the effects to the specific action of ether, and not to suffocation. In his notes he also wrote:

I have made no experiments on the nitrous oxide myself—to ascertain whether the heart continues to act after death—but probably it does—this produces intoxication . . . There are, no doubt, many other gases which may operate like ether by destroying the functions of the brain . . . [Thomas, 1962].

Accounts of the early history of nitrous oxide anaesthesia usually do not make specific mention of the use of the gas for public entertainment before about 1830 (Robinson, 1946, p. 83). The Enthoven Theatre Collection at the Victoria and Albert Museum, however, contains a playbill (fig. 2) announcing positively the last night of M. Henry's entertainment at the Adelphi Theatre, Strand, which included the administration of nitrous oxide, or laughing gas, "to any of the Audience who may chuse to inhale it". It is dated Saturday, June 5, 1824 (see Fullmer, 1964). It is possible that M. Henry also gave his entertainment in other cities, but laughing gas may have been a very recent addition to the repertoire. The Enthoven collection contains four other playbills for the same season of M. Henry at the Adelphi. One headed "LAST WEEK"—giving the dates Monday, May 10, Thursday, 13, and Saturday, 15, 1824—mentions "THE LAUGHING GAS!! continuing to excite peals of laughter, will be repeated every evening. The excessive exhilaration caused by this gas, together with its wonderful effects, must be seen to be believed!" Lower down in the same playbill is advertised: "Part III—Novel and interesting experiments on gas! amongst which will be introduced the Inflation and Ascent of a Balloon in the theatre, and the laughing gas!!!" These latter words are repeated on another undated playbill which is headed "THE LAST WEEK"; but playbills dated March 4 and 5 announce "Part III—Novel and interesting experiments on gas" without mentioning laughing gas. The experiments on gas are particularized on the playbill of March 5 as follows: "An illustration of the necessity of Oxygen to support

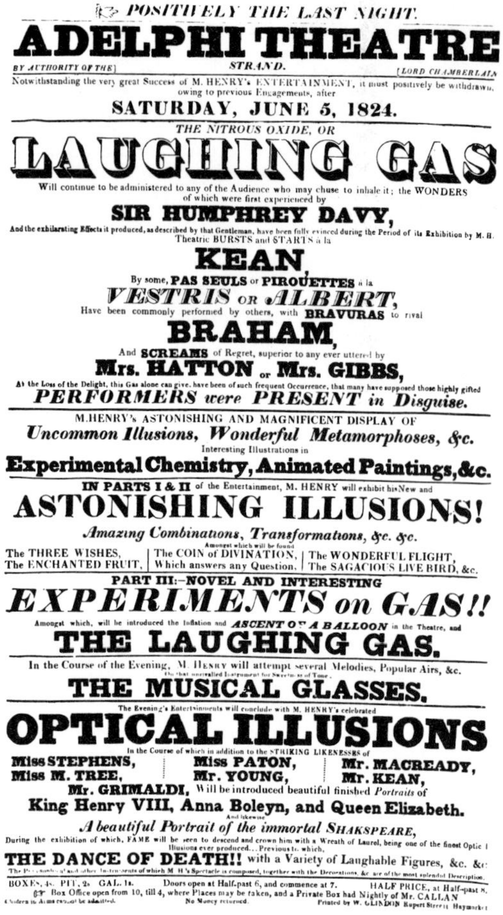

FIG. 2

Playbill of a show in London in 1824, which included a demonstration of the effects of inhaling laughing gas. (Enthoven Theatre Collection: Crown Copyright. Victoria and Albert Museum.)

combustion. The characteristic qualities regarding combustion of atmospheric air, carbonic acid gas, and oxygen—a very curious effect."

Schoenbein, a German naturalist, witnessed a demonstration of laughing gas at the Adelphi Theatre during one of his visits to England before 1839. He may have been in London as early as 1824, but 1826 is the earliest date mentioned in his *Journal* (Schoenbein, 1842, p. 350). He was in Germany in 1823, but in 1825 he became a teacher at Epsom, and he remained in England for two years (Kahlbaum, 1899). He wrote:

In some of the smaller theatres, physical and chemical experiments are sometimes made, more for the entertainment than for the edification of the audience, and I once saw such a performance. It was at the Adelphi Theatre and they wanted to demonstrate the very odd properties and the physiological effects of the laughing gas.

When the curtain was raised, you could see on the stage, in a wide semicircle, a dozen or more large caoutchouc bladders with shining metal taps, filled with the laughing gas. The "Experimentator" appeared in a simple dress suit, and made a short opening speech in which he described the properties of the gas, and its preparation, in a way which would have done credit to a professor of chemistry. At the end of his lecture he asked for someone from the audience to come on the stage and to inhale from one of the bladders. A tall daring fellow jumped over the orchestra and on to the stage, and grabbed one of the bladders. But the audience didn't like him and greeted him with cries of "Off! Off!" At first he did not comply, but when the cries grew louder he went away. A second candidate appeared, but he too was shouted off. When the third met with the same undignified reception, the "Experimentator" interceded and asked the audience firmly but politely not to be so fickle and to let the show go on. This appeal had the desired effect and they proceeded. The volunteer—sitting in a chair—put the tap to his mouth, compressed his nose, and inhaled the laughing gas while the "Experimentator" held the bladder. The tap was then closed while the subject breathed out through the nose. The tap was opened again, the nose compressed, and some more gas inhaled through the mouth. He continued in this way until the bag was emptied. Now the "Experimentator" retired; but the "luft-trunken" man remained sitting in his chair for a few minutes, while he stared straight ahead, holding his nose. You can imagine how this comical posture sent the audience into roars of laughter which increased when the intoxicated man leapt smartly from his chair and then made astonishing bounds all over the stage.

When the audience had had its fill and the man had sobered up, a voice called out: "All nonsense and humbug!" "All nonsense and humbug!" echoed immediately from hundreds of throats. "No! No!" came the emphatic reply. When the protests continued, the "Experimentator" appeared and shouted at the top of his voice: "Ladies and Gentlemen". When he obtained a hearing he assured the audience that the experiment was genuine, and he invited the man who had first voiced his doubts to try the experiment himself. The man responded with alacrity and displayed his incredulity by demanding to empty the largest bladder. His request was immediately complied with, and the effect of the gas upon the disbeliever was so great that he beat around him like a madman and assaulted the "Experimentator". This performance confirmed the sceptics in their doubts and brought forth fresh demonstrations of disbelief.

The description of the subject breathing in through the mouth and out through the nose is unusual. It is not clear whether this was a deliberate avoidance of rebreathing, or whether it was because the flow resistance of the tap was so great that it was a relief to exhale freely through the nose.

The Enthoven collection at the Victoria and Albert Museum has been searched for Adelphi Theatre playbills dated 1826 and mentioning laughing gas, but none was found. There is, however, an Adelphi Theatre playbill dated Wednesday, February 22, 1826, announcing that "M. Henry will have the honour of repeating his Third Annual Entertainment of 'Table Talk . . . Odd Sayings and Queer Doings' . . ." (G. W. Nash (1965), personal communication). It is possible that he had good reason for omitting further demonstrations of laughing gas.

Schoenbein continued:

My chemical readers may be interested to know that this gas is nowhere inhaled more often than in England, because its marvellous effects were first discovered in this country by Sir Humphry Davy. Once when I stayed in the country with a friend, who was an amateur chemical experimenter, we discussed laughing gas and decided to make a good supply of it ourselves. One fine afternoon, a large party met in the garden to inhale the intoxicating gas in the open air. Some young men inhaled it first, and they all showed undoubted signs of wellbeing and pleasure. When another man of more mature age had his doubts, he decided to take a large quantity of the gas for himself. After breathing a lot of gas, he began to dance and devastate the adjoining flower-bed in his ecstasy—to the delight of his audience. Maybe it will become the custom for us to inhale laughing gas at the end of a dinner party, instead of drinking champagne, and in that event there would be no shortage of gas factories.

This account implies that the inhalation of laughing gas was relatively frequent in England, but the sceptical reactions of the audience at the Adelphi Theatre and at the party suggest that its properties were not widely known.

In 1826, Bostock produced a new textbook of physiology in which he stated that: "Of gases, which although not capable of supporting life are still respirable, the one that is least injurious to the system appears to be nitrous oxide." He continued with a brief account of the experience of Davy and his friends, and observed that

the experiment has been now so frequently repeated, that although in certain constitutions the peculiar excitement cannot be perceived and, in some instances there seems to be a sedative effect produced, yet no doubt can remain of the general truth of the fact.

In a footnote he added:

Thenard Chem. t.iii. p. 674 gives an account of its effects upon M. Vauquelin. I may add that I experienced the same feelings in my own person: the first inspiration of the oxide produced a sensation like that of fainting, which quickly proceeded to insensibility.

In the following year, Brande (1827), in his series of lectures on chemistry delivered at the Royal Institution, and reported fully in the *Lancet,* commented:

It is a very curious fact, in regard to this gas, that it may be breathed for some time, and that it produces effects analogous to intoxication, making persons incoherent in their talk, rambling in their walk, and so on, in the same way as if they had drunk spiritous liquor, and it has been supposed that persons may inhale it without inconvenience; but I have seen ill effects from having inhaled it, such as pain in the head, giddiness, and so on, so that I should advise you never to do it: and I speak this, because in some schools of chemistry I know it is customary to allow pupils to breathe it, but it is a foolish experiment, and you may be content with a statement of the facts.

An illustration, by George Cruikshank, of the effects of inhaling nitrous oxide during a class experiment is shown in figure 3.

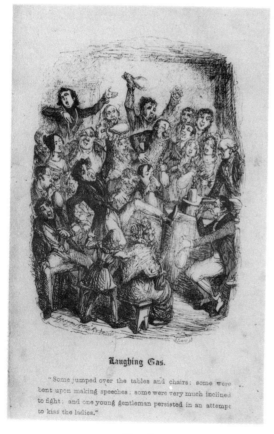

Laughing Gas.

"Some jumped over the tables and chairs; some were bent upon making speeches; some were very much inclined to fight; and one young gentleman persisted in an attempt to kiss the ladies."

FIG. 3
An illustration by Cruikshank of the effects of inhaling nitrous oxide (Scoffern, 1839).

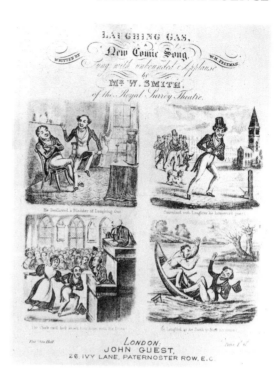

FIG. 4
An illustrated song sheet thought to have been printed *circa* 1830. (By courtesy of the Wellcome Trustees.)

The illustrated song sheet shown in figure 4, of "Laughing Gas, a New Comic Song, sung with unbounded Applause by Mr. W. Smith of the Royal Surrey Theatre", also provides evidence of the exhilarating properties of nitrous oxide having been brought before the public eye around this time. According to the title page this song was entered at the Stationers' Hall, but an extensive search of the records maintained there has not revealed any such entry. Mr. Smith is known to have been singing in the Royal Surrey Theatre in 1825, but the date of his performance of this song is not known. It is thought to have been printed *circa* 1830 (G. W. Nash, 1965, personal communication). The eleven verses of the song tell the tale of

Poor Jeremy Jones . . .
He was thin as a leaf,
And his flesh was worn from his bones with Grief . . .
A wag who heard of poor Jeremy's case,
Told him he'd very soon alter his Face;
Invited him home and while there, alas!
He swallowed a Bladder of Laughing Gas.

Some of his subsequent adventures are illustrated. Of particular interest is the apparatus shown at top left which is authentic. It depicts a gas-holder from which gas was expelled by water displacement, water being poured into the funnel and the bag being connected to the nozzle shown on the left. The function of the small cistern at the top of the apparatus was to enable gas to be collected under water. The amount of gas left in the container at any time could be seen by observing the water level in the sight tube. The idea was developed from the gas-holder designed by James Watt for Thomas Beddoes and used by Humphry Davy (see Smith, 1965), and it was described by Pepys (1802), mainly as a convenient means of storing oxygen. A detailed description of apparatus almost identical with that shown in the song sheet was given by Henry (1815, p. 124), and he prefaced his description by saying: "When large quantities of gas are required (as at a public lecture), the gas-holder . . . will be found extremely useful."

Dieffenbach (1829) referred to the work of Nysten, in France, on transfusion and infusion. Nitrous oxide, among other gases, was injected into animals intravenously, and was rapidly absorbed into the blood, even large quantities having no effect. This experiment had been suggested independently by one of the reviewers of Davy's *Researches* . . . (*Annals of Medicine*, 1800).

Curtis (1829) tried administering nitrous oxide to a patient who was subject to severe attacks of asthma. Doses of three to four quarts were rebreathed from a bladder, and the patient felt much improved. A second patient, who wheezed and had difficulty in breathing whenever she had a cold, was said to have been cured by nitrous oxide inhalations. With both patients, particular note was made of the increased circulation seen in the extremities.

Hudson (1832) suggested that nitrous oxide might be used as a stimulant in cases of cholera, on the grounds that the state of excitement would not be followed by sedation. There is no record of this treatment having been tried at the time, although it was mentioned again in a report from America thirty-four years later (*Lancet*, 1866).

Back and Morgan (1834), of Guy's Hospital, administered nitrous oxide in an unsuccessful attempt to allay severe spasms in a young man suffering from hydrophobia. The method of administration was not described. Instead of allaying the spasm, the nitrous oxide appeared to aggravate it and keep up a constant state of excitement in the patient. This report brings to mind the more recent trials of nitrous oxide in the treatment of tetanus (Lassen et al., 1954, 1956), which were discontinued because of the resulting bone marrow changes.

Stanley (1842) reported a case of poisoning by inhalation of impure nitrous oxide. Three young men prepared some nitrous oxide for their own enjoyment. One of them convulsed after inhaling it and took a while to recover. This was thought to have been due to the inhalation of impurities resulting from overheating the ammonium nitrate.

These glimpses of nitrous oxide are enough to let us see that, in the United Kingdom, it was introduced into the medical student's curriculum, in at least some hospitals, very early in the century; that its preparation was demonstrated, and that it was sometimes inhaled at lectures on chemistry. It was also inhaled for both private and public entertainment, and doctors knew sufficient about nitrous oxide to consider using it therapeutically.

In the United States travelling showmen, otherwise described as itinerant lecturers, are reported to have toured the country demonstrating the effects of nitrous oxide from the early 1830's (Robinson, 1946). One of these was Samuel Colt, designer of the first revolver to be mass produced. In 1832, at the age of 18, he toured the east coast between Canada and Maryland demonstrating the effects of laughing gas in halls. He had recently returned from a long voyage, and he described himself as Dr. S. Coult of Calcutta, London and New York. An advertisement of a demonstration given at Portland on October 13, 1832, read as follows:

NITROUS OXIDE GAS FOR LADIES AND GENTLEMEN
Dr. S. Coult respectfully informs the Ladies and Gentlemen of Portland and vicinity, that he will administer the NITROUS OXIDE, or Exhilarating Gas, on Monday evening at the City Hall. Exhibition to commence at 7 o'clock precisely. The peculiar effects of this singular compound upon the animal system, was first noticed by the English Chemist, Sir Humphry Davy. He observed that when inhaled into the lungs it produced the most astonishing effects upon the nervous system; that some individuals were disposed to laugh, sing, and dance; others, to recitation and decla-

mation, and that the greater number had an irresistible propensity to muscular exertion, such as wrestling, boxing, etc., with numerous fantastic feats. In short, the sensations produced by it are highly pleasurable, and are not followed by debility. . . . Dr. C. has exhibited the extraordinary powers of the gas in many cities of the United States, to audiences composed of Ladies and Gentlemen of the first respectability—and many Ladies have inhaled the gas at select Exhibitions. Those Ladies who may be anxious of witnessing the Exhibition, in this city, may be assured, that the City Hall embraces every accommodation for their comfort, and that not a shadow of impropriety attends the Exhibition,, to shock the most modest. He will attend, on reasonable terms, to any applications for private Exhibitions to select parties of Ladies and Gentlemen . . . [Cary, 1961].

Although Stodart (1802), Barton (1808) and "Syntax" (1820a) mentioned the relief of pain afforded by inhalation of nitrous oxide, no one except Davy hinted at its possible use as an anaesthetic during surgical operations. But it was due to the knowledge of nitrous oxide being kept alive that inhalation anaesthesia was first introduced. That it lived and remained alive was probably due to the initial impact of Davy's *Researches.* . . .

One cannot expect Davy to have visualized anaesthesia as we know it today, but there can be no justification for presuming that he did not mean what he wrote. "As nitrous oxide in its extensive operation appears capable of destroying physical pain, it may probably be used with advantage during surgical operations"—this has a clear enough meaning, and it is immaterial whether he imagined that the patients would be unconscious, semiconscious or just analgesic. The thoughts behind the additional clause, ". . . in which no great effusion of blood takes place", are less obvious. Cartwright (1952, p. 327) has made the reasonable suggestion that Davy may have thought that loss of blood would influence the effect of the gas rather than that he was concerned, in this context, with the increased danger of haemorrhage. Whatever Davy's full thoughts on the matter may have been, it would seem that, in the absence of supporting experimental evidence, his convictions were not sufficient for him to attempt conversion of his contemporaries to the idea. It was born and published before it was immediately acceptable.

Be that as it may, if Davy or any of his contemporaries had explored the possibilities of his suggestion, anaesthesia might have started on a

surer and, perhaps, a more seemly footing. Instead of developing haphazardly and empirically, it could have grown directly from the enthusiastic investigations into the properties of nitrous oxide, carried out in a new research Institution where material and intellectual resources had been concentrated. Watt had already designed what was virtually rudimentary anaesthetic apparatus. The nitrous oxide generators, "hydraulic bellows", gas-holders, bags, mouthpieces and non-return valves were already there. Even flexible tubes supported by brass wire spirals were mentioned (Beddoes and Watt, 1794). There was a background of relevant physical, chemical, animal and human experimentation. The use of oxygen with nitrous oxide had been tried and the greater safety of this was appreciated. With Clayfield's (1800) mercurial air-holder, spirometry and primitive methods of gas analysis had already been applied to the measurement of nitrous oxide uptake and lung volumes. These basic problems were being thought about, deeply. The Pneumatic Institution could have evolved into the first Anaesthetic Research Institution. The stage was set, but the actors went away.

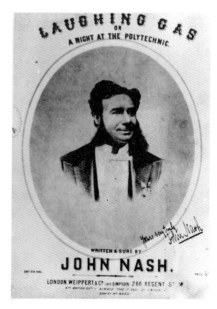

FIG. 5

Title page of a song sheet about nitrous oxide thought to be dated *c.* 1860. By courtesy of The Wellcome Trustees.

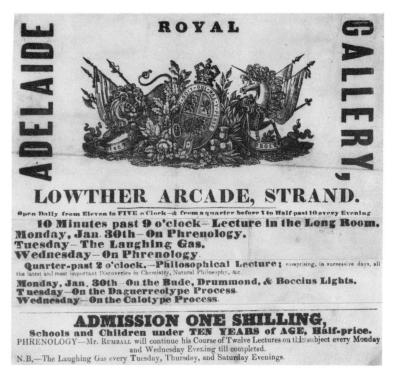

FIG. 6

Royal Adelaide Gallery hand-bill mentioning laughing gas. Thought to be dated 1837. (In possession of the author; photography by C. H. Redman of the Royal College of Surgeons of England.)

APPENDIX

Nitrous oxide for entertainment.

The use of nitrous oxide for entertainment purposes did not stop with the advent of inhalation anaesthesia. Figure 5 shows the title page of a song entitled *Laughing Gas; or a Night at the Polytechnic*. The verses describe the adventures of young Humphrey Brown from Gloucestershire who fell asleep in the lecture room of the Regent Street Polytechnic which, at that time, was something of a mixture between a Schoolboys' and a Manufacturers' Exhibition, and a Science Museum. It was well described in *Punch* (1865). Topical references in the song appear to date it about 1860.

Before the Regent Street Polytechnic was launched, there used to be a similar popular scientific exhibition at the Adelaide Gallery, Lowther Arcade, Strand. After a while "science" gave way more and more to popular entertainment, as described by Smith (1849). Walford (1897) and Pritchard (1961). Figure 6 shows a handbill from the Royal Adelaide Gallery which advertises "The Laughing Gas" at "10 minutes past 9 o'clock—Lecture in the Long Room, on Tuesday" (probably January 30, 1837), and "The Laughing Gas every Tuesday, Thursday, and Saturday Evenings".

The first volume of *Punch* (1841) also contains a reference to laughing gas in relation to medical students in a series entitled "The Physiology of the London Medical Student". This was later republished in book form as *The London Medical Student* (Smith, 1861).

The Adelaide Gallery was opened in 1830. It was originally intended as a place of amusement and instruction combined, where 20-minute lectures could be given on various aspects of science and practical demonstrations of models being worked by steam and clockwork and so on. But it became a place for amusement and dancing only, for the Strand in those days was hardly suitable for serious-minded people. It was not surprising that the gallery quickly failed in its original objects. Its secretary, Charles Payne, resigned in the late 1830s and was persuaded by Sir George Cayley to become manager of the "Royal Gallery of Arts and Sciences" in Regent Street. This was opened in 1838 and received a Royal Charter in 1839. It was from this that the Regent Street Polytechnic later grew (see Pritchard, 1961).

According to Smith (1849), the Adelaide Gallery ". . . was at first devoted to the diffusion of knowledge. . . . Then came a transition stage in the existence of the Adelaide Gallery, at first stealthily brought about. The oxy-hydrogen light was slyly applied to the magic lantern; and laughing gas was made instead of carbonic acid. By degrees music stole in; then wizards; and lastly talented vocal foreigners from Ethiopia and the Pyrenees. Science was driven to her wit's end for a livelihood, but she still endeavoured to appear respectable. The names of the new attractions were covertly put into the bills, sneaking under the original engines and machines in small type. . . . But during this time a mania for dancing had been gradually coming on, and at last burst forth. . . . And at last all the steam engines were cleared away, and the Adelaide Gallery was devoted entirely to the goddess of the 'twinkling-feet', and called a Casino."

This evidence indicates that the date of the handbill could not have been before 1830, but must have been before 1849. It was felt that it was probably dated around the time that Charles Payne moved from the Adelaide Gallery to the new Institution in Regent

Street. The handbill mentions specifically "Monday, Jan 30th". The only years between 1830 and 1849 in which January 30 fell upon a Monday were 1837, 1843 and 1848, so 1837 was considered to be the likely date.

Figure 6 shows a few pasted-up extracts from the whole handbill, which measures 20″ × 15″ and contains much small print. Three items mentioned provide clear evidence that it was dated after 1837. A Philosophical Lecture on the Daguerreotype process was advertised for Tuesday at "Quarter-past 2 o'clock", and another on the Calotype process for the following day. No. 30 on the list of "Magnificent Transparent Dissolving Views" is "Her Most Gracious Majesty, Queen Victoria". William IV did not die until June 20, 1837. The Daguerreotype process was published in 1839 and Talbot took out a patent for his Calotype process in 1841. The date of the handbill, therefore, must be either 1843 or 1848.

ADDENDUM

Dr. D. R. Nagle has drawn my attention to the administration of nitrous oxide by William Wright in 1829, for the relief of deafness: "The inhalation of the nitrous oxyde gas, excites in most persons ... great acuteness of hearing, but it shortly goes off: I have administered it medically, in small quantity, to one or two persons who were deaf, and desirous of trying the experiment, but it had only the temporary effect of increasing the hearing for an hour or so" (Wright, 1829).

ACKNOWLEDGMENTS

This study started with Duncum (1947) and frequent reference was made to this source. Background reading included Cartwright (1952)—particularly relevant to this instalment—Robinson (1946), Sykes (1960, 1961), Leake (1947), and Keys (1945). Research was carried out in a number of libraries, often with the help and encouragement of their librarians. Both Mr. W. Le Fanu of the Royal College of Surgeons of England, and Mr. P. Wade of the Royal Society of Medicine, for example, recommended an approach to Mr. K. D. C. Vernon of the Royal Institution. He, in turn, suggested writing to Professor June Z. Fullmer of the Department of Chemistry, Delaware, who drew attention to the Adelphi Theatre playbill and to Schoenbein (1842). The latter was obtained from Bern through the Brotherton Library, Leeds University, and I am greatly indebted to Miss M. Schoenel for translating relevant passages. Mr. G. W. Nash searched the Enthoven Collection at the Victoria and Albert Museum, and later drew my attention to the existence of the illustrated song sheet (fig. 4), which Mr. E. Gaskell of the Wellcome Historical Library kindly unearthed. Dr. M. P. Crosland drew my attention to the relevant chemical literature. Mr. W. Hill of the Wills Library, Guy's Medical School, gave much assistance in the search for evidence of the teaching of nitrous oxide to medical students at the start of the last century. Dr. R. A. Butler, now at the Department of Anesthesia, Philadelphia, sought out Barton's thesis. Mr. G. Carnall of the Department of English Literature, Edinburgh, drew attention to the reference to nitrous oxide in *The Tour of Dr. Syntax through London*.

REFERENCES

Annals of Medicine (1800). Sect. I: Analysis of books pp. 227–258. "On Researches, Chemical and Philosophical . . ." by H. Davy.

Anon (1818). Miscellanea. V: Effects of inhaling the vapour of sulphuric ether. *Journal of Science and the Arts*, 4, 158.

Ashhurst, J. (1897). Surgery before the days of anaesthesia (reprinted from the *Scientific American*). *Brit. J. dent. Sci.*, 40, 735.

Babington, W., and Allen, W. (1802). *A syllabus of a course of chemical lectures read at Guy's Hospital*. London: W. Phillips.

Back and Morgan (1834). Hydrophobia—inhalation of nit. oxide gas. *Lancet*, 2, 703.

Barton, W. P. C. (1808). *Thesis: a dissertation on the chymical properties and exhilarating effects of nitrous oxide gas; and its application to pneumatick medicine;* submitted as an inaugural thesis for the degree of Doctor of Medicine. Philadelphia.

Beddoes, T. and Watt, J. (1794). *Considerations on the medicinal use of factitious airs, and on the manner of obtaining them in large quantities*, 1st ed., Part II, p. 26. Bristol: Bulgin and Rosser.

Black, J. (1803). *Lectures on the Elements of Chemistry delivered in the University of Edinburgh by the late Joseph Black, M.D., Professor of Chemistry in that University. Now published from his manuscripts by John Robinson, M.D.* Vol. II, p. 746. Edinburgh: Mundell & Son.

Bostock, J. (1804). *An Essay on Respiration*, Parts I and II, p. 148. Liverpool: Longman and Rees.

—— (1826). *An Elementary System of Physiology*, Vol. II. London: Baldwin, Cradok and Jay.

Brande (1827). Lectures on chemistry. XVII: On muriatic acid, hydriodic acid, and nitrous oxide. *Lancet*, 1, 455.

Cartwright, F. F. (1952). *The English pioneers of anaesthesia: Beddoes, Davy and Hickman*. Bristol: Wright.

Cary, L. (1961). *The Colt Gun Book*, p. 9. Greenwich, U.S.A.: Faucett.

Chapman-Houston, D., and Cripps, E. C. (1954). *Through a City Archway: the story of Allen and Hanburys 1715–1954*, p. 56. London: Murray.

Clayfield, W. (1800). Description of a mercurial air-holder suggested by an inspection of Mr. Watt's machine for containing factitious airs. *Tilloch's Philosophical Magazine*, 7, 148.

Curtis, J. (1829). Nitrous oxide gas, as a remedy in chronic diseases of the chest. *Lancet*, 2, 376.

Davy, H. (1800a). A letter from Mr. Davy, Superintendent of the Pneumatic Institution, to Mr. Nicholson, on Nitrous Oxide, or gaseous oxide of azote, on certain factors relating to heat and light, and on the discovery of the decomposition of the carbonate and sulphite of ammoniac. *Nicholson's Journal*, 3, 515.

—— (1800b). *Researches, Chemical and Philosophical; chiefly concerning nitrous oxide, or dephlogisticated nitrous air, and its respiration*. London: J. Johnson.

Dieffenbach (1829). Foreign department: transfusion and infusion. *Lancet*, 2, 324.

Duncum, B. M. (1947). *The development of Inhalation Anaesthesia: with special reference to the years 1846–1900*. London: Oxford University Press.

Faraday, M. (1819). Miscellanea. 8: Nitrous oxide. *Journal of Science and the Arts*, 6, 361.

Fayle, J. (1884). *The Spitalfields Genius: The story of William Allen, F.R.S.*, p. 42. London: Hodder and Stoughton.

Fullmer, J. Z. (1964). The great laughing gas experiment. *Chemistry*, **37**, 6.

Fulton, J. F., and Stanton, M. E. (1946). *The Centennial of Surgical Anesthesia; an annoted catalogue of books and pamphlets bearing on the early history of surgical anesthesia*. New York: Henry Schuman.

Henry, W. (1815). *The Elements of Experimental Chemistry*, 7th ed., Vol. I. London: Baldwin, Cradock and Joy.

Hudson, J. (1832). Nitrous oxide in cholera. *Lancet*, **2**, 629.

Kahlbaum, G. A. (1899), in Kahlbaum and Darbishire, (1899).

—— Darbishire, F. V. (1899). *The letters of Faraday and Schoenbein 1836–1862, with notes, comments and references to contemporary letters*. London: Williams and Norgate.

Kendall, J. (1954). *Humphry Davy: "Pilot" of Penzance*, p. 55. London: Faber and Faber.

Keys, T. E. (1945). *The History of Surgical Anesthesia*. New York: Schuman.

Lancet (1866). The progress of medicine and the collateral sciences: protoxide of nitrogen in cholera. **1**, 69.

Lassen, H. C. A., Bjorneboe, M., and Ibsen, B. (1954). Treatment of tetanus with curarization, general anaesthesia and intratracheal positive pressure ventilation. *Lancet*, **2**, 1040.

—— Henrikson, E., Neukirch, F., and Kristensen, H. S. (1956). Treatment of tetanus: severe bone marrow depression after prolonged nitrous oxide anaesthesia. *Lancet*, **1**, 527.

Leake, C. D. (1947). *Letheon: the cadenced story of anesthesia*. Austin: University of Texas Press.

Macintosh, R. R., and Pratt, F. (1940). *Essentials of General Anaesthesia with special reference to Dentistry*. London: Blackwell.

Medical and Chirurgical Review (1800–1801). "Researches, Chemical and Philosophical . . ." by H. Davy. **7**, 268, 332.

Monthly Review (1801), **35**, 33.

Pepys, W. H. (1802). Description of a new gas-holder. *Tilloch's Philosophical Magazine*, **13**, 153

Pritchard, J. I.. (1961). *Sir George Cayley, the inventor of the aeroplane*. London: Parrish.

Punch (1841), p. 201. The physiology of the London medical student. 6: Of the grinder and his class.

—— (1865), December 16, p. 236. A wonderful shillingsworth.

Read, J. (1947). *Humour and Humanism in Chemistry*. London: Bell.

Robinson, V. (1946). *Victory over Pain*. New York: Henry Schuman.

Schoenbein, C. F. (1842). *Mittheilungen aus dem reisetagebuche eines deutschen naturforschers*. Basel.

Scoffern, J. (1839). *Chemistry no Mystery; or a lecturer's bequest*. Being the subject matter of a course of lectures, delivered by an old philosopher, and taken in shorthand by one of the audience, whose name is not known. Arranged from the original

manuscript by J. Scoffern. London.

Shaw, P. (1889). Personal recollections of the discovery of anaesthetics. *Manchester Odont. Soc.*, **1**, 217.

—— (1893). Personal recollections of the discovery of anaesthetics (reprinted from *Manchester Odont. Soc.*, **1**, 217). *Brit. J. dent. Sci.*, **36**, 721.

Smith, A. (1849). *The Casino, in Gavarni in London: Sketches of Life and Character, with illustrated essays by popular writers*. Edited by Albert Smith, p. 13. London: David Bogue, 86 Fleet Street.

Smith, Albert (1861). *The London Medical Student*. Edited by Arthur Smith. London: Routledge.

Smith, W. D. A. (1965). A history of nitrous oxide and oxygen anaesthesia. Part I: Joseph Priestley to Humphry Davy. *Brit. J. Anaesth.*, **37**, 790.

Stanley, F. (1842). Poisoning by the inhalation of impure nitrous oxide gas. *Lancet*, **1**, 395.

Stodart, J. (1802). On the effects of the respiration of the nitrous oxide; particularly an instance in which the excitation of the system produced unpleasant symptoms. In a letter from Mr. James Stodart to Mr. Nicholson. *Nicholson's Journal*, N.S.1, 225.

Sykes, W. S. (1960). *Essays on the First Hundred Years of Anaesthesia*, Vol. I, p. 125. Edinburgh: E. & S. Livingstone.

—— (1961). *Essays on the First Hundred Years of Anaesthesia*, Vol. II. Edinburgh: E. & S. Livingstone.

"Syntax" (1820a). *Doctor Syntax in Paris; or, a tour in search of the grotesque*. London: W. Wright.

—— (1820b). *The Tour of Doctor Syntax through London; or the pleasures and miseries of the metropolis: a poem*, 3rd ed., p. 208 London: J. Johnstone.

Thomas, K. B. (1962). Ether used to produce insensibility in 1821. *Brit. J. Anaesth.*, **34**, 588.

Thomson, T. (1804). *A System of Chemistry in Four Volumes*, 2nd ed., Vol. I, p. 587. Edinburgh: Bell.

Tilloch's Philosophical Magazine (1801). Royal Institution of Great Britain. **10**, 86.

Tilloch's Philosophical Magazine (1819). On the respiration of oxygen gas in an affectation of the thorax. **53**, 273.

Ure, A. (1823). *A Dictionary of Chemistry on the basis of Mr. Nicholson's, in which the principles of the science are investigated anew, and its applications to the phenomena of nature, medicine, mineralogy, agriculture, and manufacture, detailed*, 2nd ed., p. 597. London: Thomas Tegg.

Walford, E. (1897). *Old and New London, a narrative of its history, its people and its places. Illustrated with numerous Engravings from the most authentic sources. Westminster and the Western Suburbs*, Vol. III, p. 132. London: Cassell.

Wilks, S., and Bettany, G. T. (1892). *A Biographical History of Guy's Hospital*, p. 388. London: Ward, Lock, Bowden & Co.

Wright, W. (1829). *On the Varieties of Deafness and Diseases of the Ear, with proposed methods of relieving them*, p. 117. London: Hurst, Chance.

5

PARSONS SHAW, DOCTOR SYNTAX AND NITROUS OXIDE

We beg the world will not alone
Take either his or our averment
For Gospel, or award preferment,
Till it has heard what has been said
By "Syntax" self upon his head—
Him who alone can truly judge
Whose tale is true, and whose is fudge.

(*Doctor Syntax in Paris*, p. v, 1820a)

Doctor Parsons Shaw (fig. 1) was the first Dean of the Victoria Dental Hospital, Manchester, England, the opening of which was reported in the *Manchester Guardian* of July 23, 1883 (J. Miller, personal communication, 1965). (It was mentioned that on each of the three dental chairs there were two bottles, each containing fifty gallons of nitrous oxide.) In 1886 he patented the Shaw Dental Engine in which the flexible steel shaft between the driving pulley and the dental drill of earlier machines (introduced in 1870) was replaced by a device which imitated the movements of the human arm, having flexible "elbow" and "wrist" joints. Shaw was said to be a man of some small eccentricities of character, but a man of wide gifts and attainments (Simms, 1903). In 1889 he drew attention to the passage in *Doctor Syntax in Paris* (1820a) which described the use of nitrous oxide to assuage the torments of the face following dental extractions (see Part II, Smith, 1965). The complete poem describing this incident in *Doctor Syntax in Paris* (pp. 312–316) is quoted below. The lines extracted by Shaw were 4–8, 20–22 and 57–61.

Our roving pair were now exhumed,
And Madam's face became relumed.
They straight set out on their return,
But Dolly cries, "My jaws do burn!
5 I've caught the tooth-ach from the damp,
So to a doctor let us tramp."
"Here lives, my dear, a skilful man,"
Said Syntax, "called Le Charlatan;
Who in the papers advertises,
10 That he himself most wondrous wise is,
Can cure each malady that's known
Or in the country or the town;
Would, if his sage advice were followed,
And his prescriptions duly swallowed,

15 Engage Pandora's baleful box
To fasten up with triple locks;
Yet, strange to say, this very man
Himself looks sickly, pale, and wan.
But here's the shop, let us walk in."
20 Le Charlatan, with knowing grin,
Welcomed his patient, heard her case,
Received his fee, and took his place.
Poor Mrs. Syntax oped her lips,
Le Charlatan a tooth out whips.
25 'Twas black, but Mrs. Syntax said,
"It was the best one in her head";
And never owned the tooth'ach's power.
The Dentist said, "We'll draw one more;
But first, I'll prove which it should be,

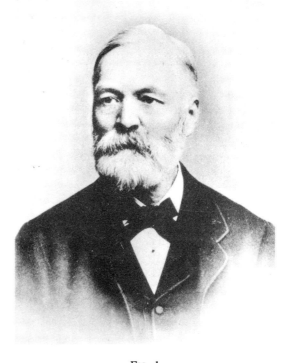

FIG. 1

Doctor Parsons Shaw, Dean of the Victoria Dental Hospital, Manchester. (By courtesy of Department of Medical Illustration, Royal Infirmary, Manchester England.)

30   By Galvanism, trust that to me."
      Le Charlatan now insulates
      His patient, and whilst thus she waits,
      Holds in his hand th' electric chain.
      "By this," said he, "I soon shall gain
35   A knowledge which is the bad tooth."
      Said she, "I wish you had in sooth
      Done so before you robbed my jaws
      Of what can never by your claws,
      Or any other's be replaced;
40   But make amends by making haste."
      Le Charlatan a piece of wire,
      Connected with the electric fire,
      Inserted into Madam's mouth,
      And laid it on full many a tooth.
45   Said he, "When you feel pain, cry out."
      Madam replied, "I shall, no doubt."
      At length the patient cried in pain,
      "Remove, remove, your cursed chain!"
      The Dentist marked the tooth which had
50   Been numbered thus among the dead.
      Without remorse, or science' puzzle,
      Advancing up to Madam's muzzle,
      As boldly as St. Dunstan did
      Towards the Devil's ugly head,
55   When he with tongs red and hot,
      Gripped hard his black and scorched snout,
      Our Dentist quickly twisted out
      The offending tooth, and Dolly rose.
      Le Charlatan observed, "Suppose,
60   Madame, you snuff some Nitrous Gas,
      To assuage the torments of your face."
      Said Syntax, "I have often heard
      Philosophers with high regard
      Speak of this nitrous inhalation,
65   And of its gay exhilaration.
      Now, as my wife and I have been
      To view a dismal, deadly scene,
      The place you call the Catacombs,
      Where millions rest in their last homes,
70   We're both in hypochandriac mood,
      And I don't think a mouthful would
      Do me much harm, although my mind,
      And not my body, is, I find,
      The seat of this my melancholy."
75   "This will dispel it, Monsieur, wholly,"
      Replied Le Charlatan; "so come
      With me into the adjoining room,
      Where you shall see the grave and wise
      Enjoy an earthly Paradise.
80   The Othman's opium is vile fare,
      Compared to this our heavenly air;
      For you must know, your Laureate Poet,
      Famed Southey, cares not who may know it,
      But 'tis his first and firm opinion,
85   That when with Angels' daring pinion
      The soul has reached the highest heaven,
      Such air as this will then be given
      To fill it with immortal bliss."
      Said Syntax, "He is right, I guess.
90   Besides, the thought's in high degree
      Poetical, and fit to be
      In golden letters hung on high,
      To catch the passing stranger's eye.
      So let us have a sweet foretaste
95   Of what we hope with souls more chaste,
      To breathe through a perpetual spring,
      When Death has dropt his venomed sting."
      Our Sage and wife were ushered in,
      And rapt in joy with bag at chin,

100   They saw a group of aged men
      Dancing like warlocks in a glen;
      A band of ancient matrons too,
      Were here enjoying raptures new,
      Like Shakespeare's witches round the kettle
105   They might be deemed; but then such mettle
      As they exhibited, gave proof
      That theirs was not to weave the woof
      Of Fate, or mankind to annoy,
      But Life and Pleasure to enjoy.
110   Syntax and spouse were soon provided
      With gas, but they with scorn derided
      Such silly capers as they saw
      Exhibited, and to each jaw
      Applied the gas, when instantly
115   They proved how futile it must be
      For man or woman to assert,
      When Pleasure rules the buoyant heart,
      That they can still the rules maintain
      Which mark the dull or irksome reign
120   Of inert Apathy or Pain.
      They tripped it on fantastic toe—
      So rapidly the moments flow
      On Pleasure's gay and downy wing,
      That they scarce heard the signal ring,
125   Which should have called them home to dine,
      And 'stead of gas to swallow wine;
      But they, cameleon-like, the air
      To a more solid dish prefer.
      Syntax at length woke by his wife
130   To the realities of life
      The sober garb of "hodden gray",
      Which mankind wear on every day,
      Paid down the fee his host demanded,
      Observing as the cash he handed,
135   "You make your visitors to pay
      For air to keep their lungs in play."
      And added, with a knowing leer,
      "You're not the only Financier
      Who has done so on larger scale,
140   As window-duties tax the gale.
      But never mind, so vale! oh vale!"
      Syntax and spouse now quick departed
      With buoyant spirits, and light-hearted.

After quoting the extract from *Doctor Syntax in Paris,* Shaw (1889) wrote:

There can be little doubt that this description was drawn from facts, and that in either London or Paris (probably in London) some person, as early as 1820, united gas administration with tooth drawing. But it is inconceivable that any man, however ignorant, after having got the idea of easing the pain *after* tooth extraction should have not thought of giving the gas *before* the operation. And it is yet more inconceivable that of the many thousands of intelligent readers of Dr. Syntax's exploits—for the work had great popularity in its day—no one caught the suggestion so broadly given.

Be that as it may, it may seem even more surprising that any dentist who had seen teeth extracted painlessly after the inhalation of nitrous oxide in 1845, should, apparently, not have considered giving his patients any form of general anaesthetic for dental extractions before 1868. A dentist who appears to have been in this position was Parsons Shaw himself. In 1889 he wrote:

. . . the most interesting and the most decisive part of my personal experience in connection with this matter was in the summer of that year (1845) while spending a fortnight in Hartford. While there I made the acquaintance of the very gentleman [Dr. Riggs] who had extracted Wells' tooth when the discovery [of nitrous oxide anaesthesia] was made, and who had taken his practice. Among the other things that he had bought was the machinery Wells had erected for making and giving the anaesthetic gas. The idea of painless tooth extraction was then so new that but few people could be induced to try it: but this gentleman held a sort of field day once a week for its administration. On not less than two occasions I was invited to attend, and assisted and saw teeth extracted without pain.

Yet, in 1868, Shaw published a textbook on the causes, prevention and cure of toothache, and the only mention of any form of anaesthesia was the ether spray:

. . . it becomes, therefore, exceedingly difficult to pursue any systematic plan in extractions, owing to the natural reluctance of the patient to suffer except to relieve present pain. Tooth extraction has been rendered much less painful since the introduction of Mr. Richardson's most admirable ether-spray apparatus.* People who previously were unable to endure this operation, are now able to sustain it. For if not altogether relieved of pain, the suffering is so much mitigated as to be quite bearable. It is not, however, altogether owing to the patient that teeth are so commonly extracted only under the impulse of severe pain; or that it becomes difficult to pursue a systematic plan in extraction. It is to be largely attributed to the general ignorance of dentists.

Shaw thus provided another example of the way in which new ideas may not catch on.

Even if "le Charlatan's" broad hint was ignored, the idea that somebody may have united gas administration with tooth drawing as early as 1820 warrants close examination. If the doggerel was based upon real life, then it would be of considerable interest to find out more about the original incident, and how "le Charlatan" arrived at the idea of using nitrous oxide in this way. The first obvious step would be to find out something about the author.

"Doctor Syntax" was a fictitious character brought into being by Ackerman, Rowlandson and Combe in 1809 (*Dictionary of National Biography*, 1887). Rowlandson contributed a series of illustrations portraying incidents in the travels of a schoolmaster (Doctor Syntax) to Ackerman's

Poetical Magazine. William Combe wrote doggerel verse to accompany each illustration.* The first series of illustrations with accompanying doggerel was published in book form in 1812 under the title *The Tour of Doctor Syntax in Search of the Picturesque*, and it was extremely popular. Thus encouraged, Rowlandson and Combe collaborated to produce similar works called *The Dance of Life, The Dance of Death*, and, in 1820, *Doctor Syntax in Search of Consolation*, followed by *Doctor Syntax in Search of a Wife* in 1821. They were all published by Ackerman, and William Combe remained anonymous.

"Doctor Syntax" became so popular that many imitations of the Rowlandson-Combe style appeared on the market, and the anonymity of William Combe led to some confusion as to their authorship. Towards the end of 1820 Combe tried to clarify the position by prefacing the third edition of *Doctor Syntax in Search of Consolation* with a list of works which had been written by the original author. *Doctor Syntax in Paris; or, A Tour in Search of the Grotesque*, which was published by W. Wright in the same year,† was not included. Shortly before Combe died in 1823, Ackerman asked him for a complete list of all his works. This he provided, except that he omitted certain works which had been written for others under confidential agreement (Cole, 1852; Hotten, 1868). *Dr. Syntax in Search of the Grotesque* was not mentioned in this list, so it seems unlikely, although not impossible, that it was written by William Combe.

As a young man William Combe travelled widely and had many adventures, but by 1820 he was eighty years old and, as a debtor, he had spent at least forty years under the rules of the King's Bench Prison. His persistent anonymity may have been related to this fact. If he had written *Doctor Syntax in Search of the Grotesque* it is unlikely that his description of the incident with "le Charlatan" would have been based solely upon personal experience. Although a "prisoner",

---

* Introduced in 1866.

* In writing this doggerel Combe satirized the writings of the Rev. William Gilpin (1724–1804) who was the Headmaster of Cheam School, Surrey, for twenty-five years ("Peterborough", 1964). The present Headmaster of Cheam School has been unable to throw any light on *Doctor Syntax in Search of the Grotesque* (M. Stannard, 1965, personal communication).
† The date of publication is given erroneously as 1826 in the current British Museum Catalogue.

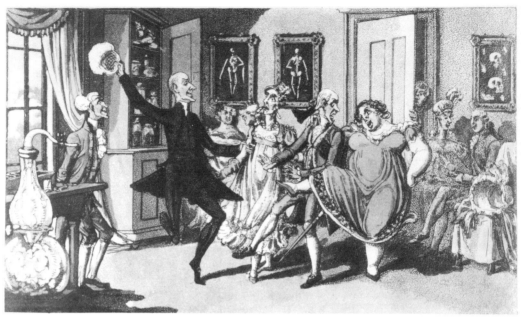

FIG. 2

"Doctor Syntax" and his wife making an experiment in pneumatics (*From Doctor Syntax in Paris;
or, a Tour in Search of the Grotesque,* facing page 315).

however, he used to enjoy excellent society and he lived in the midst of an extensive library (Hotten, 1868), so he could have been well informed about nitrous oxide.

An attempt to find some clue as to authorship by identifying the illustrator of *Doctor Syntax in Search of the Grotesque* proved disappointing. My opinion is that the illustrations (see figure 2) are not up to the same standard and probably not by the same artist as those accompanying the doggerel known to have been written by William Combe. This is supported by Grego (1880) who referred to *Doctor Syntax in Paris* as an imitation. He made no mention of it in relation to illustrations done by Rowlandson around 1820, but he acknowledged that he had not been able to prepare a complete catalogue of Rowlandson's works. Tooley (1954),* on the other hand, while acknowledging the text as an imitation appears to attribute the plates to Row-

landson, although the evidence for doing so is not stated.

Abbey (1956) states that the work originally came out in eight parts. The six plates in Parts 2–4 were by Charles Williams, under the pseudonym of "Argus", but none of the other twelve plates was signed. "Doctor Syntax" and his wife making an experiment in pneumatics (see figure 2) was published in Part 8. The front wrapper of the first part was lettered within an engraved border as follows:

No. 1 2/6 / Doctor Syntax / in Paris; / or, / a tour in search of / the / Grotesque / A Poem. / By Doctor Syntax, / Author of "Syntax in London, or the Pleasures / and Miseries of the Metropolis" / To the public / Eighteen lines advertising puff / London / Printed for W. Wright etc. . . .

The front wrapper of the fourth part was lettered:

No. IV. Price 2/6d / The original / Doctor Syntax / in Paris: / or, / a tour in search of / the / Grotesque. / Being a / Humorous Delineation / of the / Pleasures and Miseries / of the / French Metropolis. / By the celebrated Doctor Syntax / illustrated by a number of excellent and / curious engravings by artists of celebrity / To be completed in eight parts / Note / This is the only genuine Syntax / London: / Printed for W. Wright etc. . . .

---

* Tooley (1965, personal communication) has since confirmed that the note in his book (Tooley, 1954) was not meant to attribute the illustrations directly to Rowlandson but only to group the "Syntax" series and the imitations together. He has no evidence as to the actual author of the illustrations.

The alleged relationship between *Dr. Syntax in London* and *Dr. Syntax in Paris* is of interest in view of the fact that they both refer to nitrous oxide. The mention of "artists of celebrity" implies that it cannot be assumed that all the illustrations were by Charles Williams. Abbey's conclusions about authorship were that:

The author of the text is unknown, but, although this is manifestly in plates and general style a Syntax imitation, the text might conceivably be genuinely by Combe. It will be noticed, however, that the early wrappers used for Parts 1, 2, 3, 6, 7 & 8 only claim Doctor Syntax as the author of *Syntax in London* (also published in 1820, but by J. Johnstone) while the new setting for the wrappers of Parts 4 & 5 more boldly claim this is the only genuine Syntax. This is as likely to be the usual effrontery of the day as an indication that Combe did have a hand in this book and the *Syntax in London*.

William Wright, of No. 46 Fleet Street, does appear in London directories between 1820 and 1824, where he is described variously as "Bookseller" or "Bookseller and Publisher" (A. H. Hall, Guildhall Library, personal communication, 1965). By 1826 he had moved to Paternoster Row (E. Gaskell, Wellcome Historical Medical Library, personal communication, 1965). He does not appear to have been connected with John Wright, Publisher, of Bristol, who came from Tewkesbury, was apprenticed in Bristol in 1821, and created his own company in 1825 (L. G. Owens, personal communication, 1965).

That "the torments" of "To assuage the torments of your face" (line 61) referred to pain is reinforced by lines 115–119:

They proved how futile it must be
For man or woman to assert,
When Pleasure rules the buoyant heart,
That they can still the rules maintain
Which mark the dull or irksome reign
Of inert Apathy or Pain.

Lines 9 and 10 et seq. alert us to the possibility that somewhere a Quack may have mentioned nitrous oxide in an advertisement announcing his various skills:

Who in the papers advertises,
That he himself most wondrous wise is.

Payne (1924) referred to the blatant advertisements of dental charlatans at the end of the eighteenth century and early in the nineteenth century. He also suggested that the English dentists of that day were a long way behind their French confreres, which may favour "le Charlatan", if he ever existed, as having practised in Paris rather than in London.

Galvanism had been used for the treatment of toothache certainly as early as 1756. Lovett (1756) wrote: "The tooth-ach, if proceeding from a Defluxion of Rheum, is presently assuaged, or totally removed by this remedy" (p. 126). He gave a particular instance of such a cure: "A man, 57 years old, deaf for 32 years past from a wound under the left eye, and much afflicted with a violent tooth-ach, was cur'd of this complaint immediately . . ." (p. 127). He also gave instructions on how to connect the wires:

If it be an under tooth, bring the end of the connecting wire under the chin and tooth and lay the end of another wire to the top of the tooth; then bring the other end of it to the excited apparatus, and the circuit will not only be compleated, but the electrical aether will pass the right way: if an upper tooth, bring the end of the connecting wire to the top of the forehead, as near as may be over the tooth; then lay one end of the iron style to the bottom of the tooth, and, bringing the other end of the excited apparatus on which the phial is suspended, the aether, as before, will pass through the tooth [p. 131].

The use of electrical phenomena to entertain a patient following the extraction of a tooth was mentioned by Lindsay (1933), and her account referred to the reign of George III (1760–1820):

An eighteenth-century dentist, James Spence, protégé of John Hunter, rose to be dentist to George III through his influence. The vitriolic Foote gives an account of the shop of James Spence, before the practitioner rose to eminence as dentist to the King, and when he practised in Grays Inn Lane—now vanished. Foote, suffering from the toothache, sought Spence's shop, which he states was in "the vilest neighbourhood" . . . he speaks of the neatness and cleanliness, the professional appearance of Spence, the appointments of the place and everything shining and clean. Teeth were exhibited "as white and polished as ivory, the only wonder was how they came to lose their destined homes and how they were found where I saw them". He speaks of the painted hand in the window, with its ruffles of lace, holding a tooth. After the extraction "that sort of explanation which ever takes place between the professional man and his patient. . . . I was most kindly introduced into a back room." Here he found that Spence was a most ingenious experimenter in electricity; he displayed to Foote's delight dancing figures, attracting air and feathers, firing a gun, after which entertainment he shook hands with his patient and said, "Young gentleman, we professional men never take anything from one another."

It is not surprising, therefore, that "le Charlatan" should have used galvanic apparatus, or that he should have ushered his patient into a side room after extracting two of her teeth. What is almost as startling as the use of nitrous oxide to assuage the torments of the face, however, is his use of galvanism as a diagnostic tool (lines 30–48).

Duchenne (1871) made no reference to the use of electricity for diagnostic purposes. Donaldson (1960) stated that: ". . . no record has been found of a pulp tester invented before 1900". The literature on this subject was reviewed by Hilding (1946) and the earliest reference appears to be Magitot (1867). Magitot, who was not born until 1833, wrote:

Un autre moyen a été egalement proposé; il consiste à faire passer un courant électrique dans toute l'étendue d'une des arcades dentair d'un des petits appareils d'induction si frequement employés aujourd'hui en médecine : au passage d'un courant d'ailleurs assez faible pour ne causer par lui-même aucune douleur, la dent cariée sera le siege d'une sensation aigue et nettement localisée.

In view of the early reports of the cure of toothache by electricity, and the evident popularity of electrical machines at the time, it would not be surprising if a number of casual experimenters had discovered that electrical stimulation of an inflamed dental pulp was painful—provided that it was still viable. But it is surprising that apparently the first recorded mention of the application of this observation to dental diagnosis, *and* the first recorded mention of the use of nitrous oxide to relieve pain associated with dental extraction, should be made together in the doggerel of an imitation "Doctor Syntax". Herein may lie a clue as to the identity of "le Charlatan", if he ever existed as a particular person in real life, or, if he was a fictitious character, to his inventor.

Lines 62–65 confirm that the exhilarating property of nitrous oxide was part of the general knowledge of the time:

> Said Syntax, "I have often heard
> Philosophers of high regard
> Speak of this nitrous inhalation,
> And of its gay exhilaration".

The reference to Southey (lines 80–88), however, implies that the author may have had a fairly detailed knowledge of Davy's early experiments on the respiration of nitrous oxide. Southey was one of the participants in the experiments on

the inhalation of nitrous oxide which were carried out in Bristol twenty-one years before *Doctor Syntax in Paris* was published. Beddoes (1799) reported Robert Southey's experiences following the inhalation of nitrous oxide in these words: "In a second experiment, he felt pleasure still superior—and has since poetically remarked, that he supposes the atmosphere of the highest of all possible heavens to be composed of this gas." This was quoted in the contemporary reviews of Beddoes' (1799) *Notice of some Observations . . .* in *Tilloch's Magazine* (1799), the *Monthly Review* (1799) and *Nicholson's Journal* (1800). This particular quotation was not given by Davy (1800), although in a letter to Davy of August 3, 1799, Southey wrote:

. . . you still, I suppose, go on working with your gaseous oxide, which, according to my notions of celestial enjoyment, must certainly constitute the atmosphere of the highest of all possible heavens. I wish I was at the Pneumatic Institution, something to gratify my appetite for the delectable air, and something for the sake of seeing you [Davy, 1858, p. 37].

These quotations may be compared with lines 80–88:

> The Othman's opium is vile fare,
> Compared to this our heavenly air;
> For you must know, your Laureate Poet,
> Famed Southey, cares not who may know it,
> But 'tis his fixt and firm opinion,
> That when with Angels' daring pinion
> The soul has reached the highest heaven,
> Such air as this will then be given
> To fill it with immortal bliss.

In passing, it may be noted that the reference to the window tax in line 140 ("As window-duties tax the gale") was probably a topical one. This tax was reduced only three years later, in 1823. It was not abolished until 1851 (*Encyclopaedia Britannica*, 1926).

The fact that there was also a mention of nitrous oxide in another imitation *Syntax* published in the same year ("Syntax", 1820b; see Part II, Smith, 1965) suggests that laughing gas may have been a topical subject, and that a thorough search of the general literature of the period might well reveal further references to it.

Whoever wrote *Doctor Syntax in Paris* was probably widely read, and one might expect him to have known how to seek information on any subject that particularly interested him. If he had searched the volumes of *Nicholson's Journal* which were published around the time that the effects of inhaling nitrous oxide became known, he could have come across Stodart's letter describing the relief of pain in the side of his face (Stodart, 1802; see Part II, Smith, 1965), and the review of Beddoes' *Notice* . . ., which quoted Southey's reactions to inhaling nitrous oxide. It is possible, although perhaps less likely, that he read about the relief of Davy's toothache in the *Annals of Medicine* (1800; see Part II, Smith, 1965), or in Davy's own account of his researches (Davy, 1800; see Part I, Smith, 1965), where he could also have read Davy's suggestion that nitrous oxide might be used with advantage during surgical operations. All the references to nitrous oxide in *Doctor Syntax in Paris* could have been the outcome of imaginative writing based upon careful reading. One cannot assume that a "le Charlatan" ever existed who actually used nitrous oxide in the way described; but he may have done.

Doctor Syntax in Paris might have been written by someone who joined in the experiments in Bristol in 1799–1800, or by someone who had connections with that circle of predominantly literary friends.

At first sight Samuel Taylor Coleridge could be taken as a likely author. Beddoes (1799) reported:

Mr. S. T. Coleridge inhaled the gas. He felt suddenly diffused with warmth, particularly about the face—warmth and distension of the eyes; thrilling in the cheeks, arms and hands. He definitely recollects a most delightful glow some years past, on entering a warm room from the cold, and the present exactly resembles it. He had a propensity to laugh, which, however, he restrained.

As mentioned in Part I (Smith, 1965) Coleridge became an opium addict, and he would have been in a good position to have made the comparison between opium and the "heavenly air" (lines 80–81). He also concerned himself with pain. In a letter to Davy of December 2, 1800, he wrote:

. . . I have not received your book. I read yesterday a sort of medical review about it. I suppose Longman will send it to me when he sends down *Lyrical Ballads* to Wordsworth. I am solicitous to read the latter part. Did there appear to you any remote analogy between the case I translated from the German Magazine and the effects produced by your gas? Did Carlisle ever communicate to you, or has he in any way published his facts concerning *pain*, which he mentioned when we were with him? It is a subject that *exceedingly interests* me. I want to read something by somebody expressly on *pain*, if only to give an arrangement to

my own thoughts, though if it were well treated, I have little doubt it would revolutionize them [Davy, 1858, pp. 83–84].

Galvanism also caught Coleridge's imagination and he mentioned the subject to Davy in letters dated October 9, 1800; February 3, 1801; May 20, 1801; and October 31, 1801 (Davy, 1858, pp. 80–91). Coleridge was all his life interested in galvanism and electricty, and in the theory and practice of medicine, and he was not above doggerel in private (K. Coburn, 1964, personal communication). There is, however, quite a strong objection to thinking that Coleridge might have written *Doctor Syntax in Paris*. He disapproved of Malthus. In an earlier part of *Doctor Syntax in Paris* there is a section which implies that the author approved of Malthus.

The Carlisle referred to in Coleridge's letter quoted above was probably Sir Anthony Carlisle (1768–1840). In 1800 Carlisle made the discovery that water is decomposed by voltaic electricity (Nicholson, 1800), and it was probably the publication of this discovery that particularly attracted the attention of Davy to this subject (Gregory, 1930). Professionally, Carlisle was a surgeon at Westminster Hospital from 1793, but he had many other interests. He was admitted to the Royal Academy when quite young and in 1808 he became its Professor of Anatomy. He would have been in a good position to have known the artists of his day. He was in the habit of writing to the newspapers, especially to *The Times*, about such subjects as military flogging and quackery. In 1820 he delivered the Hunterian Oration on "The Anatomy of the Oyster", after which he was christened "Sir Anthony Oyster". He published a pamphlet on "Man-Midwives" in which he denounced the attendance of manmidwives as indelicate and hinted that something worse might follow from it (see Petigrew, 1838; Clarke, 1874). It may be coincidence that "manmidwife" and "obstetric stuff" are mentioned in the introductory doggerel to *Doctor Syntax in Paris*, but on present evidence one could not rule out the possibility that Carlisle was its author. It would, however, be easy to add many names to a list of possible authors, and a major research effort would be needed to sort them out.

It is unlikely that there will be an easy solution to the problem of identifying "le Charlatan" and finding out how he came so close to discovering nitrous oxide anaesthesia without actually doing so. He may never have existed, except in doggerel form and in the imagination, in which case the main interest becomes focused on his inventor. The riddle of "le Charlatan" may never be solved, but posing the problem and attempting its solution may uncover more of the early history of nitrous oxide, and of the factors which influenced the growth of the idea and of the practice of anaesthesia.

ACKNOWLEDGMENTS

The riddle of "le Charlatan" has been the subject of discussions and correspondence with many people whose helpful comments have been appreciated. In particular, I would like to mention Mr. W. R. Le Fanu and Mr. Cornelius of the Royal College of Surgeons of England who put me on the track of William Combe and made several useful suggestions; Mr. P. Wade of the Royal Society of Medicine; Mr. K. D. C. Vernon of the Royal Institution; Professor Kathleen Coburn of Victoria College, Toronto (an expert on Coleridge); Mr. G. Carnall of the Department of English Literature, Edinburgh (an expert on Southey and his time); Professor June Z. Fullmer of the Department of Chemistry, Ohio Wesleyan University, who gave freely of her knowledge of the early history of nitrous oxide; Mr. J. F. Physick of the Victoria and Albert Museum who drew my attention to Abbey (1956); Mr. F. J. Salfeld of the *Daily Telegraph*; Professor A. E. W. Miles of the London Hospital Medical College; Mr. E. Gaskell of the Wellcome Historical Medical Library; Mr. A. H. Hall of the Guildhall Library; Mr. L. G. Owens, director of John Wright and Sons Ltd.; Mr. G. Wilson of the Manchester University Medical Library who provided information on Dr. Parsons Shaw, which was extended by Professor J. Miller of the Welsh National School of Medicine; Dr. D. W. Hill of the Royal College of Surgeons; Mr. Bruce Hammond of the Medical Research Council, Mill Hill; and the Thomson and Ronalds Library at the Institution of Electrical Engineers.

REFERENCES

Abbey, J. R. (1956). *Travel in Aquatint and Lithography, 1770–1860 from the library of J. R. Abbey*, Vol. 1: World, Europe and Africa, pp. 94–95. London: privately printed at the Curwen Press.

Annals of Medicine (1800). Sect. I: Analysis of Books, pp. 227–258. "On Researches, chemical and philosophical . . ." by H. Davy.

Beddoes, T. (1799). *Notice of some Observations made at the Medical Pneumatic Institution.* Bristol: Biggs and Cottle.

Clarke, J. F. (1874). *Autobiographical Recollections of the Medical Profession*, p. 293. London: Churchill.

Cole, R. (1852). William Combe and his works. *Gentleman's Magazine*, N.S. 37, 467.

Davy, H. (1800). *Researches, Chemical and Philosophical; chiefly concerning nitrous oxide, or dephlogisticated nitrous air, and its respiration.* London: J. Johnson.

Davy, J. (1858). *Fragmentary remains, literary and scientific, of Sir Humphry Davy, Bart.* London: Churchill.

Dictionary of National Biography (1887). William Combe (1741–1823), Vol. II, p. 430. London: Smith, Elder and Co.

Donaldson, J. A. (1960). The development of the application of electricity to dental surgery up to 1900. *Brit. dent. J.*, **109**, 121.

Duchenne, G. B. (1871). *A Treatise on Localized Electrization, and its applications to pathology and therapeutics;* translated from the 3rd edition of the original by Herbert Tibbits. London: Robert Hardwick.

Encyclopaedia Britannica (1926). Window Tax, 13th ed., Vol. 28, p. 713: London: Encyclopaedia Britannica.

Grego, J. (1880). *Rowlandson the caricaturist*, Vol. 2, pp. 249, 366. London: Chatto and Windus.

Gregory, J. C. (1930). *The Scientific Achievements of Sir Humphry Davy*, p. 37. London: Oxford University Press.

Hilding, B. (1946). Electrical excitation of teeth and its application to dentistry. *Stockholm Svensk Tandläkere-Tidskrift*, **39**, Supplementum.

Hotten, J. C. (1868). *Dr. Syntax's Three Tours: In Search of the Picturesque, Consolation, and a Wife*, by William Combe. The original edition, complete and unabridged, with the life and adventures of the author, now first written by John Camden Hotten. London: Hotten.

Lindsay, L. (1933). *A Short History of Dentistry*, pp. 50–51. London: John Baile, Sons and Danielsson.

Lovett, R. (1756). *The subtil medium prov'd: or, that wonderful power of nature, so long ago conjectured by the most ancient and remarkable philosophers, which they call'd sometimes aether, but oftener elementary fire, verify'd.* London: J. Hinton.

Magitot, E. (1867). *Traité de la carie dentaire*, p. 163. Paris.

Monthly Review (1799). Notice of some observations made at the Medical Pneumatic Institution, **30**, 405.

Nicholson, W. (1800). Account of the new electrical apparatus of Sig. Alex. Volta, and experiments performed with same. *Phil. Trans.*, **4**, 179.

Nicholson's Journal of Natural Philosophy, Chemistry and the Arts (1800). Accounts of the strange effects produced by the respiration of the gaseous oxide of azote. **3**, 446.

Payne, J. L. (1924). Milestones in the history of British dentistry. *Brit. dent. J.*, **45**, 138.

"Peterborough" (1964). *The Daily Telegraph*, December 31.

Pettigrew, T. J. (1838). *Medical Portrait Gallery: biographical memoirs of the most celebrated physicians, surgeons, etc., who have contributed to the advancement of medical science*, Vol. 1, p. 13. London: Fisher.

Shaw, P. (1868). *Odontalgia, commonly called toothache; its causes, prevention and cure*, p. 165. Manchester: Palmer and Howes.

—— (1889). Personal recollections of the discovery of anaesthetics. *Manchester Odont. Soc.*, **1**, 217.

Simms, W. (1903). A little bit of history. *Manchester Medical Students' Gazette*, 17.

Smith, W. D. A. (1965). A history of nitrous oxide and oxygen anaesthesia. Part I: Joseph Priestley to Humphry Davy. *Brit. J. Anaesth.*, **37**, 790.

—— (1965). A history of nitrous oxide and oxygen anaesthesia. Part II: Davy's researches in relation to inhalation anaesthesia. *Brit. J. Anaesth.*, **37**, 871.

Stodart, J. (1802). On the effects of the respiration of nitrous oxide; particularly an instance in which the excitation of the system produced unpleasant symptoms. In a letter from Mr. James Stodart to Mr. Nicholson. *Nicholson's Journal*, N.S. **1**, 225.

"Syntax" (1820a). *Doctor Syntax in Paris; or, a Tour in Search of the Grotesque.* London: W. Wright, 46 Fleet Street.

—— (1820b). *The Tour of Doctor Syntax through London; or, the Pleasures and Miseries of the Metropolis.* A poem. 3rd ed., p. 208. London: J. Johnston.

Tilloch's Philosophical Magazine (1799). Medical Pneumatic Institution. **5**, 301.

Tooley, R. V. (1954). *English Books with Colour Plates. 1790 to 1860. A bibliographical account of the most important books illustrated by English artists in colour, aquatint and colour lithography.* London: Batsford.

6

THE CRUCIAL EXPERIMENT, ITS ECLIPSE, AND ITS REVIVAL

> I make no claim to any merit in the matter myself; but it is a great pleasure to remember that at the request of Wells, I gave the gas and produced the first anaesthetic condition for a surgical operation.
> (Colton, 1868)

The story of the introduction of inhalation anaesthesia for the relief of pain during surgical operations has been confused by the clamour of the rival claimants to its discovery, and their supporters; but it has been told many times. In re-telling it here, prominence is given to the tale of nitrous oxide anaesthesia. The question of who "discovered" surgical anaesthesia is played down. Re-evaluation of all the evidence has not been attempted. This would entail a major research effort which should, for preference, be carried out in America.

Gardner Quincy Colton.

The researches of Humphry Davy at Thomas Beddoes' Pneumatic Institution (see Part I, Smith, 1965a) stimulated interest in nitrous oxide in Europe and America. His scientific observations were repeated and praised; but the greatest applause was for the effects of inhaling the gas, which he had discovered and then persuaded volunteers to experience and comment upon—including Boulton and Watt, Kinglake, Joseph Priestley's son, Coleridge, Southey, Roget and Wedgewood. In the course of time others were to provide facilities for breathing the gas as an entertainment, and among them was Gardner Quincy Colton (fig. 1).

Colton had entered the College of Physicians and Surgeons, New York, in 1842, when he was twenty-eight years old, and he studied under Dr. Willard Parker*; but after two years he became

---

* Dr. Willard Parker (1800–84) graduated M.D. from Harvard in 1830, presenting an inaugural dissertation entitled "A Thesis on Nervous Respiration". He was a renowned teacher and he became Professor of Surgery in 1832. He may have been the first in America to operate successfully upon an abscessed appendix (Warbasse, 1907; *Dictionary of American Biography*).

short of money and had to leave. For a livelihood he took up lecturing on popular scientific subjects, including the effects of breathing nitrous oxide (McNeille, 1898; Fulton, 1930; Waters, 1944; Duncum, 1947, p. 94). According to Fulton (1930) he learned of the exhilarating effects of nitrous oxide during his early studies, and Willard Parker has certainly been quoted as having referred to the inhalation of nitrous oxide by medical students as early as 1831 (Wells, 1935). Even if Willard Parker was partly responsible for Colton learning about the gas, however, apparently he did not feel

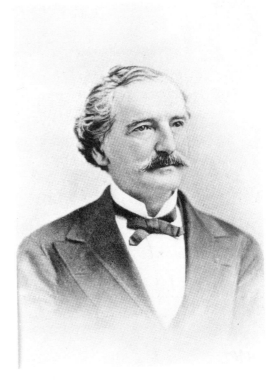

strongly in favour of Wells's use of it for the production of anaesthesia, because later he was a member of an active group which met in his house in New York to support Morton's claims to the "discovery" of anaesthesia (Veits, 1946). The following advertisement, which Colton placed in the *Hartford Daily Courant* on December 10, 1844, bears a striking resemblance to the bill which advertized Samuel Colt's nitrous oxide demonstration in Portland twelve years before (see part II, Smith, 1965b).

A Grand Exhibition of the effects produced by inhaling Nitrous Oxid, Exhilarating or Laughing Gas! will be given at Union Hall, this (Tuesday) Evening, Dec. 10th, 1844.

Forty Gallons of Gas will be prepared and administered to all in the audience who desire to inhale it.

Twelve Young Men have volunteered to inhale the Gas, to commence the entertainment.

Eight Strong Men are engaged to occupy the front seats, to protect those under the influence of the Gas from injuring themselves or others. This course is adopted that no apprehension of danger may be entertained. Probably no one will attempt to fight.

The effect of the Gas is to make those who inhale it either Laugh, Sing, Dance, Speak, or Fight, and so forth, according to the leading trait of their character. They seem to retain consciousness enough not to say or do that which they would have occasion to regret.

N.B. The Gas will be administered only to gentlemen of the first respectability. The object is to make the entertainment in every respect a genteel affair.

Mr. Colton, who offers this entertainment, gave two of the same character last Spring in the Broadway Tabernacle, New York, which were attended by four thousand ladies and gentlemen, a full account of which may be found in the *New Mirror* of April 6th, by N. P. Willis. Being on a visit to Hartford, he offers this entertainment at the earnest solicitation of friends. It is his wish and intention to deserve and receive patronage of the first class. He believes he can make them laugh more than they have for six months previous. The entertainment is scientific to those who make it scientific.

Those who inhale the gas once are always anxious to inhale it a second time. There is not an exception to this rule.

No language can describe the delightful sensation produced. Robert Southey (poet) once said that "the atmosphere of the highest of all possible heavens must be composed of this gas".

For a full account of the effect produced upon some of the most distinguished men of Europe, see *Hooper's Medical Dictionary*, under the head of Nitrogen.

Mr. Colton will be the first to inhale the Gas.

The History and the properties of the Gas will be explained at the commencement of the entertainment.

The entertainment will close with a few of the most surprising Chemical Experiments.

Mr. Colton will give a private entertainment to those Ladies who desire to inhale the gas. None but Ladies will be admitted. This is intended for those who desire to inhale the Gas, although others will be admitted.

Entertainment to commence at 7 o'clock. Tickets 25 cents—for sale at the principal Bookstores and at the Door. [Taken from Wells, 1935.]

Perhaps the most noteworthy differences between the two advertisements are that Colt's mentioned Davy and that Colton's gave the quotation from Southey; "No language can describe the delightful sensations produced. Robert Southey (poet) once said 'the atmosphere of the highest of all possible heavens must be composed of this gas'."* Colton also gave *Hooper's Medical Dictionary* as a source of reference on "the effect produced upon some of the most distinguished men of Europe". At that time the seventh edition (1839) of *Hooper's Medical Dictionary* would have been available. The sixth edition (1831) was published in the year before Colt's first demonstration of laughing gas. Neither edition mentioned the effects upon distinguished men of Europe. After referring to the parts played by Priestley and Davy, and giving a fairly full account of the physical properties of nitrous oxide, it said

When mingled with atmospheric air, and then received into the lungs, this gas generates highly pleasurable sensations: the effects it produces on the animal system are eminently distinguished from every other chemical agent. It excites every fibre to action, and raises the faculties of the mind, including a state of great exhilaration, an irresistible propensity to laughter, a rapid flow of ideas, and unusual vigour and fitness for muscular exertions, in some respects resembling those attendant on the pleasantest period of intoxication, without any subsequent languor, depression of the nervous energy, or disagreeable feelings; but more generally followed by vigour, and a pleasurable disposition to exertion which gradually subsides.

Colt and Colton were born in the same year, and their paths may well have crossed. It is also possible that Colton may have come across references to nitrous oxide in Willard Parker's

---

* See Cartwright, 1952, p. 321. Southey's comment was quoted in *Tilloch's Magazine*, 1799; *Monthly Review*, 1799; *Nicholson's Journal*, 1800; Barton (1808), and *Medical Repository* (1800). See appendix for an account of one of Colton's first performances.

library,* which contained about four thousand volumes when he died (Warbasse, 1907).

Horace Wells and the crucial experiment.

One of the young men who volunteered to inhale the gas at Colton's "Grand Exhibition" on

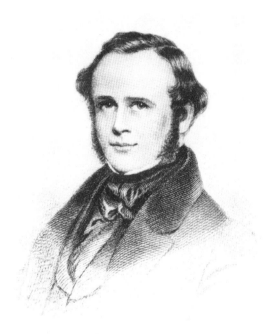

* This library was donated to the Medical Society of the County of Kings (Warbasse, 1907), but the collection has not been kept separate from other volumes in the library of the Academy of Medicine of Brooklyn, and until recently no catalogue of its contents had been located (Draper, W., 1964, personal communication). The catalogue has now been found and some of the chemical and physiological works listed do mention nitrous oxide (Draper, W., 1965, personal communication). Unfortunately the catalogue does not contain a list of periodicals which Dr. Parker might have had. Beddoes (1799), Davy (1800) and Hooper (1831) are not listed (Draper, W., 1966, personal communication), but Colton, as a medical student, would have had access to the New York Hospital Library (Draper, 1957), and possibly to other medical libraries.

December 10, 1844, was Samuel Cooley. Also in the audience was a local dentist, Horace Wells (fig. 2), who noticed that Cooley bruised and abraised his knees against the furniture without seeming aware of the injury. This observation led directly, on the following day, to the performance of the crucial experiment of operating on a patient while he was under the influence of nitrous oxide. The instigator and the subject of this experiment was Horace Wells. He invited Colton to bring some of his gas to the surgery so that he could breathe it immediately before a colleague, Dr. Riggs, extracted a troublesome tooth. The experiment was painless and when Wells recovered he was said to have exclaimed: "A new era in tooth pulling".

Wells's experiment may have resulted from more than just an inspiration of the moment fired by the observation of Cooley's behaviour. According to a deposition made subsequently by Dr. L. P. Brockett (Smith, 1858, p. 18), the possibility of using nitrous oxide during surgical operations had already crossed Wells's mind.

. . . in 1840, in the month of July or August, I called at Dr. Wells's office and found him engaged in some experiment, which led to a conversation between Dr. Wells and myself respecting nitrous oxyd gas. Dr. Wells first spoke of the gas, and inquired of me if I had seen it administered. I replied that I had seen two or three persons inhale this gas, and described the effects upon them under its influence. We conversed upon this subject for some time, and Dr. Wells remarked that he believed that a man might be made so drunk by this gas or some similar agent, that dental and other operations might be performed upon him without any sensation of pain on the part of the patient.

Confirmatory evidence was given by Wells's wife, although it suggests that the thoughts were more recent than 1840:

For some months previous to the delivery of a course of chemical lectures by Mr. G. Q. Colton, in the city of Hartford, December, 1844, Dr. Wells turned his attention to the discovery of some means of rendering the human system insensible to pain under dental and surgical operations, and made several experiments in mesmerism with reference to that object. Towards the close of Mr. Colton's course of lectures, I went with my husband to witness an exhibition of the effects of inhaling nitrous oxyd, or laughing gas. It was in the evening at Union Hall, in this city. My husband and several others took the gas in my presence, the effect of which on the parties occasioned much amusement to those present. When we came out of the lecture room to return home, I reproached my husband for taking the gas and making himself ridiculous before a public assembly. He replied to me that he thought it might be used in

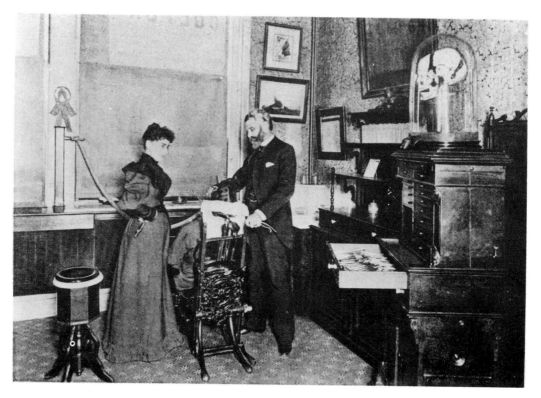

FIG. 3

Laird W. Nevius, associate of G. Q. Colton, administering nitrous oxide (from Nevius, 1894, facing p. 101). By courtesy of The Wellcome Trustees.

extracting teeth, and in surgical operations, so as to prevent pain; and said he meant to try the experiment himself the next day. And accordingly, he took the gas and had a tooth extracted the next day, and declared that he did not experience any pain. It was a wisdom tooth, and had troubled him a considerable length of time. [Smith, 1858, p. 20.]

Mrs. Wells's comment about her husband's wisdom tooth having troubled him for a considerable length of time adds a little weight to a report given by Shaw (1889) (see Part III, Smith, 1965c). Shaw told how he was a dental student in Boston in 1844, and how one day in December that year he received an invitation to attend the private seance of a Mr. Colton, who was in the habit of going round the country lecturing on nitrous oxide and administering it to those who chose to come upon his platform. That Colton sometimes held preliminary meetings to which he invited the leading professional and business men of the locality was confirmed by Nevius (1894), who was

an associate of Colton, and Colt before him certainly advertised private Exhibitions (Cary, 1961). Quoting Shaw verbatim:

When Mr. Colton found I was a dental student he told me of an incident that had happened at the last place he had visited, which was Hartford in Connecticut. While there, so he told me, a dentist had an aching tooth out without pain, under the influence of the gas. Colton mentioned this merely as a curious incident, and he certainly then had no idea that a great discovery had been made. . . . From what I subsequently learned in Hartford, from other sources, it appears that the full particulars of the incident mentioned to me by Mr. Colton were these. Dr. Horace Wells, of that city, had gone to one of his private meetings and inhaled the gas. While under its influence Wells noticed that he suffered nothing from an aching tooth which had been giving great and continuous pain for some time. That was the suggestive starting point in the anaesthetic discovery. At the public exhibition in the evening Dr. Wells noticed that one of the subjects bruised himself a good deal against a form. Wells asked the man if he felt pain at the time, to which he answered that he felt nothing. This was the second step in the discovery. Dr. Wells then got Mr. Colton to administer the gas the next day, and a brother dentist removed the offending tooth from his mouth. No pain was felt and the discovery was made complete.

Shaw's version of the story does not seem to have been recorded anywhere except in his own writings (Shaw, 1889, 1893). As they were published some forty-five years after the event, they should be regarded with reserve, but doubtless he had already told the story many times.

Waters (1944) described the developments in American dentistry which may have alerted Wells to the advantages of pain relief during dental extractions.

Technical skill in the preparation of false teeth had advanced to such a point that the removal of useless teeth in preparation for artificial replacements was frequently desirable and always painful. Being under the necessity of inflicting such suffering in his daily practice and realising that if the useless teeth could be removed without pain, many more patients would be candidates for the prosthetic replacements, Wells was in a position to appreciate the practical value of this effect of nitrous oxide.

Wells was, in fact, intimately involved in the technicalities of making false teeth. He went into partnership with W. T. G. Morton in Boston, and on January 2, 1844, they published the following advertisement

Messrs Wells and Morton, Dentists, No. 19 Tremont Row, are determined to make their valuable invention extensively known, and duly appreciated in the shortest possible time; with this end in view we now propose to insert teeth of gold (until further notice) without compensation until the expiration of one year; then if the patient is perfectly satisfied that our invention is really valuable and superior to any other mode of constructing gold plates, we shall expect a small compensation which may previously be agreed on, otherwise we shall ask nothing. All we shall require, when the teeth are inserted, will be just enough to pay for the materials used, which will be but a trifle. If by this means we are enabled to introduce our improvement more extensively than in the ordinary way, our object will be attained.

The partnership lasted only a few weeks and Wells returned to Hartford (Wells, 1935).

A disastrous demonstration.

The "new era in tooth pulling" did arrive much later, but Wells played a sad and disappointing part in it. Colton taught him how to make the gas, and with the assistance of Dr. Riggs he used it for dental extractions in fifteen patients. The procedure was to administer the gas from an animal bladder through a wooden tube, while the patient's nose was compressed between finger and thumb. In 1845 he gave a demonstration to students and staff at the Massachusetts General Hospital in Boston. W. T. G. Morton was present. It was greeted with derision, and Wells and his method were discredited as humbug. In his own words,

I was then invited to extract a tooth for a patient in presence of the medical class, which operation was performed, but not entirely successful, as the bag was removed too soon; and as the man said he experienced some pain, the whole was denounced as an imposition, and no-one was inclined to assist me in further experiments. [Wells, 1847.]

The introduction of ether and chloroform and the eclipse of nitrous oxide.

In the following year, 1846, William Thomas Green Morton (1819-68) gave a demonstration of the use of ether in the same hospital (Bigelow, 1847), and this was acclaimed "no humbug".

It was not appreciated at the time that Morton had been preceded by Crawford William Long (1815-78) (see Young, 1942). Soon after starting in general practice in Georgia, Long was asked to prepare some nitrous oxide so that friends could experience its exhilarating effects, but as he had no suitable apparatus, he suggested sulphuric ether as an alternative.* Long inhaled it himself and discovered bruised and painful spots on his person which he could not recall inflicting, and he was satisfied that they were received while under its influence. He noticed also that his friends appeared to receive falls and blows without pain when etherized. In 1842 he gave it to a boy by the name of James Venable, to inhale before excising a small tumour. The operation was quite painless. Long was anxious to repeat the experiment on a number of cases before publishing his discovery, but only a very few suitable cases came his way. Meanwhile Morton demonstrated ether anaesthesia in Boston; and because of the nature and place of his demonstration, because he tried to conceal the identity of the anaesthetic agent by calling it Letheon, and to patent it, and also because his claims were contested by Wells and by Jackson (who also claimed

---

* It had been reported previously that ". . . when the vapour of ether mixed with common air is inhaled, it produces effects very similar to those occasioned by nitrous oxide" (*Journal of Science and the Arts*, 1818; also quoted by Pereira, 1839).

to have "discovered" ether anaesthesia), Morton received much publicity.

In 1847, James Young Simpson (1811-70) introduced chloroform as an anaesthetic agent.

Even if Wells's demonstration of nitrous oxide anaesthesia in Boston had not been a fiasco, the advantages of using ether and air instead of indiluted nitrous oxide, for anything but the briefest procedures, would soon have become obvious. This was apparent to H. J. Bigelow after he had tried using nitrous oxide anaesthesia for the removal of a breast tumour in 1848 (Bigelow, 1900 p. 96).

The patient . . . was made to respire nitrous oxide gas through a valved mouthpiece and a flexible tube leading through a bladder to two large copper reservoirs filled with the gas. After several inspirations, the patient's lips and the most vascular part of the tumour began to assume a purple colour. She remained quiet, however, and in a short time was evidently insensible, though the muscles were not perfectly relaxed. . . .
During the above operation, the patient inhaled about sixty quarts of gas, which was delivered under moderate pressure.

Bigelow commented that

. . . Anaesthesia by nitrous oxide was then abandoned, not only in view of the livid surface and muscular rigidity, both doubtless due to asphyxia, but also on account of the preparation of the gas on a large scale, and especially from the bulk of the apparatus required for its administration. This will continue to prevent the extensive employment of the nitrous oxide in surgical operations while agents so much more portable are at command. For the extraction of teeth, dental practitioners may prefer to keep on their premises a reservoir of nitrous oxide rather than a permanent odour of ether, but the amount consumed in surgical operations alters the question.

Wells became disheartened and his health soon deteriorated. He gave up dentistry and went to Paris where his claims were brought before the Academy (see also Part IV, Smith, 1966), which had already recognized C. T. Jackson as the discoverer of the principle of anaesthesia and W. T. G. Morton as the first to apply it. He then returned to America. He continued to fight for the recognition of nitrous oxide anaesthesia, but started to experiment with chloroform. Early in 1848, the Paris Medical Society voted that to Horace Wells was due all honour of having successfully discovered and successfully applied the use of vapours or gases whereby surgical operations would be performed without pain. They also elected him

an honorary member, but he was never to know it. He had become mentally unstable and he committed suicide before the news reached America (Robinson, 1946).

For a while nitrous oxide ceased to be used as an anaesthetic, although Colton, among other activities,* continued to tour the country giving "Grand Exhibitions" of its effects.

John Snow (1813-58).

News of the use of ether during surgical operations soon arrived in England and John Snow was quick to take an interest. Before long he had investigated its properties, designed his own vaporizer and used it in clinical practice. Then he transferred his interest to chloroform. He experimented with many possible anaesthetic agents, and thought deeply about the results he obtained, but I have found no record of Snow having used nitrous oxide. This was not because he did not know about it. He knew that Davy had expressed the opinion that nitrous oxide might probably be used to prevent pain during surgical operations (Snow, 1847b), and that Horace Wells used it for dental extractions (Snow, 1858, p. 313). He had probably read Nunneley's (1849) conclusion, after trying it on animals, that "the nitrous oxide could never be employed as an anaesthetic, and that inhalation of it is not as harmless as is generally stated", but he does not appear to have left any record of his own views. Much of Snow's basic work on inhalation anaesthesia, however, is relevant to nitrous oxide anaesthesia, and this account would be incomplete without some mention of it.

The first publication to Snow's name (1839), written within a year of qualifying and about half way between the death of Hickman and the discovery of chloroform anaesthesia, was a contribution to a debate on poisoning by charcoal fumes. Snow was convinced that carbon dioxide exercised a deleterious effect, independently of the diminution of oxygen associated with its inhala-

* Quoting Nevius (1894): "In 1847, at Pittsburgh, Pa, he made the first application of electricity (on a small scale) to the propulsion of cars. In 1849 he went to California, and was appointed the first Justice of the Peace for San Francisco. Returning to New York in 1851, he invested his 'pile of gold' in the salt works of Syracuse, New York, and lost the whole. The salt had lost its savour. He then resumed his lectures upon chemistry, natural philosophy, etc."

tion, but he thought that some of the facts and arguments brought forth in support of that opinion, of which he gave examples, were objectionable. He described a series of animal experiments, using small birds and mice, in which he tried to avoid the usual sources of error. He placed the animals in a very large bottle of 2,000 cubic inches capacity, after first filling the bottle with known gas mixtures. Using 75 parts of air with 20 parts of carbon dioxide and 5 parts of oxygen (i.e. 20 per cent oxygen, 20 per cent carbon dioxide and 60 per cent nitrogen), he found that small birds died and that a mouse lived for $1\frac{1}{2}$ hours before expiring. Using 85 parts of air with 12 parts of carbon dioxide and 3 parts of oxygen (i.e. 20 per cent oxygen, 12 per cent carbon dioxide and 68 per cent nitrogen), he found that a bird lived for $2\frac{1}{2}$ hours before dying and that a mouse, although feeble, lived after remaining in the bottle for 14 hours. Then he put 16 per cent of oxygen in the jar, without carbon dioxide, and with lime water to absorb any carbon dioxide produced. He found that a sparrow died after 6 hours in the jar. When he repeated the experiment using 12 per cent oxygen, a sparrow convulsed after 35 minutes, and although he removed it immediately, it died. Finally he demonstrated that the combined effects of carbon dioxide and oxygen lack were more fatal than either alone. From "narrowly" watching the animals he also considered that carbon dioxide acted as a "stimulant to the lungs". These experiments were subsequently reported in greater detail (Snow, 1846). They did not lead Snow to the idea of using "suspended animation" during surgical operations (see Part IV, Smith, 1966). There was nothing new in the observation that carbon dioxide had an effect independent of the diminution of oxygen (e.g. Bostock, 1826), but apparently the earlier experiments were not generally known and Snow approached the subject afresh and satisfied himself that it was so. These experiments were an appropriate prelude to his anaesthetic researches which he started some seven or eight years later.

In some ways Snow's experimental approach using volatile anaesthetics was similar to Davy's with nitrous oxide. Although Snow was perhaps less brilliant, he was thorough and he had by then reached a greater maturity. He was already an experienced physician. He knew the humane application of the drugs he was investigating and, indeed, the desire to understand how best to use them was probably one of the driving forces behind his researches. He was able to take the final step of applying experimental results to anaesthetic practice, and this, together with his methodical approach, probably accounted for much of his confidence and skill as a clinical anaesthetist.

Benjamin Ward Richardson (1828-96) described one of Snow's goals and his method of seeking it:

His grand search was for a narcotic vapour which, having the physical properties and practicability of chloroform, should, in its physiological effects, resemble ether in not producing paralysis of the heart.

First he ascertained the boiling point of the substance under investigation; then the point of salination of air at different temperatures; next the effects of inhalation of the vapour by inferior animals: and finally the quantity required to be inspired with the air breathed, to produce insensibility. When he had obtained any substance which would produce insensibility favourably on animals, he pushed it, in one or two experiments, to its extreme in animals of different kinds. Then having produced death by inhalation, both by giving rapidly a large dose, and by giving a small dose for a long period, he observed the mode of death, whether it occurred primarily by cessation of the heart, or by cessation of respiration. If the agent seemed to promise favourably from these enquiries, he commenced to try it on man; and the first man was invariably his own self. [Richardson, 1858, p. xxix.]

Snow adopted this approach from the beginning of his anaesthetic researches. It is apparent in his first book, *On the Inhalation of Ether in Surgical Operations* (Snow, 1847a), which was completed when he had administered about eighty human anaesthetics. Even at this early stage he had a clear understanding of the essential problems and processes of inhalation anaesthesia. He described five degrees of anaesthesia (p. 1). He noted how long it took an average man to pass through the first four degrees of anaesthesia when inhaling ether vapour at a given concentration, and the rate at which ether was evaporated in the vaporizer. He pointed out that not all this ether was absorbed because some was expired. He appreciated that when inhalation of ether was discontinued, the rate of recovery was rapid at first and then became progressively slower (p. 2). Although he did not call it by that name, he described the state of ether analgesia (Artusio, 1954, 1955) seen when patients recovered their mental faculties before the end of operation (p. 3) (see also Péan, cited Buxton, 1885). He even suggested that if a patient was kept for some time in this stage of etherization, by breathing very diluted vapour, an immunity from pain might result (pp. 4-5) (see also Snow, 1858, pp. 36, 318).*

He emphasized that knowledge of the strength of ether vapour was essential for the correct determination of the state of the patient at all times (p. 15), and he designed apparatus to meet this requirement (pp. 15-23). He stressed the importance of using tubing wider than the trachea for connecting the vaporizer to the inhaler, in order to minimize resistance arising from friction of the air against the interior of the tube. He recommended an internal diameter of $\frac{3}{4}$ inch, although he pointed out that $\frac{5}{8}$ inch was ample for admitting air to the vaporizer, because air expanded to nearly twice its bulk in passing over the ether.† He described how to manipulate the expiratory valve so that the concentration of ether inhaled could be increased steadily during the induction of anaesthesia, and irritation of the air passages avoided (p. 31).

Although he noticed that arterial blood was often less bright than usual when ether was being administered (p. 44), he was satisfied that the insensibility produced by ether was not due to the privation of air.

Although etherization and asphyxia resemble each other in some respects, yet the rapidity with which frogs are affected by ether, whilst they are so very slowly asphyxiated by privation of air, proved that they differ widely, and shows clearly enough that the effects of ether are not due to its excluding part of the oxygen of the air by the space that it occupies, as might at first, perhaps, be supposed. That such is not the way in which ether acts I have ascertained in a more direct way . . . by supplying the oxygen so displaced, when I found that the peculiar effects of ether were produced in animals just as readily as before [p. 82].

---

* Coleman (1862) also demonstrated the state of analgesia by extracting one of his own molars painlessly after a few breaths of chloroform.

† Note that the ratio between these diameters is 1.2 to 1. The ratio of their fourth powers is 2.1 to 1. Hagen published his discovery, that the volume of fluid flowing through a tube of given length varies as the fourth power of the diameter of the tube, in 1839. Poiseuille published the same observation in 1840 (see Macintosh, Mushin and Epstein, 1958, p. 161).

Snow also realized that the volume uptake of ether would affect the concentration of oxygen in the lungs.

If hydrogen, nitrogen, or any neutral gas which does not support life, were mixed with air, in even half the quantity that the vapour of ether is commonly mixed with it, the oxygen of the air, over diluted, would fail to be imbibed into the blood in exchange for carbonic acid, and the patient would suffer asphyxia. . . . The oxygen is often reduced by the vapour of ether to 10 or 11 per cent of what the patient breathes, whilst if it were reduced but to 16 per cent by a gas which is not absorbed, no increased efforts of respiration would prevent asphyxia from quickly supervening. That nothing of the kind takes place during the inhalation of ether depends on the circumstance that the vapour is absorbed as fast as it reaches the air cells of the lungs, leaving the oxygen in its usual proportion per cent; and to get enough of it the patient usually enlarges his respiratory movements instinctively, as he would do if situated on a high mountain, where the air is much rarified [p. 83].

Objection might be taken to parts of this analysis, when considered in detail, but there can be no doubt that Snow was thinking along the right lines. The assumption of the inevitability of asphyxia when inhaling as much as 16 per cent oxygen was probably based upon his experiments with small birds (Snow, 1839, 1846) which are notoriously susceptible to hypoxia.* The effect of the volume exchange of nitrous oxide between the alveoli and the pulmonary circulation, upon the concentrations of other alveolar gases, does not appear to have been mentioned until 1955, when Fink described the "diffusion anoxia" that may occur on breathing air following prolonged nitrous oxide anaesthesia. Under these circumstances the nitrous oxide eliminated from the pulmonary circulation into the alveoli dilutes the air inspired.

From this work alone (Snow, 1847a), it can be assumed that if nitrous oxide anaesthesia had been introduced in Great Britain during Snow's lifetime, and before the discovery of the anaesthetic effects of ether and chloroform, he would have defined the essential problems of its administration and would have gone some way towards their solution. We can assume that he would have differentiated between the effects of hypoxia and of nitrous oxide, and determined the concentration

---

* It may also be because the Dutch chemists, Deiman and Trootzwick, used birds in their experiments that they concluded that the inhalation of nitrous oxide was not compatible with life (see Davy, 1799; Murray, 1819).

of nitrous oxide and the time required to produce unconsciousness; that he would have considered the limits of safety and the use of oxygen; and that he would have attempted to devise apparatus for the administration of nitrous oxide at known concentrations.

When nitrous oxide anaesthesia took root in this country, however, Snow had been dead for ten years, and then another twenty-four years passed before Hewitt (1889) introduced the use of nitrous oxide and oxygen anaesthesia in Great Britain. The relative contributions of oxygen deprivation and of nitrous oxide to the anaesthetic state were in doubt for many years, and the question is still argued in relation to the induction of anaesthesia using 100 per cent nitrous oxide. Even today many of the dental nitrous oxide and oxygen anaesthetic machines in use are of doubtful accuracy.

Snow may have recognized the hypoxia that was associated with the use of nitrous oxide, and dismissed this gas as altogether inferior to the alternatives of ether and chloroform, even for short surgical procedures with ambulant patients. It is possible that when Richardson later denounced nitrous oxide as "the best known, least wonderful, and most dangerous of all substances that has been applied for the production of general anaesthesia" (*Lancet*, 1868), he may have been reflecting Snow's opinion as previously expressed in conversation, but there is no evidence to support or refute this. One cannot be sure how Snow would have reacted if an enthusiastic revival of nitrous oxide anaesthesia had occurred during his lifetime. He might have accepted very brief nitrous oxide and oxygen anaesthesia as expedient, but one can be sure that the matter would not have rested there.

Snow gave his first anaesthetics in the out patient department of St. George's Hospital, for cases of tooth drawing. He used ether, and the superiority of his mode of administration, using his own vaporizer, led directly to his introduction to Liston at University College Hospital, for whom he administered it with equal success (Richardson, 1858, p. xv). Soon, however, he abandoned ether in favour of chloroform. Although he regarded ether as the safer anaesthetic he was confident in his safe use of chloroform, and he is quoted as saying, in self-defence, "an

occasional risk never stands in the way of a ready applicability" (Richardson, 1858, p. xxxv).

There is a modern ring to Snow's remarks about dental anaesthesia. The number of teeth extracted at a time varied from one to nineteen, but it was

... thought better, as a general rule, to make more than one operation when the number of teeth to be extracted exceeded ten, in order that the mouth might not contain too many wounds at one time, and that the loss of blood might not be too great. [Snow, 1858, p. 314.]*

Snow observed fainting in the immediate post-operative period (Snow, 1858, p. 314).

... chloroform ... is occasionally followed by a feeling of faintness, especially if the patient remains in the sitting posture. ... Some amount of faintness and depression usually accompanies the sickness caused by chloroform, and is in fact a consequence of it, being, like the sickness, most frequent after a full meal. This depression is usually relieved by vomiting. I have met a few cases in which there has been more decided faintness, and once or twice absolute syncope after chloroform, which was not attributable to loss of blood. In these cases, however, the patients were in a sitting posture, and they recovered from the syncope immediately upon being placed horizontally.† The patients most subject to faintness after chloroform are those who are subject to this affection at other times, being often persons in a state of anaemia, or having the symptoms of fatty degeneration of the heart. Faintness is, however, very much more rare after operations with chloroform than without it. The only cases in which I have seen it follow the use of chloroform in the horizontal position, and where there was no considerable loss of blood, have been two or three operations on the rectum, performed before breakfast.

He also had some pertinent comments to make on the nature of syncope.

It is necessary to point out the difference between ordinary syncope and cardiac syncope. One of the best examples of ordinary, or what may be called anaemic syncope, is that which occurs in a common blood letting, whilst the patient is in the sitting posture. When the blood vessels, especially the veins,

---

* See also Buxton, 1898.

† Although chloroform is used rarely today, comment made previously by Sibson (1848) may be quoted in the same vein. "In three out of four fatal cases the chloroform was given in the sitting posture. This requires much greater power in the heart to carry on the circulation than the recumbent. Chloroform should not, if possible, be administered in the sitting posture. In three out of four cases, the chloroform was administered by the operator: this should never be."

which at all times contain the greater part of the blood in the body, do not accommodate themselves fast enough to the diminished quantity of blood, the right cavities of the heart are supplied with less and less of the circulating fluid; and in a little time are not supplied at all, when the heart ceases to beat, in accordance with the observation of Haller, that it does not pulsate when it is not supplied with blood. The moment the heart ceases to supply blood to the brain there are loss of consciousness and stoppage of respiration; but on the patient being placed in the horizontal position the blood flows readily into the right cavities of the heart from the great veins of the abdomen and lower extremities; the heart immediately recommences its contractions; the brain is again supplied with blood, and respiration and consciousness return.

The blood may remain in the ordinary quantity; but if the blood vessels do not keep up their usual support, and exert sufficient pressure on their contents, the same kind of syncope will soon occur as that from blood letting. The late Sir George Lefevre related the case of a lady who fainted whenever she left her bed, and assumed the upright posture; no cause could be found for this until it was ascertained that she suffered from varicose veins of the legs: bandages to these extremities prevented the fainting. . . . The faintness which often occurs on first rising, when a person has long kept the recumbent posture from any local cause, is probably of the same kind; the veins not having had to support the weight of the usual column of blood for some days or weeks, lose their tone, we may presume, and yield when they are all at once subjected to the weight of a column of blood extending from the lower extremities to the heart, so that this organ ceases to be properly supplied with the circulating fluid.

In cardiac syncope, on the other hand, the cavities of the heart, or at all events the right cavities of this organ, are always full, whether the syncope depend on paralysis of the heart by a narcotic, or inherent weakness of its structure, or on its being overpowered by the quantity of blood with which it is distended. After death from this kind of syncope, if the blood has not been displaced by artificial respiration or other causes, the right cavities of the heart and the adjoining great veins will be found filled with blood. . . . In death by anaemic syncope, on the contrary, all the cavities of the heart are found empty, or nearly so.

The syncope occasioned by some kinds of mental emotion is of the ordinary or anaemic kind, and consequently the condition of the brain must act first on the blood vessels, and not directly on the heart. . . .

Fear probably occasions each kind of syncope in different cases. . . .

Pain is also capable of causing both kinds of syncope.

Snow was also well aware of the dangers of leaving the patient in the sitting position following a faint.

A gentleman named Walter Badger, twenty-two years of age . . . died instantly at Mr. Robinson's, the dentist, in Gower Street, on June 30th, 1848, whilst commencing to inhale chloroform with the intention of having some teeth extracted. . . . Mr Robinson unfortunately allowed his patient to remain seated in the operating chair; and it was only when Dr. Waters had been sent for and arrived from a neighbouring street that he was laid upon the floor.

Colton repeats Wells's crucial experiment and forms the Colton Dental Association.

Colton used to tell the tale of Wells's experiment at his lectures and one day in 1862, in New Britain, Connecticut, seventeen years after Wells's fiasco in Boston, a lady in the audience asked him to repeat the experiment on her, which he did. The lady's dentist, Dunham, was delighted with the result. He asked Colton to show him how to prepare the gas and within a year he had given it successfully to over 600 patients. Colton and Dunham then joined forces for three weeks and two days with another dentist, Joseph H. Smith, who had a practice in New Haven. Colton was so encouraged by this trial that he set up an Institution in New York devoted exclusively to extracting teeth with the gas, which he called The Colton Dental Association.* The "new era" had arrived in America where the use of nitrous oxide soon spread, mainly for dental extractions, although there were sporadic reports of its use for major surgery—e.g. for amputation of the breast (*Brit. med. J.*, 1865, 1866b), re-amputation of a stump (*Brit. med. J.*, 1866a), amputation of a leg (*Brit. med. J.*, 1866b), and amputation of a foot (*Brit. med. J.*, 1866c).

The first brief published account of Colton's use of nitrous oxide for dental extractions was by Latimer (1863), and Samuel Lee Rymer drew the attention of the Odontological Society of Great Britain to this in December 1863. It amounted to a description of only two cases.

The first case was a lady of some twenty years and nervo-sanguine temperament. She had some ten or twelve fangs to be removed. Dr. Colton administered the gas as for ordinary entertainments, save that the patient was sitting and the inhalation was continued much longer. Two minutes were required to induce complete anaesthesia, then half the fangs were quickly removed, and three minutes from the commencement of inhalation, the patient was completely conscious. After waiting a few minutes for the bleeding to subside, inhalation was commenced and continued the same time as before with the same results. There was no indication of excitement, and the anaesthesia was perfect.

---

* This has been taken from Colton's own account as quoted by Duncum (1947, pp. 273–4). It differs in its details from the version given by Nevius (1894).

A gentleman of some forty-five years, and nervo-bilious temperament next took the chair. He had been suffering intensely for some time with periodontitis, and was, consequently, very nervous. The first attempt to bring him under the influence of the gas was frustrated by the exhibition of some little excitement after which he inhaled about thirty seconds. A second attempt, however, was more successful, and in one minute and forty-five seconds from the commencement of inhalation, the tooth was removed painlessly, though a most difficult one to extract. This patient was conscious that the tooth was being removed, but felt no pain.

Some supplementary information was given in an advertisement which appeared in the *Dental Cosmos* of November 1863 (cited by Rymer, 1864) in which it was announced that Dr. Colton had associated himself with two eminent dentists, Dr. John Allen and Son, and that they had devoted their exclusive attention to the extraction of teeth by use of the gas. The advantages of nitrous oxide over ether were summed up as follows:

First—*It is perfectly harmless* and there is no danger of giving too much. Second—The insensibility induced is perfect and complete in *all cases* where a sufficient quantity is given. Third—The effects all pass off within three minutes from the commencement of the inhalation, leaving the patient feeling as well as before. Fourth—The danger and disagreeableness of inhaling ether and chloroform are all avoided.

It was added that "to accomplish these results the gas must be made *very pure,* and be properly administered, and that Dr. Colton has already exhibited it for the extraction of more than 4,000 teeth, and with very decided success."

The first note to be published by Colton did not appear until April 1864. It opened: "There are probably a thousand dentists in the country now using the nitrous oxide gas as an anaesthetic for the extraction of teeth." The remainder of the contribution was devoted to explaining that three deaths which had been reported were not due to nitrous oxide, and to emphasizing the safety of the gas. The note ended:

While I claim that nitrous oxide is a very safe anaesthetic if made pure and properly administered, I admit that there may be rare cases and conditions of the system in which it would be injudicious to give it.

He gave no indication as to how he considered that it should be administered.

Not all reports from America were so enthusiastic. Foster (1864), for example, under the heading "Nitrous oxide is not an anaesthetic", wrote:

When I say nitrous oxide is not an anaesthetic, *per se,* I mean strictly so; that without the dangerous narcotising power of carbonic acid gas, which is exhaled into the bag, and is rebreathed again and again in ever increasing proportions, *its present effects would not be produceable.*[*] Nitrous oxide may be given pure and with the greatest caution; it does not affect the statement just made; the principle is the same. Nitrogen does not support combustion or respiration. Free oxygen supports both, but the two gases chemically united, as in nitrous oxide, do not support respiration, but slightly if at all.

Samuel Lee Rymer's experiments with nitrous oxide in London.

Rymer experimented with nitrous oxide anaesthesia in London, basing his methods on what little he could learn of the American practice. He published his observations in January 1864, and gave the following description of the method of administration:

The usual method of inhaling the nitrous oxide is from a bladder filled with the gas, and to which is attached a tube of wood. The mouth-piece is held by the right hand of the person inhaling the gas, the nostril being closed with the left. The tube is placed in the mouth, and the gas breathed from and into the bladder.

For a practical purpose, such as the extraction of a tooth, the orifice of the tube must be much larger than for common experiments—in other respects, the inhalation is conducted after the same manner, except that it ought to be under the direction of a professional man, and it is desirable that two persons should be in attendance on the patient—one to administer the gas, and the other to extract the tooth.

Rymer reported only five administrations of nitrous oxide, to three subjects and one patient. An upper bicuspid tooth was extracted from the patient, aged 16, with complete success. He opined that

. . . transient anaesthesia may, in almost all cases, be produced by the *proper* inhalation of the gas: by which I mean not only the exhibition of pure nitrous

---

* Davy tried the control experiment of presenting a bag of common air "to Mr. Hammick, and he observed that it produced no effect" (Beddoes, 1799, p. 11). In 1802, Woodhouse did the same thing and found that many of his subjects "were affected with quickness of the pulse, dizziness, vertigo, tinnitus aurium, difficulty in breathing, anxiety about the breast, etc." (Barton, 1808, p. 4). Barton (1808, p. 5) repeated the experiment upon himself and concluded that the symptoms were due to the accumulation of azotic and carbonic acid gases.

oxide quickly, but the exercise of some discretion in allowing its exhibition at all—thus excluding persons suffering from diseases of the vital organs.

His final comment was: "I have only to add that the *uniform* success claimed by Dr. Colton is a matter of perplexity. . . . "

Subsequently Rymer (1868) admitted that the experiments were discontinued because, apart from the inconvenience of manufacturing the gas, "Dr. Odling* advised them, if they proceeded at all, to do so with the utmost possible caution, because he considered its exhibition was attended with the greatest danger".

No more interest appears to have been taken in nitrous oxide anaesthesia in London until it was re-introduced by Dr. Evans, an enthusiastic American dentist who had a thriving practice in Paris. He had received personal instruction on how to prepare and administer the gas from Colton, who visited the International Exhibition and the first International Congress of Medicine in Paris in 1867. Dr. Evans found the new method so satisfactory that he visited London in 1868 in order to make it known to his fellow practitioners in England. Before returning to Paris he even went so far as to present £100 to the Odontological Society of Great Britain for research into and development of nitrous oxide anaesthesia.

APPENDIX

The following account of Colton's "Exhibition of Laughing Gas" in New York was given under the heading of "Diary of Town Trifles" (*New Mirror*, 1844).

There is a certain curiosity to know "how the thing went off", even though the show in question was a bore to the spectator. Perked up people think that only such curiosity as would sit well upon George Washington should be catered for in print, but I incline to think that almost any matter which would be talked about by any two people together would be entertaining to one man reading by himself. So I think I may put down what I saw at a show that was advertised as an "EXHIBITION OF LAUGHING GAS".

The youngest subscriber to the *Mirror* may possibly require to be told that nitrate of ammonia, like himself, has a soul that fire will burn out of it. When the lamp over which it is held gets too hot "to be stood" any longer, up rises a little whitish cloud which has most of the properties of common air, but which has a sweet taste and an agreeable odour, and

will pass into any human soul's body upon very slight invitation. Once in, however, it abuses the hospitality extended to it, by immediately usurping all the functions of the body, and behaves, in short, extremely like another more notorious enemy, who "when admitted into your mouth steals away your brains". The stimulus of this intoxicating gas to the nervous system is very surprising. Sir Humphry Davy administered it to Southey the poet, whose feelings are thus described: "He could not distinguish between the first effects and a certain apprehension, of which he was unable to divest himself. His first definite sensations were a fulness and a dizziness in the head, such as to induce the fear of falling. This was succeeded by a laugh which was involuntary, but highly pleasurable, accompanied by a peculiar thrilling in the extremities—a sensation perfectly new and delightful. For many hours after this experiment, he imagined that his taste and smell were more acute, and is certain that he felt unusually strong and cheerful. In a second experiment, he felt pleasure still superior, and has since poetically remarked that *he supposes the atmosphere of the highest of possible heavens to be composed of this gas!*"

There were between three and four thousand people assembled in the Tabernacle. A platform in the centre was hemmed in with benches, and it was advertised that "twelve strong men" would be there to prevent injury to the spectators. It was mentioned in the advertisement also that the gallery would be reserved for ladies, though I thought that the inviting of ladies, to be present at the removal of all restraint from men's tongues and actions, was a strong mark of confidence in the uppermost qualities of our sex. After some impatience on the part of the audience, the professor appeared with his specimen of "the highest possible heaven" in an India-rubber bag. The candidates for a taste of it were many and urgent, crowding up from below like the applicants to St. Peter, and the professor seemed somewhat embarrassed as to a selection. A thick-necked and bony youth got possession of the bag, however, and applied his mouth to the stopper. After inhaling its contents for a minute or two he squared away and commenced pummelling the professor in the most approved butcher-boy style—which was probably *his* idea of the "highest possible heaven". The "twelve strong men" rushed to the rescue, the audience applauded vociferously, and the lad returned to his senses, having been out of them perhaps three minutes. A dozen others took their turn, and were variously affected. I was only very much delighted with one young man, who coolly undertook a promenade over the close-packed heads of the audience. The impertinence of the idea seemed to me in the highest degree brilliant and delightful. There was one corsair-looking man who rushed up and down the stage, believing himself on the deck of some vessel in pursuit of another, and that was perhaps the best bit of acting. One silly youth went to and fro, smirking and bowing, another did a scene of "Richard the Third", and a tall good-looking young man laughed heartily, and suddenly stopped and demanded of the audience, in indignant rage, what they were laughing at! There was nothing else worth even putting down among trifles, and I was glad when it was over. The only imaginable entertainment in such an exhibition would be to watch the effect of self-abandonment on those whose

---

* Professor of Chemistry at St. Bartholomew's Hospital.

characters we know when under restraint. Among acquaintances it would be charming—particularly if the subjects were ladies. I should recommend to the professor to advertise himself as open to invitations to administer his "highest possible heaven" to small and select parties. It would be better than a masquerade and not so unlawful.

Cartwright (1952, p. 320) inferred that Colton was extremely well informed of the literature on nitrous oxide, because, in his advertisement in the *Hartford Daily Courant*, he mentioned Southey's description of his sensations after breathing the gas, which was published by Beddoes (1799). From present evidence, however, it is not certain whether Colton introduced the *New Mirror's* commentator to Southey's remarks, or whether the commentator introduced Colton to them after the performance in the Tabernacle. Either of them could have obtained the quotation from the *Medical Repository* (1800), or from the other periodicals already mentioned. (There may have been other topical sources which have not yet come to light.) The above quotation is complete and as published by Beddoes (1799), and repeated in the other periodicals, except for the spelling of "superiour", for the use of italics, and for the final exclamation mark. The accuracy of the quotation suggests that Colton either read it out to his audience or knew it by heart, and that the commentator was able to take it down verbatim, or that the commentator had a printed version available for reference. The complete version may have been given in the notice advertising Colton's "Exhibition" in New York, but I have seen no reproductions of this. It may be noted, however, that the passage quoted subsequently in the *Hartford Daily Courant*, was the passage printed in italics in the *New Mirror*, except that Colton substituted *must be* for *to be*.

ACKNOWLEDGEMENTS

This study started with Duncum (1947). Other general sources have been acknowledged in previous instalments. I would like to thank Mr. E. Gaskell of the Wellcome Historical Medical Library for selecting the illustrations for this instalment, and for other assistance; Mr. Wesley Draper of the Library of the Academy of Medicine of Brooklyn for information on Willard Parker's library; Dr. R. A. Butler of Philadelphia for information on Barton's (1808) thesis; and Mrs. Gillian O'nions for the extract from the *New Mirror* (1844).

REFERENCES

Artusio, J. F. (1954). Di-ethyl ether analgesia: a detailed description of the first stage of ether anaesthesia in man. *J. Pharmacol. exp. Ther.*, **111**, 343.

—— (1955). Ether analgesia during major surgery. *J. Amer. med. Ass.*, **157**, 33.

Barton, W. P. C. (1808). Thesis: *A dissertation on the chymical properties and exhilarating effects of nitrous oxide gas; and its application to pneumatick medicine*; submitted as an inaugural thesis for the degree of doctor of medicine, p. 57. Philadelphia.

Beddoes, T. (1799). *Notice of some observations made at the Medical Pneumatic Institution.* Bristol: Biggs and Cottle.

Bigelow, H. J. (1847), cited Boot, F.: Surgical operations performed during insensibility, produced by the inhalation of sulphuric ether. *Lancet*, **1**, 6.

—— (1900). *Surgical Anesthesia: addresses and other papers.* Boston: Little Brown & Co.

Bostock, J. (1826). *An Elementary System of Physiology*, Vol. II. London: Baldwin, Crodok and Jay.

British Medical Journal (1865), **2**, 335. Anaesthesia by nitrous oxide.

—— (1866a), **1**, 81. Progress of medical science. Reamputation for intense neuralgia in a stump: anaesthesia by nitrous oxide gas.

—— (1866b), **1**, 633. Progress of medical science. Nitrous oxide as an anaesthetic.

—— (1866c), **2**, 151. Anaesthetics.

Buxton, D. W. (1885). The practice of artificial anaesthesia, local and general, with especial reference to the modes of production, and their physiological significance. *Brit. med. J.*, **2**, 531.

—— (1898). *Trans Anaesth. Soc.*, **1**, 127.

Cartwright, F. F. (1952). *The English pioneers of anaesthesia: Beddoes, Davy and Hickman.* Bristol: Wright.

Cary, L. (1961). *The Colt gun book*, p. 9. Greenwich, U.S.A.: Fawcett.

Coleman, A. (1862). Anaesthesia: considered especially in reference to operations in dental surgery. *Trans. Odont. Soc. (Lond.)*, February 3.

Colton, G. Q. (1864). Nitrous oxide gas an anaesthetic. *Dental Cosmos*, **5**, 490.

—— (1868). Letter. *Brit. J. dent. Sci.*, **11**, 253.

Davy, H. (1799). Extract of a letter from Mr. H. Davy. *Nicholson's Journal*, **3**, 93.

—— (1800). *Researches, Chemical and Philosophical; chiefly concerning nitrous oxide, or dephlogisticated nitrous air, and its respiration.* London: J. Johnson.

Dictionary of American Biography (1934). Parker, Willard (Sept. 2, 1800–April 25, 1884), Vol. 14, p. 242. London: Milford. Oxford University Press.

Draper, W. (1957). Medical Libraries of New York State. *N.Y. St. J. Med.*, **57**, 584.

Duncum, B. M. (1947). *The Development of Inhalation Anaesthesia; with special reference to the years 1846–1900.* London: Oxford University Press.

Fink, B. R. (1955). Diffusion anoxia. *Anesthesiology*, **16**, 511.

Foster, C. W. (1864). Nitrous oxide not an anaesthetic. *Dental Cosmos*, **5**, 614.

Fulton, J. F. (1930). Gardner Quincy Colton (Feb. 7, 1814–Aug. 9, 1898), in *Dictionary of American Biography*, Vol. 4, pp. 321–322. London: Humphrey Milford. Oxford University Press.

Hewitt, F. (1889). On the anaesthesia produced by the administration of mixtures of nitrous oxide and oxygen (preliminary notice). *Lancet*, **1**, 832.

Hooper, R. (1831). *Lexicon Medicum; or Medical Dictionary*. The sixth edition, considerably improved. London: Longman.

Journal of Science and the Arts (1818). Miscellanea. V: Effects of inhaling the vapour of sulphuric ether. **4**, 158.

Lancet (1868) **1**, 507. Medical Annotation. A new anaesthetic (?).

Latimer, J. S. (1863). *Dental Cosmos*, **5**, 16.

Macintosh, R., Mushin, W. W., and Epstein, H. G. (1958). *Physics for the Anaesthetist, including a section on explosions*, 2nd ed. Oxford: Blackwell.

McNeille, C. S. (1898). Dr. Gardner Quincy Colton: obituary. *Dental Cosmos*, **40**, 874.

Medical Repository (1800). Dr. Beddoes Medical Pneumatic Institution. **3**, 423.

Monthly Review (1799). Notice of some observations made at the Medical Pneumatic Institution. **30**, 405.

Murray, J. (1819). *A System of Chemistry in Four Volumes*, Vol. II, 4th ed., pp. 235–244.

Nevius, L. W. (1894). *The Discovery of Modern Anaesthesia. By whom was it made? A brief statement of facts*, p. 94. New York: Nevius.

New Mirror (1844). New York. Diary of town trifles. April 6th, p. 8.

Nicholson's Journal of Natural Philosophy, Chemistry and the Arts (1800). Account of the strange effects produced by the respiration of the gaseous oxide of azote. **3**, 446.

Nunneley, T. (1849). On anaesthesia and anaesthetic substances generally: being an experimental inquiry into their nature, properties and action, their comparative value and danger, and the best means of counteracting the effect of an over dose. *Trans. Provincial Med. Surg. Assoc.*, **16**, 167.

Pereira, J. (1839). *The elements of Materia Medica; comprehending the natural history, preparation, properties, composition, effects and uses of Medicines*. London: Longman, Orme, Brown, Green and Longmans.

Richardson, B. W. (1858). Memoir in Snow, J. (1858).

Robinson, V. (1946). *Victory over Pain*. New York: Henry Schuman.

Rymer, S. L. (1863). *Brit. J. dent. Sci.*, **11**, 543.

—— (1864). Remarks upón the use of nitrous oxide in dental operations. *Dent. Rev.*, N.S., **1**, 1.

—— (1868). *Brit. J. dent. Sci.*, **11**, 202.

Shaw, P. (1889). Personal recollections of the discovery of anaesthetics. *Manchester Odont. Soc.*, **1**, 217.

—— (1893). Personal recollections of the discovery of anaesthetics (reprinted from *Manchester Odont. Soc.*, **1**, 217). *Brit. J. dent Sci.*, **36**, 721.

Sibson, F. (1848). On death from chloroform. *Lond. med. Gaz.*, **42**, 108.

Smith, T. (1858). *An examination of the question of anaesthesia arising on the memorial of Charles Thomas Wells, presented to the United States Senate, second session, thirty-second congress, and referred to a select committee, of which the Hon. Isaac P. Walker is chairman. Prepared for the information of said committee*. New York: John A. Gray.

Smith, W. D. A. (1965a). A history of nitrous oxide and oxygen anaesthesia. Part I: Joseph Priestley to Humphry Davy. *Brit. J. Anaesth.*, **37**, 790.

—— (1965b). A history of nitrous oxide and oxygen anaesthesia. Part II: Davy's researches in relation to inhalation anaesthesia. *Brit. J. Anaesth.*, **37**, 871.

—— (1965c). A history of nitrous oxide and oxygen anaesthesia. Part III: Parsons, Shaw, Doctor Syntax and nitrous oxide. *Brit. J. Anaesth.*, **37**, 958.

—— (1966). A history of nitrous oxide and oxygen anaesthesia. Part IV: Hickman and the "introduction of certain gases into the lungs". *Brit. J. Anaesth.*, **38**, 58.

Snow, J. (1839). On the effects of carbonic acid. Debate on poisoning by charcoal fumes. *Lancet*, **2**, 93.

—— (1846). On the pathological effects of atmospheres vitiated by carbonic acid gas, and by a diminution of the due proportion of oxygen. *Edin. Med. Surg. J.*, **65**, 49.

—— (1847a). *On the inhalation of the vapour of ether in surgical operations: containing a description of the various stages of etherization, and a statement of the result of nearly eighty operations in which ether has been employed in St. George's and University College Hospitals*. London: John Churchill.

—— (1847b). Inhalation of vapour of ether in surgical operations. *Lancet*, **1**, 552.

—— (1858). *On chloroform and other anaesthetics: their action and administration*. Edited, with a memoir of the author, by Richardson, B. W. London: Churchill.

Tilloch's Philosophical Magazine (1799). Medical Pneumatic Institution. **5**, 301.

Veits, H. R. (1946). Natham P. Rice, M.D., and his trials of a public benefactor, New York. *Bull. Hist. Med.*, **20**, 232.

Warbasse, J. P. (1907). Willard Parker and his medical library. *Long Island med. J.*, **1**, 122.

Waters, R. M. (1944). Nitrous oxide centennial. *Anesthesiology*, **5**, 551.

Wells, C. J. (1935). Horace Wells. *Curr. Res. Anesth.*, **14**, 176.

Wells, H. (1847). *A history of the discovery of the application of nitrous oxide gas, ether and other vapours, to surgical operations*. Hartford: Gaylord Wells.

Young, H. H. (1942). Crawford W. Long: the pioneer of ether anaesthesia. *Bull. Hist. Med.*, **12**, 191.

Brit. J. Anaesth. (1966), **38**, 212

7

HENRY TURTON, WILLIAM LLOYD POUNDALL AND HALLAM

I believed myself to be the first Dentist in England who had successfully extracted teeth under the influence of laughing gas.

(Poundall, 1870)

In the previous instalment (Part V, Smith, 1966), it was implied that the use of nitrous oxide for dental anaesthesia petered out after the failure of Wells' demonstration in Boston; that it was not used again for this purpose in America until Colton re-introduced it in 1862; and that it was never used in England until Rymer tried Colton's methods about two years later. The last two statements, however, are not strictly true.

On February 19, 1870, William Lloyd Poundall of 1, London Terrace, Derby, wrote the following letter to the editor of the *British Journal of Dental Science* (Poundall, 1870), to which I have seen no subsequent reference:

> Having called at the Dental Hospital on Tuesday last, February 15th, with the view of witnessing the administration of nitrous oxide, in conversation with one of the junior Dental Surgeons, I stated that I believed myself to be the first Dentist in England who had successfully extracted teeth under the influence of laughing gas. As this gentleman took considerable interest in the case, perhaps you may think it merits insertion in your Journal. Although I have to furnish the case from memory, its accuracy in its general bearings may be relied upon. In the year 1856, or 1857 (the former year I think), a Mr. Turton, then residing in Burton-upon-Trent, wished to know whether I would remove a tooth from him under its influence—I consented to do so. The gas was prepared by the patient, and bottled under water. A tube and a stop-cock was attached, with an ivory tube for the mouth, similar to the end of an enema syringe. Mr. Turton was accompanied by his friend Mr. Hallam, chemist and druggist, of Burton. The gas was inhaled, and a bicuspid tooth removed without pain. The patient then became pugilistically inclined, and we had to take care of him and ourselves also, after which he laughed hysterically, and then thoroughly recovered. At a future time I extracted a badly decayed upper wisdom tooth for the same gentleman under its influence. On this occasion he was placed in a semi-recumbent position, and the disagreeable symptoms were less marked.

Although Mr. Turton appears to be the one who took the initiative, there is no indication of where he got the idea. Mr. Hallam should have been in a position to advise on the preparation of nitrous oxide and to have provided the necessary materials and facilities, but he may have been no more than an interested friend. The incidents evidently made an impression on Mr. Poundall, but there is no evidence that he tried to develop the idea. Apart from the mention of disagreeable symptoms, his letter did not express his own views, or those of Mr. Turton and Mr. Hallam, on the success of the experiment. The fact that a second tooth was subsequently removed under the influence of nitrous oxide does not necessarily mean that the first "anaesthetic" was an unqualified success. The description of the apparatus and the mode of administration is unsatisfactory, and the story requires corroboration.

No record has been found of Mr. Poundall having had a practice in Burton-upon-Trent (Stanesby, K. F., Burton-upon-Trent Public Library, 1964, personal communication), but it has been confirmed that he was resident in Derby between 1850 and 1874 and a list of relevant entries in local directories is given in Appendix A (Bletcher, E., Derby Central Library, 1964, personal communication). He was certainly resident in Derby in 1857 but no directory is available for the year 1856. Burton-upon-Trent is, of course, only eleven miles from Derby and Poundall may well have seen patients there. Alternatively, Turton and Hallam may have attended Poundall's surgery, complete with their bottle(s) of nitrous oxide.

Evidence that Poundall visited at least one patient as much as eighteen miles from Derby, is provided by a surviving letter (fig. 1) addressed to Mr. Poundall on April 13, 1869, and asking

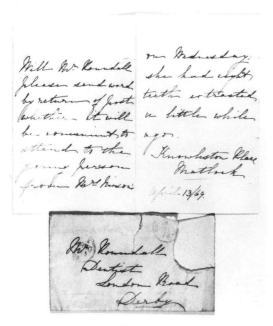

FIG. 1

A letter addressed to William Lloyd Poundall, in 1869, asking him to attend a "young person" in Matlock. (By kind permission of Mr. Alfred Poundall.)

him to attend "the young person from Mrs. Nixson's" at Knowleston Place, Matlock. Furthermore, Poundall knew Derby and its environs well; his wife, *née* Walker, was a Burton girl; and he was born at Alfreton and there were relatives at Stoke-on-Trent and at Chesterfield (Poundall, A. B., 1965, personal communication).

Mr. Turton does not appear in any of the Burton-upon-Trent directories of that period, but Francis White and Company published a *History Gazetteer and Directory of the County of Derby with the Town of Burton upon Trent Staffordshire* in which, in 1857, there was the following entry: "Turton, Henry. Engineer. High Street" (Stanesby, K. F., 1964, personal communication). Another source quotes Henry Turton's address as "Station Street" (*Burton Daily Mail*, 1964).

It has also been confirmed that a Mr. Hallam was a chemist and druggist in Burton at the time in question. The firm of Francis Hallam existed in the High Street until about 1950, and a Hallam was in charge of the business until

about 1912 (Stanesby, K. F., 1964, personal communication).

From his obituary it can be learned that Francis Hallam died in 1891 at the age of 57 years, and that about thirty years before he had joined his brother, C. M. Hallam, in business as a chemist and druggist "at a shop in the High Street* which Mr. Hugh Brooks had not long left. Ten years later the partnership was dissolved, and Mr. F. Hallam commenced business on his own account at the shop adjoining Messrs. Ordish and Hall's".†

If the thirty years quoted is taken literally, the brothers would have started their joint business in 1861, when Francis Hallam would have been 26–27 years old. There is nothing to indicate what they were doing previously. In 1856, Francis Hallam would have been 21–22 years old, so it would seem likely that Henry Turton's friend would have been Charles M. (Milne?) Hallam who died before Francis and who was probably the elder brother.‡

Further attempts to gain information about Messrs. Turton and Hallam were unsuccessful, so attention was again directed to William Lloyd Poundall. He wrote two more letters to the *British Journal of Dental Science* on different subjects (Poundall, 1879, 1882). The second gave his address as 2 Palmeira Terrace, West Brighton, which has been confirmed in local directories of 1883 and 1884. He then moved to

---

* This was at 20 High Street (Stanesby, K. F., 1964, personal communication).

† Ordish and Hall's were at 23 High Street. Francis Hallam was at 22 High Street, and he was the grandfather of Miss Margaret E. Hall (Hall, M. E., 1964, personal communication), to whom I am indebted for the obituary notice and for all the additional data about the Hallams.

‡ Charles Hallam built a house at Barton-under-Needwood, near Burton, named Errisberg House, which is now a Home for Old People. His daughter, Susan, married a Mr. Mee who was an architect for the brewery company of Worthingtons, and he also organist at Barton Church. They had two daughters, whose cousin, Mr. C. Shepherd, can remember one of them showing him a box, or a drawer, of old papers and saying: "I don't know what I'm going to do with all these, there will be no-one interested after my death." He thought that her estate was inherited by some distant relation. If the papers still exist it is remotely possible that they may contain relevant information. Mr. Shepherd also thought that the other children of Charles Hallam died without issue (Hall, M. E., 1964, personal communication).

Hove (Musgrave, C. W., The Royal Pavilion Public Library, 1964, personal communication). Subsequent addresses have been obtained from the *Dentists' Register* which was first published in 1879.† (Appendix A.)

In 1882 he moved to Wallington, Surrey, and finally, in 1891, to Fleet, Hants. Entries in his name ceased after 1898 and a search at Somerset House confirmed that he died on March 12, 1898 in Fleet, at the age of 74 years.

Although William Lloyd Poundall did not appear in the *Dentists' Register* in 1899, Poundall, Alfred Ben, of 20 Compton Street, Brunswick Square, London, W.C., appeared in his place. He registered on November 1, 1899, and passed his L.D.S., R.C.S. in 1897. His name continued to appear until 1916, when his address was given as 63 Queens Road, Wimbledon, S.W. In 1923 the name William Lloyd Poundall reappeared. His address was given as 34 Thurloe Square, London, S.W.7. He was registered on April 29, 1922, as "Dentist, 1921". No qualifications were mentioned and the name did not appear again after 1925. At first sight it looked as if Alfred Ben Poundall was William Lloyd Poundall's son, and as if the second William Lloyd Poundall was his grandson, but a search at Somerset House revealed that the second and third Poundalls were both sons of William Lloyd Poundall. Alfred Ben Poundall died at the age of 46 years on April 10, 1917, and William Lloyd Poundall the second at 62 years of age on August 11, 1925. They were both born in London Terrace, Derby.

As Poundall is an unusual name, a search through all the telephone directories of England and Wales (1964) was tried in the hope of tracing descendants of the above two gentlemen. Only five Poundalls were found. Four of them lived in or near Derby. The fifth lived in Sussex and his initials were W. L.

Mr. W. L. Poundall the third confirmed that William Lloyd Poundall the first was his grandfather, but he was unable to throw any light on the two anaesthetics administered in 1856. He thought that his mother might have been able to help, but she died during the Second World War. He did, however, mention a cousin of the same surname whose "father was also a dentist and a

very good one". He thought that he lived in North London, but he did not know his address, and his name was not in the telephone directory.

At this stage it seemed that the only way of continuing the search would be to examine likely electoral registers, street by street. Such a search was just about to be instituted when Mr. W. L. Poundall provided the name of the firm for which he thought his cousin used to work. I telephoned the Head Office, expecting no more than confirmation that Mr. Poundall used to work for the firm, and, perhaps, an address. In fact I was put through to him, and to my astonishment I was soon listening to a further account of the two dental extractions under nitrous oxide anaesthesia which had been performed over a century ago. This was read from a small booklet which William Lloyd Poundall had written in 1881 (fig. 2). Mr. Alfred Poundall happened to have the booklet with him, having shown it to his own dentist only a week or so earlier.

Mr. Alfred Poundall very kindly searched old family papers in the hope of finding further evidence, but without success. He wrote (Poundall, A. B., 1964, personal communication): "... so I have only hearsay to pass on".

As I recall; the patient was an engineer who had lived in America; he suggested the use of nitrous oxide for a tooth extraction to a friend who arranged a discussion on ways and means with my grandfather [fig. 3]. Between them they had to improvise the apparatus and produce the gas.
I have no idea of the size of the wine bottle. I understand it was very necessary to extract the tooth quickly on both occasions which would seem to indicate that anaesthesia was not carried out to its full extent.
I believe that the patient's nose may have been closed by clip for the second operation instead of by finger and thumb as was used for the first extraction. I do not know how the mouth was closed during inhalation, but it was intended to create a closed circuit of the gas.
It certainly seems that Mr. Turton was the prime mover in this, but I would think it possible that Mr. Hallam and my grandfather could have heard of nitrous oxide.

He added (Poundall, A. B., 1965, personal communication): "... grandfather ... was one of the many dentists who supported Sir John Lubbock's petition, 1878, to Parliament praying for an Act to be passed rendering an examination in dental surgery compulsory".

---

† William Lloyd Poundall registered on December 3, 1878, as Lic.Den.Surg., R.Coll.Surg.Eng., 1872.

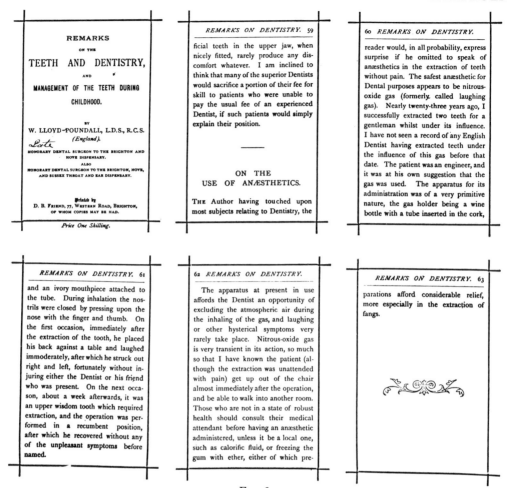

FIG. 2

The title page and an extract from the booklet written by William Lloyd Poundall in 1881.
The booklet was a revision and an extension of a previous pamphlet which the author wrote
"with the intention of imparting to unprofessional persons information which he believed to
be indispensable". (By kind permission of Mr. Alfred Poundall.)

The account given in William Lloyd Poundall's booklet of 1881 indicates that the date of the incident was 1858. He was, however, in some doubt about the precise date when he wrote the letter which was published in 1870, and he may have been in no less doubt eleven years later. All that can be said is that Mr. Turton was anaesthetized some time between 1856 and 1858. In other respects the two accounts agree nicely. In the letter (Poundall, 1870) the patient was referred to as a Mr. Turton, whereas in the booklet he was referred to as an engineer.* The two accounts taken together tally well with the entry in Francis White and Co.'s directory: "Turton, Henry. Engineer. High Street."

The first account (Poundall, 1870) stated that: "The gas was prepared by the patient, and bottled under water. A tube and a stop-cock was attached, with an ivory tube for the mouth." If the bottle was kept inverted under water, the tube could have been passed into it as far as it would go, and

---

* William Lloyd Poundall's brother-in-law, Tom Walker, was the first Croydon Borough Engineer, and Mr. Alfred Poundall "always imagined that this was Turton's field of engineering" (Poundall, A. B., 1965, personal communication).

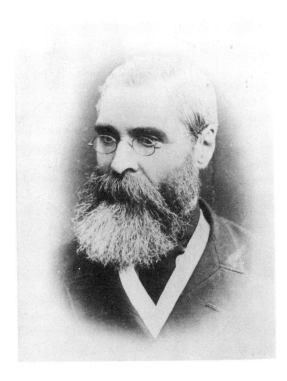

FIG. 3

William Lloyd Poundall, L.D.S., R.C.S., 1824–98. This photograph was taken in Fleet, when he would have been at least 67 years old. (By kind permission of Mr. Alfred Poundall.)

breathing from and into the bottle would have been quite possible, provided that it was wide enough. (The experiment has been tried in the laboratory. With a narrow bottle the changes in hydrostatic pressure during breathing would be excessive.) This arrangement would have been consistent with the idea that "it was intended to create a closed circuit of the gas". The use of such a system was also reported by Barton (1808) who witnessed: "A number of young gentlemen . . . breathing . . . from glass jars furnished with long tubes and stop-cocks, and inverted over water in a pneumatick tub . . ."

The second account (Poundall, 1881), however, described the gas holder as "being a wine bottle with a tube inserted in the cork and an ivory mouth-piece attached to the tube". In order to inhale nitrous oxide from a corked bottle, it would be necessary to admit gas or liquid to take its place. (There is no mention of the use of a reservoir bladder, nor of valves.) A second tube may have been inserted for this purpose, and if it admitted air, there would have been dilution of the nitrous oxide according to the relative sizes of the wine bottle and Mr. Turton's breaths, and the dilution would have increased with each breath. Possibly the most efficient way of using such a system would be for the patient to breathe right out, take in a deep breath of nitrous oxide, and then hold it for as long as possible. The experiment has been tried in the laboratory, and it is described in Appendix B. At first the subject claimed to have known what was happening throughout the experiment, although he realized that he came very near to losing consciousness; but after listening to a tape recording of the experiment, and to the account of it given by colleagues, he thought that he might have lost consciousness for a brief period. One cannot know how much pain he would have experienced if a tooth had been extracted, but the margin of analgesia would have been small. It might also have been difficult to have gained access to the tooth.

It may have been that the bottom was knocked out of the wine bottle and that a system was used like that described by James Wylde in his book, *The Magic of Science*, which was published first in 1861. It is quoted below. Turton may have got the idea from a similar but earlier account or demonstration.

EXPERIMENT 26.—*To procure Laughing Gas.*—Put two ounces of nitrate of ammonia, which you must obtain from an operative chemist, into a retort or Florence flask with a bent tube. Place this on the ring-stand, and let the stem of the retort or flask dip into the pneumatic trough, or in a basin. Instead of using cold water in these, a solution of two ounces of sulphate of iron or green vitriol dissolved in a gallon of warm water should be employed, the object being to purify the gas as it passes through the liquid. A gas jar open at one end and corked at the other, is now filled with the water in the trough, and arranged so that the stem of the retort shall dip under its lower edge. A gentle heat is now to be applied to the retort by means of the spirit lamp till the salt contained in it melts. Laughing gas will then pass over and will gradually fill the glass jar, of course driving out the water. When no more gas passes over, remove the retort from the ring-stand, and let the jar of gas stand over the water for some time, so that any gases present, which if breathed might do you serious injury, may be absorbed. You will observe that the process is exactly like that used for making oxygen, with the exception of our last-named precaution, which you must never fail to observe.

EXPERIMENT 27.—*To breathe Laughing Gas.*—Never try this experiment, unless, at least, two persons are present beside yourself; and secure the person who is about to breathe the gas to a post, by a rope fastened around the waist. Have ready a cork, which will just fit the neck of the glass jar you have filled with gas, and into this cork fit a piece of pewter tube, which must pass through a hole bored into the cork. To this a piece of india-rubber piping, about three feet long should be attached, ending in a small piece of metal tube, which will serve as a mouth-piece. Our diagram, fig. 18 [fig. 4], will explain the construction of the arrangement. On the right, you observe the pneumatic trough, in which the jar of gas stands. From the jar the india-rubber tube passes, and through this, the person taking the gas, inhales it into his lungs . . . the person taking the gas should place the mouth-piece in his mouth, close the nostrils with his fingers, and inhale the gas into his lungs, until you observe a peculiar appearance in his eyes, say after a few seconds of time. Remove now the pipe from his mouth; and leave him to give way to his feelings . . . the writer gives here an account of a scene which he witnessed a short time ago.

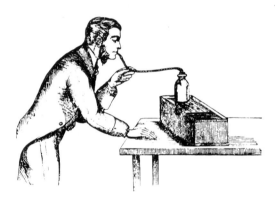

FIG. 4

A subject inhaling nitrous oxide from a glass jar having openings at both ends, in which the gas had been collected under water, as described in the text. (From Wylde, J. (c. 1872), p. 16. By courtesy of The Polytechnic, Regent Street, London, W.1. Photographed at the Leeds General Infirmary.)

Several persons having desired to take the gas, each in turn was fastened by a rope to a strong pillar. Some, after breathing the gas, commenced the most extravagant laughter; others were desirous of fighting; one stripped off his coat, and would have done serious damage to the faces of his neighbours had they not kept out of the way; and one young man attempted to kiss the ladies present, showing no symptoms of choice as to age or beauty. Altogether the effects are always highly amusing: each person seems to exhibit the peculiarities of his character in their most exaggerated form. In most cases the effect soon wears off; but we must warn those friends who are of a highly sanguine or nervous temperament, either not to partake of it at all, or to do so to a very moderate extent. We do not advise its use by the fair sex, under any circumstances.

Using this method it is probable that the subject would inspire only a single breath of the gas.

The fact that Mr. Alfred Poundall made a particular point of mentioning that the patient had been to America suggests that that was where he got the idea: but his use of a bottle instead of a bladder or a bag makes it unlikely, though not impossible, that he got the idea from attending one of Colton's "Grand Exhibitions".

APPENDIX A

RESIDENCES OF WILLIAM LLOYD POUNDALL (1824–98)
From Derby Directories (and from Mr. Alfred Poundall)

1844 Druggist, Alfreton, Near Derby.*
1850 (Glover) Poundall, W. L., Surgeon Dentist, Corn Market.
1852 (Freebody) Poundall, William Lloyd, Chemist, 54 Carrington Street.
1855 (Kelly) Poundall, William Lloyd, Dentist, 20 Victoria Street.
1855 (Kelly) Poundall William Lloyd, Chemist, Park Street.
1857 (White) Poundall, William Lloyd, Surgeon Dentist, 20 Victoria Street.
1858 (Glover) Poundall, William Lloyd, Chemist & Druggist & Surgeon Dentist, 20 Victoria Street.
1861 Dentist, 91 Devonshire Street, Derby.*
1869 Dentist, London Road, Derby.*
1871 (Wright) Poundall, William Lloyd, Dental Surgeon, 5 London Terr. & Street.
1874 (Wright) Poundall, William Lloyd, Dental Surgeon, 1 London Terr., London Street.

From Brighton Directories
1883, 1884 Palmeira Terrace.
1885, 1886, 1887 39 Church Road, Hove.

From The Dentists' Register
1879 5 Landsdown Terrace, East Brighton.
1883 2 Palmeira Terrace, West Brighton.
1888 Wallington, Surrey.
1891 Derby Lodge, Fleet, Hants.

APPENDIX B

Experiment to demonstrate the effects of breath-holding following a single deep inspiration of nitrous oxide from a bottle.

Method.

A subject sat comfortably in a dental chair, wearing a nose-clip and breathing through his mouth. After making a maximum expiration, a tube connected to the bottom of an aspirating bottle, which had been filled with nitrous oxide, was placed in his mouth. The top of the aspirating bottle was at the same time opened to room air by removing a cork from a small tube which had been inserted through the bung. The capacity of the aspirating bottle, plus the tubing between it and the subject's mouth, was 6.25 l. The subject then took a slow deep inspiration and held his breath. An observer called out as the subject carried out each respiratory manoeuvre, and he gave a running commentary of subsequent events. A second observer counted aloud, speaking the numbers at irregular intervals (averaging about 2 seconds) and

* Poundall, A. B., 1965, personal communication.

starting from the time that the subject began to hold his breath. As the subject heard each number counted, he responded by operating the striker of a hand bell with his right index finger. The running commentary, the spoken numbers and the ringing of the bell, were recorded on magnetic tape.

The Subject.

Age 46 years. Height 182 cm. Weight 86kg. Predicted surface area 2.08 sq. m. Approximate vital capacity 5 l. During previous experiments he had been able to respond to spoken numbers while breathing 80 per cent nitrous oxide from a non-rebreathing system, for 70 sec; while breathing 100 per cent nitrous oxide after breathing room air, for 50 sec; and while breathing 100 per cent nitrous oxide after pre-oxygenation, for 60 sec.

Results (February 26, 1965).

During a preliminary control period the subject was able to hold his breath without distress for 72 sec following a single deep inspiration of room air.

The following times are given from the time of the end of the single deep breath of nitrous oxide, which took 12 sec.

Response to Spoken Numbers.

0–34 sec	Appropriate and immediate.
35 sec	Delay in one response.
38 sec	An extra bell-strike in the absence of a spoken number.
43–54 sec	No response to four spoken numbers.
60–64 sec	Numerous inappropriate bell-strikes (these were remembered by the subject).
65–67 sec	Two appropriate responses.
68–80 sec	Only inappropriate bell-strikes.
80–98 sec	Two appropriate responses to six numbers spoken. No response to remaining four (the subject may have been momentarily unconscious for parts of this period).
99 sec	Regular appropriate responses resumed.

Additional Data derived from the record (and from the subject's memory).

25 sec	Expiration (remembered as a deliberate small release of lung contents to ease discomfort without losing control).
28 sec	Lips cyanosed.
32 sec	Intermittent expirations (remembered as small).
37 sec	Small intermittent inspirations (remembered as small).
40 sec	Jactitation. (Remembered as a struggle to keep the glottis closed. This was probably not a true jactitation. Small regular jerking (rhythmic) movements were described after the experiment, but they were not recorded and their timing is uncertain.)
48 sec	Muscular spasm of back (remembered as a struggle to keep the glottis closed and the chest expanded).
50 sec	Stamping feet (memory uncertain).
69–72 sec	Stamping movements (not remembered).
86 sec	Eyes opened for the first time (this was remembered; first the left eye was opened and then the right).
90 sec	Facial movements continuous throughout (the time at which they started was not recorded; later they were described as grimaces).

95 sec	Breathing (one or two breaths remembered).
115 sec	Small breath.
120 sec	Small breath.
135 sec	Eyes open and normal breathing resumed.

These results suggest that there may have been moments of unconsciousness between 68 and 86 sec after taking the breath of nitrous oxide. There were no unpleasant sequelae.

ACKNOWLEDGEMENTS

I am indebted to Mrs P. C. L. Waddelow for permission to publish all the information that the late Mr Alfred Poundall was about to provide about his grandfather. I was led to him by his cousin the late Mr. W. L. Poundall. I wish to thank Mr. K. F. Stanesby, Borough Librarian and Keeper, Burton-upon-Trent; Mr. Ernest Bletcher, Borough Librarian, Derby; and Mr. C. W. Musgrave, O.B.E., Director of the Royal Pavilion Museums and Public Libraries, Brighton, who searched local records and made local enquiries. Mr. A. V. Parker, Director of Hallams Ltd., was instrumental in persuading Mr. A. T. Moss to make an appeal on my behalf in the *Burton Daily Mail*. I thank them for hereby putting me in touch with Miss Margaret E. Hall who provided information about the Hallams. Miss E. Hergt, of Errisberg House, also made local enquiries on my behalf. Mrs. Gillian O'Nions helped with the search in Somerset House. Dr. C. Prys-Roberts, Dr. M. Hargreaves and Mr. B. Gough assisted in the experiment outlined in Appendix B. Mr. E. R. McColvin, Librarian of The Polytechnic, Regent Street, drew my attention to James Wylde's *Magic of Science*.

I am indebted to Mr. A. L. Pegg, Department of Photography, Leeds General Infirmary, for the reparation of figures 1, 3 and 4; and to Mr. C. H. Redman, Department of Photography, Royal College of Surgeons of England, for preparing figure 2.

REFERENCES

Barton, W. P. C. (1808). Thesis: *A dissertation on the chymical properties and exhilarating effects of nitrous oxide gas; and its application to pneumatic medicine;* submitted as an inaugural thesis for the degree of Doctor of Medicine, p. 34. Philadelphia.

Burton Daily Mail (1964). A Burtonian's diary. Saturday, November 1, p. 3.

Poundall, W. L. (1870). Letter to *Brit. J. dent. Sci.*, **13**, 208.

—— (1879). Letter to *Brit. J. dent. Sci.*, **22**, 56.

—— (1881). *Remarks on the teeth and dentistry, and the management of teeth during childhood.* Brighton: D. B. Friend.

—— (1882). Letter to *Brit. J. dent. Sci.*, **25**, 114.

Smith, W. D. A. (1966). A history of nitrous oxide and oxygen anaesthesia. Part V: The crucial experiment, its eclipse and its revival. *Brit. J. Anaesth.*, **38**,

Wylde, J. (c. 1872). *The Magic of Science: A Manual of Amusing and Instructive Scientific Experiments*, 3rd ed. London: Griffin. (1st ed., 1861; 2nd ed., 1872).

Brit. J. Anaesth. (1966), **38**, 551

8

1868—NITROUS OXIDE ANAESTHESIA TAKES ROOT IN GREAT BRITAIN

There were various claimants to the honour of first using nitrous oxide as an anaesthetic; but to Dr. Evans was undoubtedly due its introduction and successful administration in this metropolis.

(James Parkinson, 1868)

T. W. Evans and his introduction of nitrous oxide anaesthesia to London—March 31, 1868.

Thomas Wiltberger Evans (fig. 1) trained as a dentist in Philadelphia. In 1847 he joined C. S. Brewster, a successful fellow countryman, in Paris, and he has left a vivid description of dentistry there at that time.

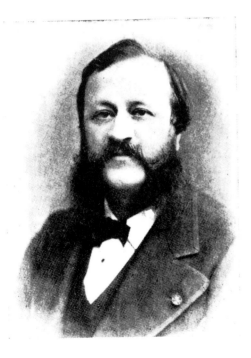

FIG. 1

Thomas Wiltberger Evans (1823–97).
By courtesy of The Wellcome Trustees.

Those persons who made it their business to treat diseases of the teeth were ranked as barbers, cuppers and bleeders, just as, a hundred years before, surgeons were, everywhere in Europe. Physicians and surgeons considered the care of the teeth as unworthy of their attention and science; the rectification of those irregularities of dentition that gave rise to defects in speech, or disfigure the mouth, they knew nothing about; and extractions were left to be performed by mountebanks at street corners, or fakirs at fairs, where the howls of the victims were drowned by the beating of drums, the clash of cymbals, and the laughter and applause of the delighted and admiring crowd. This *al fresco* practice of dentistry was to me one of the most curious and *foreign* features of street life in the old Paris of 1847.

If the dentist was sent for to attend a patient he was expected to enter the house by the back stairs, with the tailor and butcher-boy and the other purveyors to the establishment [Evans, 1905, p. 18.]

In 1848, Charles Louis Napoleon Bonaparte, soon to become Emperor Napoleon III, called for the services of Dr. Brewster, and Evans tells us: "It so happened, when the message came, that Dr. Brewster was ill and unable to respond to this call himself. It fell to me, therefore, by good fortune, to take his place professionally, and to visit the Prince" (Evans, 1905, p. 2). Evans used his opportunity. He wrote:

It was my privilege to render considerable services to the Emperor, I was richly repaid in many ways: but more especially by the direct support and encouragement he gave me in the practice of my art, and the social consideration accorded to me, and, through me, to my profession. Indeed the immense importance of this can hardly be understood by one not acquainted with the character of the men who practised dentistry when I came to Paris, and the contempt with which they were spoken of and regarded. [Evans, 1905, p. 18.]

Evans had no need to enter by the back stairs.

A biographer (*Dictionary of American Biography*) described his rise to fame thus:

. . . he remained with Brewster until 1850, when he opened his own office. . . . A friendship with Napoleon III, begun during professional services and assiduously cultivated, laid the foundations of a large private fortune and the most distinguished dental practice of the nineteenth century. A high degree of professional skill, and a tactful wife enabled him not only to become the dentist to all the important Royal Families of Europe, but also, to many of them, a personal friend. As his success grew, Evans's conceit, ever present, became boundless. He came to consider himself not only a successful dentist, but an author and a diplomat.

His biographer acknowledged, however, that: "If Evans was naïve, ambitious, and vain, as his *Memoirs* and contemporary testimony both reveal him, he was also generous and charitable", and that:

His role in the history of American dentistry is considerable. He was one of the first to experiment with vulcanite as a base for artificial dentures and in promoting the use of nitrous oxide as an anaesthetic. . . . His own distinguished reputation established the prestige of American dentistry in Europe . . . the bulk of his fortune was used in establishing the Thomas W. Evans Museum and Dental Institute, now the Dental School of Pennsylvania.

Neither his *Memoirs* nor his biography, however, mention his particular role in re-introducing

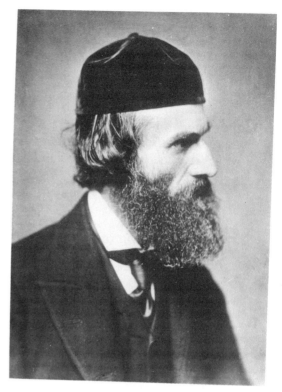

FIG. 3
Joseph Thomas Clover (1825–82). By courtesy of The Wellcome Trustees.

nitrous oxide anaesthesia to England in 1868.

Some experiments with nitrous oxide anaesthesia had already been carried out in London by Samuel Lee Rymer (fig. 2) and published in 1864, but in the words of Clover (fig. 3) ". . . they were not so successful as to induce anyone to adopt the practice of giving it". Clover (1868g) continued: "In March last, Dr. Evans, of Paris, assisted by his nephew, administered nitrous oxide to some patients at the Dental Hospital, London, in the presence of several medical men who were invited to witness its effect."

Evans had been introduced to the practice of nitrous oxide anaesthesia personally by Colton, who visited Paris to exhibit at the Paris Universal Exhibition of 1857. Evans was United States Commissioner to the Exhibition (Evans, 1868a). In his report upon the dental exhibits he wrote (Evans, 1868b):

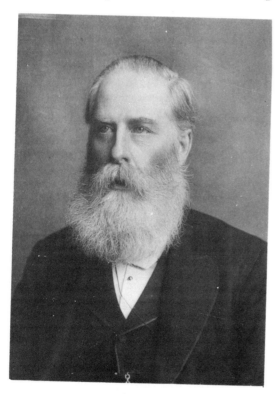

FIG. 2
Samuel Lee Rymer (1833–1909). (See also Part V, Smith, 1966.) By courtesy of The Royal Society of Medicine.

I have observed in the United States Collection in the Exposition of the *Société de Secours aux blesses* an apparatus for the production and administration of nitrous oxyde gas, exhibited by Dr. J. Q. Colton of New York. It is but just to observe that through the efforts and researches of Dr. Colton, the attention of surgeons has already been directed to the protoxyde of azote or nitrous oxyde gas. . . . Dr. Colton has re-established by thousands of experiments the superiority of the protoxyde of nitrogen gas over other anaesthetics in Dental Surgery, particularly in operations which may be promptly effected. The gas has recently been even employed with success in Paris under my own direction, in the gravest surgical operations. . . . Much and ingenious apparatus has been constructed in America for the preparation and inhalation of this valuable anaesthetic substance.

Evans did not confine his interest to the practical problems of administering nitrous oxide. He later devoted some thought to its physiological action, and he even attempted measurement of its uptake from a non-rebreathing system (Evans, 1869):

But it is to be observed that, when the condition of anaesthesia has been produced by the inhalation of nitrous oxide, the blood is by no means fully saturated with the gas.

I have endeavoured to ascertain about how much nitrous oxide it is necessary to introduce into the blood to develop the anaesthetic state—to produce insensibility. In practice, five or six gallons are required, on the average, to put to sleep an adult. Some of this is wasted—nearly the whole quantity is expired during administration. How much really remains in the system—has been absorbed—when the inhalation is suspended?

Placing a large bell-glass in a pneumatic trough, after filling it with a given quantity of gas, I have caused the gas to be inspired in such a way as that the products of expiration should be received into another glass over the same trough. These products, when the inhalation has been properly conducted, will consist of nitrous oxide, carbonic acid, watery vapour, and the residuum only of atmospheric air in the lungs at the commencement of the experiment. This last component may be balanced by the residuum of nitrous oxide in the lungs at the end of the experiment. If, therefore, we removed the carbonic acid from the second glass, the difference between the volumes of

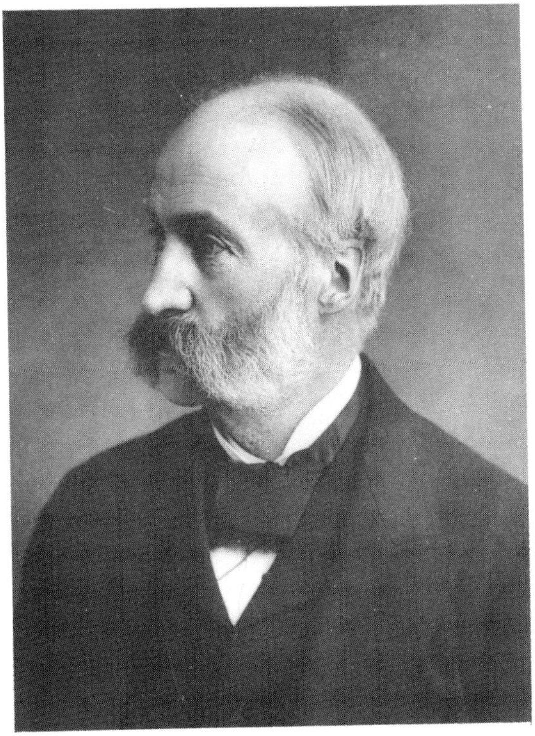

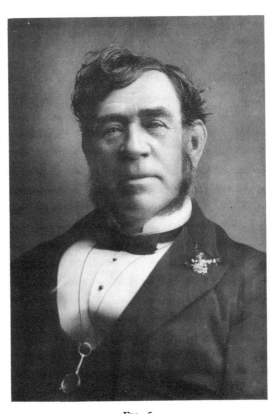

FIG. 4

Thomas Underwood (1818–1900). He served his apprenticeship under Robert Hepburn (fig. 5) (Lindsay, 1955a). By courtesy of the Royal Society of Medicine.

FIG. 5

Robert Hepburn (1810–1901). By courtesy of the Royal Society of Medicine.

gas in the two jars will show very nearly the actual amount of gas absorbed by the blood at the moment the inhalation was suspended. I have found this difference rarely to exceed *three quarts*.

On March 30, 1868, Evans called on Mr. Underwood (fig. 4) in London.

. . . and mentioned that he had been prosecuting enquiries into the use of nitrous oxide as an anaesthetic, and had tried a very large number of experiments with it in his own private practice, and that his experience was verified by the extensive practice of Dr. Colton, of the United States, in the use of this gas, and offered to administer it on the following day, Tuesday, 31st March, at the Dental Hospital. [Underwood, 1868.]

He gave demonstrations at the Dental Hospital, at Moorfields Eye Hospital and in the house of Mr. Hepburn (fig. 5). They were observed with obvious interest, but they had a mixed reception, and editorials in the *Lancet* and the *British Medical Journal* expressed almost opposite opinions.

An editorial in the *British Medical Journal* (1868a) concluded:

A great caution must be enjoined in using this agent, even by Dr. Evans' method, until we have more of our own experience to guide us. But taken with all qualifications, the results are very surprising, deeply interesting, and of great promise as supplying that important desideratum—painless and rapid anaesthesia suited for dentistry and for the quicker operations of surgery, and of which the effects are entirely transient.

In the *Lancet* (1868b), on the other hand, we find:

A very opportune discussion took place at the Medical Society of London . . . on the so-called nitrous oxide gas. A question on the subject addressed to the President—Dr. Richardson [fig. 6], whose authority on such a point cannot be questioned—drew from him a clear and careful summary of its action. It was painful, he remarked, to see the childish excitement with which nitrous oxide and its effects had recently been dwelt on. The gas had been treated as an unknown, wonderful, and perfectly harmless agent; whereas in simple fact, it was one of the best known, least wonderful, and most dangerous of all substances that had been applied for the production of general anaesthesia. . . . In speaking out thus boldly to a professional audience, Dr. Richardson has not spoken a moment too soon. The ad capitandum method of applying the most potent medicinal agents against the teachings of scientific experiment and the experience of accepted observers, is a phase in physic which requires to be put down with a strong hand. Administration of nitrous oxide, or laughing gas, as it is commonly called, is becoming a pastime for amateurs. We hope these few and timely words will prevent a catastrophe. If they fail, the fault or neglect will not rest with us.

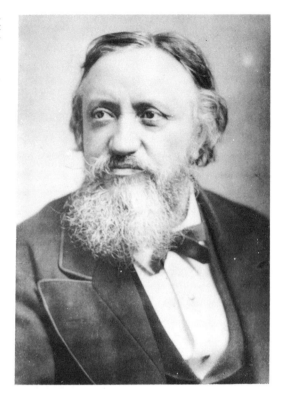

FIG. 6
Benjamin Ward Richardson (1828–96). (See also part V, Smith, 1966.) By courtesy The Wellcome Trustees.

The editorial comment in the *British Journal of Dental Science* (1868) was:

. . . but, whatever may be its ultimate fate, the Dental profession in England can never forget the liberality of Dr. Evans in devoting his time and money to the introduction among his English brethren of what he believes to be a valuable aid to their labour, and an inestimable boon to suffering humanity. Whether his enthusiasm in favour of the new agent be well grounded, time alone can show. Like a long pent up smouldering fire, it has burst into a flame in the hands of our go-ahead transatlantic brethren, and, after fascinating our susceptible neighbours in Paris, has finally landed on these shores, where it has been met with a certain amount of that cold distrust with which English medical science is apt to receive a suddenly pretentious claimant for immediate honourable recognition.

The use of chloroform for dental anaesthesia.

At that time dental operations were usually performed under chloroform anaesthesia, and Clover (1868a) had presented a paper on the subject at the previous meeting of the Odontological

Society held on March 2, 1868. He described his apparatus for delivering not more than 4 per cent chloroform, and for administering it nasally. In his opening remarks, however, he indicated the dangers of chloroform.

The experience of Dentists caused them to hail with gladness the introduction of anaesthetics, but they were soon found to be attended with inconvenience and danger. . . . Those practitioners who . . . gave the anaesthetic in strong doses not unfrequently found their patients become so prostrate as to cause the greatest anxiety, and in a few cases death was produced.

Repeatedly he emphasized the need to feel the pulse. "The faintness arising from the shock of the operation or from haemorrhage, will occur sometimes, and no amount of confidence in an instrument should cause us to relax our attention to the pulse in watching for the commencement of it." He objected to one apparatus "on the ground that it required both hands to be used, and so the pulse could not be watched". In describing his own nasal inhaler he said: "I merely exchange the face-piece of my inhaler for a nose-cap provided with valves and apply it over the nose. It is retained *in situ* by a strap which goes round the back of the head, and thus the chloroformist has his hands at liberty to watch the pulse." He also cautioned: "It is necessary, if the patient is sitting in a chair, to watch the pulse a few minutes after the operation is over."

In the discussion, Cattlin (1868a) commented:

. . . no one could have listened to his candid history of cases without observing that even under the most favourable circumstances it could not be given without danger. The chief questions for the Society to consider were, whether there was any antidote against the poisonous effects of chloroform, and if not, whether any means could be devised to lessen the danger of administering it.

Kidd (1868) ". . . thoroughly agreed with Mr. Cattlin as to the desirableness or necessity of some 'antidote' ". He also remarked that:

There was danger in Dental Operations from the patient's sitting up in the chair; the chair should be reclining.* He had investigated the subject, and had collected no less than fifteen cases of death from chloroform in newspapers and journals in Dentists' cases, and in almost every one of them one could see that death occurred . . . probably from . . . syncope after the operation was over.

---

* See also Sibson, 1848 (Part V, Smith, 1966).

Fox (1868a) stated that:

Chloroform was always administered to his patients while they were lying down on a sofa. This might seem an exceedingly inconvenient position for the Dentist to operate in, but practice and the habit of working with Mr. Clover, had enabled him to operate with success.

At the end of the meeting it was announced that on Monday, April 6, "a paper will be read by Mr. Harrison on a case of Osseous Union of the Upper and Lower Maxillae"; but the arrival of Dr. Evans and nitrous oxide anaesthesia in London at the end of the month caused a change in plan.

Monthly meeting of the Odontological Society of Great Britain held on April 6, 1868.

Evans returned to Paris, and in a letter dated April 5, (Evans, 1868c) he wrote to the President of the Odontological Society of Great Britain (Mr. James Parkinson (fig. 7)): "The results that I had in Paris were so satisfactory that I felt it my duty to make them known to my fellow-practitioners of

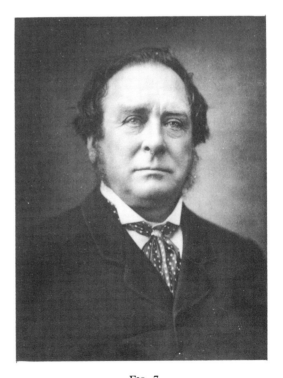

FIG. 7

James Parkinson (1815–95). (Department of Medical Photography, The University of Leeds, and United Leeds Hospitals.)

England", and "Convinced of the utility of nitrous oxide gas as an anaesthetic agent . . . I beg to offer to the Dental Hospital of London 'One hundred pounds', to be used for the purchase of apparatus and materials to manufacture the gas." He added:

> However, if, after more experience, our common hope should not be entirely realized, and the officers of the Hospital should decide to discontinue its use, they would be authorized to employ the remaining sum for the employment of any other anaesthetic that in their judgement would better fulfil the object we have in view.

Mr. James Parkinson read that letter to the General Monthly Meeting of the Odontological Society on the following day, April 6, and the ensuing discussion was taken up with the expression of individual views on Evans's demonstrations.

Underwood (1863) gave the following account of Evans's method:

> He (Evans) told him that inhalation took an exceedingly short time; that it was necessary that the operator should be as rapid as possible, as the patient would recover in the course of a very few seconds after the operation was concluded. The gas was contained in a very large bag with a gutta percha tube, having attached to it a bone or ebony mouth-piece that went into the mouth, and an ordinary stop cock which contained an inspiring and expiring valve. Dr. Evans told him that the signs of unconsciousness were pallidity of the face, snoring, extreme dilatation of the pupil and fixedness of the eye.

Underwood then described the first eleven dental anaesthetics demonstrated by Evans. The average duration of inhalation for nine of these cases was 69 seconds (47–114 seconds). The second case was a man of twenty-three from whom a second molar was extracted, and Underwood observed:

> There was pallidity of the face, but not to the same extent as in the first case. There was a decided blue cast over the face, and, in fact, these were symptoms which in the case of chloroform he should have looked upon as alarming, and should have discontinued its use. One minute was occupied; the tooth was removed, and the patient's remark was he had no pain whatever.

His comment on the tenth case was: "Mary G.—aged nineteen; second right and left molars; time one minute and five seconds; no pain. She was apparently intoxicated with three or four inhalations, and then the respiratory movements appeared to cease altogether." He mentioned also that: "One of the patients said she was perfectly aware of what was being done: she heard the administrator of the gas say, 'Now you can operate': she felt the tooth come out, but she experienced no pain whatever."

In summing up Underwood expressed his belief:

> . . . that this agent was an exceedingly valuable one, but that it must be used at present with excessive care, especially in the hands of practitioners who had not given their attention to the subject of anaesthetics. He thought that the wise course to adopt would be that a committee should be appointed, consisting of gentlemen practising as Dentists and as Surgeons, and of the chloroformists Mr. Potter and Mr. Clover, who had especially given their attention to anaesthesia; that the committee should operate upon animals, should make the most perfect experiments, and should report to the Society the result of their labours. He had no doubt that nitrous oxide would ultimately become an exceedingly valuable agent. . . . From the symptoms produced by the administration of this anaesthetic, it appeared to him that the patient was brought apparently to the verge of dissolution, and that instantly the gas was removed a reaction took place. A very small portion of the blood seemed to be affected by it, but to continue its exhibition for any lengthened time would, he should think, be exceedingly dangerous, save in the hands of one who was very experienced in the matter. He should be inclined in all operations to rely upon the first effects of the gas.

Hepburn (1868) said:

> . . . he had seen the apparatus used by Dr. Evans for generating the nitrous oxygen gas, who had fitted up a room at the Langham Hotel for the purpose of preparing it. . . . He had witnessed some experiments during the week, and would simply say that they were thoroughly successful. In some cases the operation was all over under two minutes, and, . . . the longest time for inhalation and the operation was three minutes and sixteen seconds. Some of the patients had two teeth out, and in one case three were extracted. Mr. Woodhouse operated on their friend Mr. Walker, who had written a very clear and lucid description of his sensations (see below). . . . He was also present at the Central Ophthalmic Hospital, and saw five most interesting operations performed by Mr. Haynes Walton, and Mr. Wilkinson. The whole five cases were done in under half an hour. . . . Two of the patients were children under five years of age, while one was a man of seventy-five. He was suffering from cystic tumours of the eyelids. The operation was performed on one eye without an anaesthetic. The man withered with pain; his feet turned up and he was evidently in intense agony during the operation. After the other operations were over, he was brought in again and put under the influence of this anaesthetic. The second operation was performed and the man was as quiet as a lamb. So also were the two little children and the other patients. In fact the results were perfectly marvellous. He used the word advisedly because they were none of them very apt to adopt new practices unless they were satisfied that some real advantage was to be gained. He believed it was a matter that would engage the attention of all prac-

titioners. It would do away with a great deal of time occupied, to say the least of it, in chloroform cases, and he thought it was a boon and blessing to humanity, and they could not be too grateful to Dr. Evans for the kind and generous way in which he had come to this country and had shown them these interesting experiments.

The experience of Mr. Joseph Walker, dental surgeon to the Westminster Hospital, on inhaling nitrous oxide in Mr. Hepburn's House on April 3, was reported later (*Lancet*, 1868a):

He inhaled the gas twice. On the first occasion, not being careful to exclude all atmospheric air, he experienced some unpleasant sensations of palpitations before becoming insensible, which he shortly did, and then underwent the extraction of a fang with perfect unconsciousness. On the second occasion, being careful to inhale the full strength of the gas, he became immediately insensible, and, after having another tooth extracted, became conscious very rapidly, without experiencing the least pain or uneasiness. The subsequent effects of the inhalation were a headache and a feeling of lassitude, which did not pass off entirely next day.

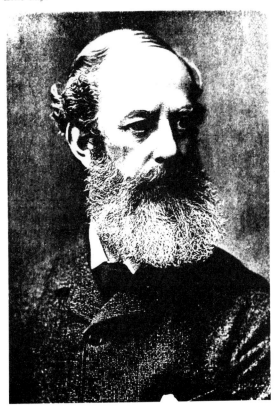

FIG. 8

Alfred Coleman (1828–1902). By courtesy of The Wellcome Trustees.

Coleman (1868a) (fig. 8) stressed the advantages which nitrous oxide gas appeared to offer and which neither chloroform nor ether procured. He gave these as the rapidity of its effects, the rapidity of recovery, the fewer disagreeable effects and the agreeable taste. After seeing further demonstrations, he confirmed Underwood's observations.

With regard to the appearance of . . . patients . . ., if he had witnessed the same symptoms in administering chloroform . . . he should certainly have felt extremely alarmed at the appearance some of the patients presented. These became suddenly livid, and [he added] as he watched the pulse in one case, it ceased for four or five seconds; that was at the time that the inhalation was discontinued. The operation was performed, and he felt the pulse return as it were a wave along the radial artery. In many cases, respiration, at the time the instrument was removed, ceased to be perceptible. The patient whilst inhaling inspired easily, but when the stage of anaesthesia was brought about, respiration, if it existed, was almost imperceptible. Such symptoms certainly would, in a patient under chloroform, appear very alarming. But perhaps, the great ground for safety in this agent might be considered to be this, that the inhalation occupied so short a time, that the moment the agent was removed, the individual was able to inspire pure air, and very soon threw off the effects of the anaesthetic.

Vasey (1868) (fig. 9) commented that he

. . . was at Mr. Hepburn's house on one occasion with Dr. Evans, and saw ten or twelve people operated on. He could fully bear out the remarks made by Mr. Underwood, for the appearance of the patient whilst under the influence of nitrous oxide was most appalling. There was a general asphyxiated condition, the whole countenance and the lips presented a most fearfully livid appearance, and one of the gentlemen, who was watching the pulse, said it was feeble, and depressed, and he felt the fluttering referred to by Mr. Coleman. It seemed to him as if Dr. Evans, from great experience, was able to tell the precise moment when the inhalation should cease and the operator perform the operation. He thoroughly supported the proposition that a committee should be appointed, so that the whole subject should be carefully investigated. . . . At the same time, he was bound to say nothing could be more successful than the results of his anaesthetics, so far as he had seen it.

Cattlin (1868b) (fig. 10) said:

. . . although he had not had any experience of the action of nitrous oxide or any anaesthetic, he had frequently witnessed its properties when inhaled as laughing gas by medical students and private friends for amusement.* Lecturers on chemistry were in the habit of giving nitrous oxide to their pupils that their classes might see the different effect it produced upon individuals of different temperaments.... The alarming symptoms produced by nitrous oxide in the cases which

* See appendix.

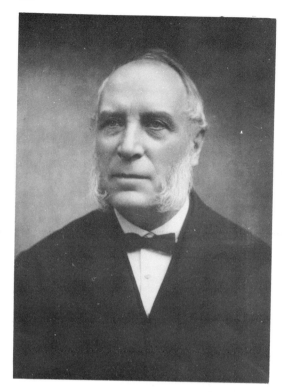

FIG. 9

Charles Vasey by courtesy of the Royal Society of Medicine.

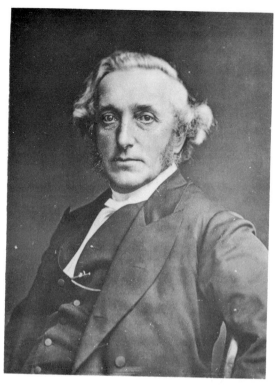

FIG. 10

William Alfred Newman Cattlin (died 1887). By courtesy of the Royal Society of Medicine.

had just been brought before the meeting . . . coupled with the great caution which Dr. Evans had properly used, showed that the profession had to deal with a dangerous agent; and while it was known that the inhalation of laughing gas at some of the hospitals had been attended with symptoms of an apoplectic character, he (Mr. Cattlin) thought the Society should suspend its sanction to the use of nitrous oxide until its action as an anaesthetic had been thoroughly investigated by a committee of the Society. Many gases were known to possess anaesthetic properties, but the main points for consideration were whether nitrous oxide was suited to dental operations, and *less dangerous than chloroform.*

Mr. Haynes Walton, having seen Evans's demonstrations at Mr. Hepburn's house in Portland Place, invited him to visit the Central London Ophthalmic Hospital which he did, "very kindly and at great inconvenience". Walton (1868a, b) gave a favourable account of the demonstrations there, but:

He felt quite sure that it (nitrous oxide) was not suited to lengthened operations . . . it may therefore be called a rapid anaesthetic. With our very limited

experience, neither Mr. Wilkinson nor myself thought it advisable to apply it to a case of cataract done on the same day.

He added:

No allusion has been made to the mode of administering it; great improvements might be introduced in this respect. First of all, the patient got frightened when the great mouth-piece was poked into his mouth. Then the gag was very unpleasant, and in the case of children, very uncomfortable. The holding of the nose seemed to frighten them very much.

Clover (1868b) contrasted the effects of laughing gas as used in former times, and the effects experienced with the protoxide of nitrogen during Evans's demonstrations. He pointed out that the difference

. . . might be explained by the fact that it used to be inhaled by means of a bladder. The patient was told to breathe out and then to inhale from the bag and breathe back again. He breathed backwards and forwards into this bag,* the result of which was that he would never at any time breathe so pure a nitrous oxide as he did in the present plan by which expired air at once escaped by the valves. There would not be such a complete arrest of oxidation in the former method as there was now. Then, generally speaking, there was no particular contrivance for obliging the patient to go on indefinitely; as soon as he got sufficiently excited, which he was expected to be, he burst away from those who were holding him, and began to breathe a little fresh air.

He went on to suggest:

. . . the instrument he (Clover) exhibited at the last meeting (Clover, 1868a) would be of great service, having a contrivance for completely covering the mouth and the nose, and for regulating the admission of air. He also exhibited a nose-piece† which would be very useful in dental operations where the mouth was required to be open. He noticed on one or two occasions the assistant of Dr. Evans called out to mind that the tube did not bend, and was rather surprised it had not occurred to him to make a coil of spiral wire inside.‡

[Clover] did not believe it would be found that the effects of the gas were different in different persons. As long as the gas was given pure, the results would be extremely uniform, and would be very much a mixture of faintness and asphyxia.

In all cases where the effects were fully produced, there would be a great failing of the pulse, and, in some instances, it would be found to be arrested. But it is likely to be a much less serious affair to have the heart stopped as the result of an agent of this kind than when chloroform had been administered for some considerable time.

He gave further details of his observations of Evans's demonstrations in the *British Medical Journal* (Clover, 1868c). He found the pulse

. . . to increase in force and frequency in every case after two or three inspirations of the gas had taken place; and as constantly its force and rapidity declined when anaesthesia was complete, which happened, on the average in less than one minute and a half. . . . In one case the pulse intermitted, and became imperceptible for five seconds just as the tooth was removed. The patient's lips were very livid, the pupils dilated, and the breathing was irregular and slow. From this apparently alarming state the man soon recovered, and in three minutes was able to walk.

Clover (1868d) also reported in detail the number of radial arterial pulsations counted during each period of five seconds in eight of the patients anaesthetized by Evans.

---

* This was not invariably the case when it was inhaled for entertainment. See Schoenbein's (1842) description of its inhalation at the Adelphi Theatre in 1824 (Part II, Smith, 1965).
† Coleman (1862) attributed the idea of nasal administration to Richardson.
‡ This idea had certainly been used as early as 1794 by Beddoes and Watt (see Part II, Smith, 1965).

At the end of that meeting of the Odontological Society of Great Britain, the following resolution, proposed by Mr. Cattlin, was agreed to:

That Mr. Tomes [fig. 11], Mr. Coleman, Mr. Underwood, with the President, Treasurer [W. A. Harrison, fig. 12] and Secretaries [John Dew and Charles J. Fox] be a committee to investigate the anaesthetic properties of nitrous oxide gas with powers to call in any other scientific aid, and to report the results of such investigations at some future meeting.

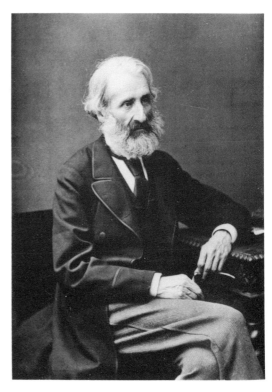

Fig. 11

John Tomes (1816–95). (Department of Medical Photography, The University of Leeds and United Leeds Hospitals.)

Meanwhile experiences and opinions were aired in the medical press, and interest in nitrous oxide anaesthesia gathered momentum.

Early trials of nitrous oxide by Coleman.

Before the end of April, Coleman's use of nitrous oxide for general surgery at St. Bartholomew's Hospital was reported as follows (*Brit. med. J.*, 1868b):

1. A boy about twelve, who took it twice (with an interval of a few minutes) whilst two tendons were

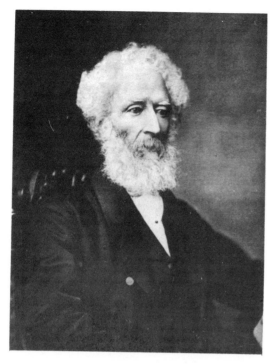

FIG. 12

William A. Harrison (1801–73). (Department of Medical Photography, The University of Leeds and United Hospitals.)

divided (Mr. Willett); 2. A boy about eleven, who had a large abscess in the groin freely opened (Mr. Paget); 3. An adult male, who had two long cuts made in the leg for a somewhat deep sinus (Mr. Paget) . . . Mr. Paget favoured us with the following opinion. . . . After seeing Mr. Coleman give the nitrous oxide . . . I cannot doubt its sufficiency for procuring total insensibility to the pain of short operations. The appearance of asphyxia is alarming; but it is so brief, that one may believe that, even if it were more profound, it might do no harm. The question of danger, however, can only be decided by the results of some thousands of cases.

Coleman (1868b) also wrote:

If . . . nitrous oxide enters and leaves the blood as such . . . then the trouble, difficulty and expense of procuring and transporting it about for anaesthetic purposes will prove very minor considerations. It is obviously evident that, by a very simple mechanical and chemical arrangement, the same gas may be employed repeatedly. The products of expiration, now wasted, need only be passed through a solution of caustic potash . . . and returned to the receiver whence the gas was inspired. . . . I need hardly say I am at once taking the proper steps for investigating so simple a suggestion as the above.

Later in the year he added (Coleman, 1868c):

I am now able to inform you that I have, in more than one hundred cases, administered the gas upon this plan; with three exceptions . . . the success has been quite equal to the method of breathing the gas only once. The amount of saving effected by the above arrangement is from two-thirds to three-fourths of the quantity of protoxide as ordinarily consumed. The agent I employ for removing the carbonic acid and aqueous vapour is quick lime recently and only partially slaked. The gas is admitted from a bag or receiver into a small india-rubber bag capable of holding about one gallon; from this it is inspired, but the expired gases pass over the lime and enter the bag by another route. I will not say that the gas respired is as pure after it has passed over the lime as it was before it entered the lungs; but it is sufficiently so to bring a second patient who may breathe it into a state of anaesthesia in nearly the same period of time as the first, and that is no longer than when the gas is breathed only once.

Early trials of nitrous oxide by Clover.

By May, Clover (1868e) was able to write:

Having witnessed the practice of Dr. Evans at the Dental Hospital, and made some experiments with nitrous oxide upon dogs and cats, with the view to trying to what extent the asphyxia may be carried without causing death, I was induced not to allow the prima facie objection that the gas was *not a true anaesthetic* to prevent my using it on the human subject. It is true that, if an animal is compelled to breathe pure nitrous oxide, it will die in a very short time; but the same may be said of any other anaesthetic. . . . The experiments I made led me to have great reliance in artificial respiration as a means of restoring animals overdosed with nitrous oxide. I have administered the gas to seventeen persons. . . . Fourteen of the cases were dental operations. Today I gave the gas at University College Hospital to three patients. . . . One of them (excision of two enlarged bursae patellae) was unconscious for seven minutes. . . . I found it much better to continue giving the gas with not more than an equal quantity of air, than to take away the facepiece, on account of the brief period which suffices to restore the patient to semiconsciousness when breathing pure air. I succeeded better with a case of amputation of the great toe, and one of operation of fistula in perinaeo: although I could have kept the patient quieter by chloroform, without greater danger. In operations lasting more than three minutes, I am not at present able to compare the gas with chloroform. For the extraction of a tooth that is not likely to be difficult to extract, I am inclined to think that it will often be preferred to chloroform. . . . Notwithstanding my confidence in chloroform,* I think there is room for nitrous oxide, since it certainly passes off much more agreeably than chloroform often does.

* The 1864 Chloroform Committee expressed its "cordial thanks to Mr. Clover, who, although not a member of the committee, attended, at their request, nearly all the meetings, administered the chloroform, and contrived, from time to time, with remarkable ingenuity, special apparatus for carrying them on" (*Med. Chir. Trans.*, 1864).

At the British Medical Association meeting at Oxford in August, Clover (1868f) referred to the apparatus which he used for administering nitrous oxide, of which he gave more details subsequently (Clover, 1868g). After describing the methods used by Rymer and Evans, mentioning that some patients struggled a good deal before they were put to sleep, and that some appeared to feel pain during the whole time of their operation, he wrote:

These partial failures were the results of the supply tube having collapsed, or from air having been sucked in accidentally. The following modification of an instrument which I have used for the last seven years, for giving four per cent of the vapour of chloroform, will be found to obviate the objections to the plan previously adopted [fig. 13]. The bag is filled with nitrous oxide, and I hang it by my side by means of a loop of ribbon; a non-collapsible tube leads from it to a face-piece which is made of sheet lead, so as to be easily moulded to the face, and edged with india rubber tubing, so that the nose and mouth may be covered by an airtight cap; two valves prevent the gas from being breathed a second time. This plan supersedes the necessity for pinching the nose; but when a patient breathes in a rapid and forcible manner, it does not always prevent a little air from being drawn in through the beard, or by the cheek falling in, during inspiration. To obviate this I have added a supplemental bag, holding about two hundred inches and connected by a three-quarter inch tube and stop-cock with the face piece. . . . As patients are apt to wake too soon, I have sometimes prolonged the anaesthesia whilst the mouth is still open, but giving the gas through the nose-cap which I have been in the habit of using with chloroform. . . . Whilst fitting the mouth-piece, the patient should breathe air only, and the gas should not be turned on till the patient breathes steadily. As long as he breathes calmly the supplemental bag should be empty, but when he begins to *pant*, the stop-cock should be opened. The gas received into the bag is so readily yielded during inspiration that there is not any air sucked in under the face-piece.

In the same article Clover included observations on the conduct of anaesthesia.

After inhaling twenty or thirty seconds, the patient begins to assume a livid appearance, this must not be taken as a sign of anaesthesia. I have often breathed the gas before a looking glass, and observed decided lividity in my lips, whilst my sense of touch was perfect. In about fifty seconds the expression of the patient suddenly alters, his eyes become unsteady and his hands slightly convulsed; I usually continue the inhalation ten or fifteen seconds after this, unless the respiration becomes very slow or stops, or unless the pulse becomes very quick or unsteady. The sudden dilatation of the pupil is another sign which should cause us to remove the gas. . . . The state of complete insensibility does not usually remain for more than half a minute after the removal of the mouth-piece, provided that the patient breathes regularly; but there is a period after this when, although there is a sensa-

tion of something being done, it is not felt as pain. I had a tooth extracted a few weeks ago after inhaling the gas. I had no knowledge of the first application of the forceps, but before the tooth was extracted I felt that it was being wiggled about, yet with no more sensation of pain than as if I had held the tooth in my fingers. . . .

He continued:

I have recorded the cases in which I have given the gas, and they amount to 384. In all these cases there has been produced an amount of lividity, which in other circumstances I should have thought dangerous to life; in the majority, convulsive twitchings of the

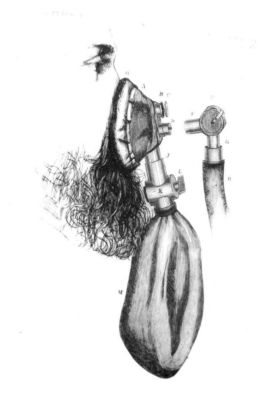

FIG. 13

Clover's apparatus for administering nitrous oxide. By courtesy of the Royal Society of Medicine.

A, the flexible metal oro-nasal mouthpiece.
a, a border of soft indiarubber tubing.
B, the expiratory valve.
C, a protective brass cap.
D, the inspiratory valve, which is attached to the supply-pipe H at F.
E, an opening for the supply of air when the gas is turned off. When the handle is moved to E the gas is turned on, and the air excluded. When the handle is moved to G the gas is cut off, and atmospheric air is admitted.
J, point of attachment of supplemental bag M.
K L, stop-cock, by which the bag is opened and closed.

hands have occurred, in a *few*, dilatation of the pupil. In several, the pulse has become quick and weak, but never imperceptible at the wrist, and the recovery has been, in all cases, rapid and complete, so that the patient required no assistance in walking away. I am aware of only three cases of sickness where vomiting occurred within a few hours of taking the gas. . . . If dangerous symptoms should arise from inhalation of nitrous oxide being continued too long, artificial respiration would be the proper remedy. The chest and abdomen should be forcibly compressed six or eight times, at intervals of a second, whilst the patient is sitting or lying; if this produce a florid colour of the face, it will suffice; if not, the patient should be placed horizontally, and Silvester's method resorted to.

Fox (1868b), who assisted Clover with some of his early animal experiments, quoted a personal note from Clover on the action of nitrous oxide:

It is possible that the presence in the blood of nitrous oxide is exciting so long as some oxygen remains, but as soon as the oxygenating property of the blood is lost the functions of the nervous system fail, and if fresh air were not soon admitted their functions would cease altogether. The functions of the brain proper cease before those of the medulla oblongata; hence we have loss of consciousness before failure of breathing, and the functions of the medulla are abolished before those of the ganglia presiding over the action of the heart, hence the heart continues to beat after breathing has ceased.

A letter from Colton and his visit to London in June 1868.

At an early stage Colton (1868) reviewed the subject in a letter to the *British Journal of Dental Science* and gave details of his own practice. "For the last three years we have used on an average, about 300 gallons a day, our patients varying from thirty to fifty each day, Sundays excepted." He gave the incidence of nausea as one in five hundred "from swallowing blood". He described what he considered the important points to observe in order to ensure successful anaesthesia:

First. Use a mouth-piece which has an aperture of a full half inch to breathe through; and five eighths is better. Second. Instruct the patient to take full, deep, and *slow* inspirations of the gas, and hold the lips and the nose so as to allow *no particle of common air to enter and dilute the gas*. By this means anaesthesia may be reached in from forty-five to sixty seconds. In certain difficult subjects, a minute and a half is required. Third. Have the patient sit in nearly an upright position, or, at any rate, with the head leaning a little forward, *and keep the head there* while the gas is being breathed. When the patient is asleep, the head can fall back for operation. The object of keeping the head forward is to allow the patient to swallow any saliva that may accumulate in the mouth. This he will do even if half asleep. With the head leaning back, the patient cannot well swallow, and he is apt to suck the saliva down the windpipe; choking

follows and you cannot carry the gas any further. The symptoms as to when the patient is "ready", although unmistakable are hardly describable—usually stertorous breathing (not always), and in delicately organised subjects a slight twitching of the fingers or the head. Feel your way carefully, and be guided by experience. You will make many mistakes by not giving enough gas or continuing it long enough. . . . In my office, where we have ten or fifteen teeth or stumps to extract for a patient, it is seldom that we have to give a second dose of gas: yet we have spent the whole time on one tooth.

In the *British Medical Journal* (1868d) it is recorded that:

On Friday, June 5th, Dr. Colton addressed a meeting of medical men and dentists at the house of Mr. C. J. Fox, detailing the history of the gas, and relating his experiences in over 27,000 cases. He then administered the gas to four patients with complete success; he repeated his address to another meeting on Wednesday, June 10th, and operated on nine patients for the extraction of teeth. It is to be noted that Dr. Colton pushes the gas much further than we have been in the habit of doing; he looks upon a sound approaching to stertorous breathing, and on the twitching of the fingers, as indications that the patient is in a profound sleep. He has administered the gas daily at the Dental Hospital to several patients; and on Monday evening met the Committee appointed by the Odontological Society to investigate the gas.

Fox (1868a) referred Dr. Colton's "pleasant stay" at his house in these words: ". . . permit me here to say that it is not easy to live for a week with a man without discovering whether he *is* or is *not* a man of truth, and straightforward unequivocal honesty. That Dr. Colton is such a man, I firmly believe." It may not be out of place to reinforce this opinion with a passage from Collyer's introduction to Colton's *Shakspeare and the Bible* (1888):

The author of this book told me once that he was nineteen years of age when he first found Shakspeare and began to read his plays . . . in no long time he read the whole thirty-seven plays, as we all did when we durst, in those days, who had been raised in the shadows of the old meeting-house and taught to believe that to read Shakspeare was a peril to the soul's health. He was soon and easily set free from this bondage "to fear", and ever since then these works of the mighty master have been his most intimate companions and friends, holding his heart captive, "entranced by their beauty and salt of truth". So he has told me more than once.

Early trials of nitrous oxide by Cattlin.

Cattlin's experiments, carried out in Brighton, were reported in two letters in June and July (Cattlin, 1868c, d).

The remarks which were made at the Medical Society of London by Drs. Richardson and Sansom . . .

have led me to institute experiments upon some of the lower animals, with the view to ascertain whether this gas does possess the anaesthetic properties imputed to it, and whether it can be safely used to produce anaesthesia in the human subject during short surgical operations.

Having witnessed its effects upon patients at the Dental Hospital of London, under skilful administration by Mr. Coleman and Mr. Potter, I have been convinced that protoxide of nitrogen does possess the power of affording immunity from pain, and I have arrived at the conclusion that, under certain conditions, it can safely be administered for one minute, but that its effects cannot be kept up beyond two or three minutes without risk unless atmospheric air be admitted from time to time when the countenance becomes congested. I am fully aware that Mr. Clover and others have maintained the anaesthetic effect of nitrous oxide for much longer periods, but in this case the unskilled cannot with impunity imitate the actions of the expert, and, until Medical men become better acquainted with the mode of administering the gas, great caution will be necessary in order to insure the safety of the patient.

Before it can come into general use it is necessary that the supply shall be equal to the demand, and that its administration shall be proved to be safe in the hands of the ordinary Medical Practitioners. The former of these requirements will probably be met by its manufacture in portable form, while experience will prove or disprove the high claims which have been set up for nitrous oxide as a safe and effectual anaesthetic agent. I have given it to the point of true anaesthesia, to the rat, rabbit, guinea-pig, dog, donkey, and pig with success, and I have been surprised how closely the symptoms produced in these animals resemble those observed in the human subject.

The conditions, according to my experience, which are necessary in order to insure the safe and effectual operation of protoxide of nitrogen are:

1. That the gas shall be moderately fresh and perfectly pure.

2. That it should not be administered for longer than one to two minutes without allowing atmospheric air to pass into the lungs.

3. That no air shall be given with the gas until the patient is profoundly under its influence.

4. That the tube through which the inhalation takes place be not of small diameter, and that great care should be taken during the operation to prevent any impediment to the free course of the gas by accidental twisting or bending of the tube.

5. That the gas shall not be forced into the lungs by too great a pressure upon the vessel in which it is contained.

The inhalers I have used have been constructed to fit each animal, upon Snow's principle, and in every case the gas has been administered in the open air.

. . . in the case of the donkey, the first experiment was very successful. The animal was rendered insensible, recovered consciousness, and was actually eating grass, all within the short space of three minutes. In the second experiment (a week afterwards), air was accidentally admitted by the side of the inhaler; consequently, the animal struggled violently, and was rendered only partially insensible to pain, although a large quantity of gas was consumed.

It was the opinion of a few Medical friends who witnessed my experiments that some of the animals were really dead; yet their complete recovery was not prolonged much beyond the time I have stated, and they have not since shown any sign of illness. . . . The pointer dog and guinea-pig are in different stages of utero-gestation, and I shall be careful to note the effect of nitrous oxide upon their offspring.

I am about to conduct experiments to ascertain the poisonous qualities of this gas, and then submit animals at the point of death to the influence of supposed antidotes, such as oxygenated air, pure oxygen, galvanism, etc.

In his second letter Cattlin (1868b) confirmed that "The pointer bitch, which was made so profoundly insensible that some of my Medical friends thought she would not recover, has lately brought forth ten healthy living puppies, and 'is doing as well as can be expected'." His repeated experiments on animals confirmed his

. . . conviction that nitrous oxide was not so dangerous an agent as many may have supposed it to be. Even with our present limited knowledge of its action, it will be found to possess some advantages over other anaesthetics for short surgical operations, and . . . I shall be surprised if it does not ultimately prove less dangerous to life and health than chloroform, although I do not expect it will supersede chloroform or other anaesthetics for very protracted operations.

Anticipating the popularity of nitrous oxide, he added:

If this anaesthetic comes into general use (and I think it will be most valuable to dentists), it will probably be administered to patients in every imaginable condition. Latterly I have been endeavouring to ascertain the effects of nitrous oxide manufactured by persons unskilled in chemical science, and with this view I directed my female servant and gardener to make some of the gas, while my son and myself also prepared some.

Early trials of nitrous oxide by Fox.

In view of the association with Clover, it is not surprising to find Fox (1868d) developing the idea of using air with nitrous oxide and writing:

From the various experiments upon animals, upon myself, and others, I am convinced that, provided a patient is first thoroughly anaesthetised with pure gas, all atmospheric air being totally excluded, it is possible subsequently to permit access of a *small* proportion of atmospheric air, without inducing excitement. My attention was first drawn to this question by observing, when giving the gas to Mr. Jackson's patient for the removal of the breast, that, having put her into a deep sleep, she did not become in the least excited or restless when the mask was entirely removed, unless it was kept off for too long. Her colour revived the *moment* air was admitted by removal of the face-piece, but restlessness did not come on for many seconds after it. It therefore occurred to me to have a gas inhaler made, with two of Mr. Clover's stop-cocks (one to admit gas, the other air), so arranged that, by a graduated scale marked upon them, I could tell exactly how evenly or to what degree each was open. . . . The two stop-cocks answered very well, but were clumsy, and I have now, with Mr. Coxeter's aid, contrived a double sliding valve, which enables me to effect my purpose admirably. Although my attention has been directed to this point chiefly with a view to utilizing the gas in general surgery, yet it is not a matter devoid of interest to the dentist, for I have found many cases that, provided the first anaesthetic sleep is quickly and thoroughly produced, the continued administration of the gas for another minute or two, with a careful admixture of atmospheric air, renders the anaesthetic state more prolonged, so that more teeth may be removed before the patient awakes. It must, however, be borne in mind that the patient, after such an administration of gas and air, is generally dull and stupid on recovering, and must be left quiet, indeed not only on such but on *all* occasions I would deprecate any endeavours to rouse the patient from the anaesthetic condition.

In a letter to the *Lancet* written at the end of the year, Fox (1869a) anticipated future techniques.

Meanwhile, I throw out these hints in order to secure the early co-operation of my medical friends* in this path of investigation, and I have no doubt, with their aid, some means will be found of prolonging the anaesthesia induced by nitrous oxide, either by the admixture of atmospheric air or some other chemical agent.

Fox (1868c) also took a prominent part in the British Medical Association meeting in Oxford where he discussed the manufacture of nitrous oxide, and, in particular, described the Sprague apparatus used by Colton. After reading this paper he suggested ". . . that as many of those present had not witnessed the effects of the gas, he should take it. Mr. Clover accordingly administered the gas to him; and, after those present had made their observations, a long and interesting discussion ensued". On the following two days Fox extracted teeth during demonstrations of nitrous oxide anaesthesia by Clover, and of nitrogen "anaesthesia" by Murray.

Comparison of the effects of inhaling nitrous oxide and nitrogen.

Broadbent and Johnson had previously suggested that the anaesthetic effect of nitrous oxide might be due to the privation of oxygen (Duncum, 1947, p. 284). This was put to the test by Sander-

son and Murray (*Brit. med. J.*, 1868c) who used nitrogen to "anaesthetise" six patients at the Middlesex Hospital. In two of these, "anaesthesia" was not produced due to air leaks. In the remaining four patients there was an

acceleration of the pulse rate of 15–20 beats per minute which was maintained during the first two or three minutes of inhalation. The breathing also accelerated. . . . None of the patients showed any marked effects until the gas had been inhaled for two minutes, when respiration became slower and laboured. Later the pulse became slower, and sometimes irregular in force and frequency, each inspiration being accompanied by a weakening of the beat, and followed by a momentary acceleration. A certain degree of pallor was observed in some of the cases; there was, however, no lividity. Insensibility was produced in the four patients in three minutes, three minutes and ten seconds, four minutes and four minutes respectively.

Sanderson (1869) compared the actions of nitrous oxide and nitrogen thus:

In man, as in animals, the action of the two gases was similar, so far as related to their effect on the heart and breathing. Both produced anaesthesia. When nitrogen was used, this did not occur until the patient was already asphyxiated, i.e. after three minutes or so of inhalation; whereas nitrous oxide rendered a patient insensible in less than a minute, i.e. before the apnoeal state had come on. In other words, nitrogen produced anaesthesia by means of apnoea; nitrous oxide independently of apnoea, by its direct action on the nervous system.

It is surprising that patients should have remained awake for as long as three minutes when inhaling nitrogen. The obvious explanation is that it was diluted with air during its preparation, or during its administration, probably as a result of mask leaks.

Preliminary report of the committee of the Odontological Society.

The preliminary report of the committee of the Odontological Society of Great Britain, which had been set up in April, was presented by Mr. Harrison on December 7, 1868 (*Trans. Odont. Soc.*, 1868). It was based upon a series of animal experiments, on 1,380 anaesthetics which had been recorded carefully by members of the committee, and on a further 1,051 cases reported to the committee by practitioners of "reliable authority". Special forms were used for recording the human anaesthetics (Fox, 1869b). In its preamble the Committee stressed "the necessity of considering this as a purely *preliminary* Report, as they were fully aware that their experience must extend over

---

* Fox was the eldest son of Charles James Fox, M.D., whose father and grandfather were also medical practitioners (Hill, 1877). He retired in 1880 and went to Canada, where he died while inhaling chloroform during an attack of asthma (Lindsay, 1955b).

as many thousands as it now does hundreds of cases, before they can venture to give decided opinions on all the points for consideration".

The conclusions drawn from experiments on dogs, cats, rabbits, guineapigs, mice and birds, were similar to Davy's (1800), as was pointed out by Smith (1869) at the time. It was found that animals died if the gas was pushed too far and that moribund animals could often be revived by giving air. What Davy was not to know, however, was: "That the pure gas . . . *was* a powerful anaesthetic—more rapid in its action, although more evanescent in its effect, than chloroform and the other anaesthetics then in general use."

The trials of nitrous oxide on patients led the Committee to the conclusion that

. . . properly administered, it is at least as safe and efficient an anaesthetic for short operations as any other now in use; but that, while it possesses certain advantages over those of other anaesthetics for such operations, it labours also under certain disadvantages when compared with them for the longer operations in surgery.

The main advantages were given as rapidity of action, rapidity of recovery, agreeableness and lack of taste, lack of irritation to the air passages, and comparative freedom from nausea and vomiting and other side effects. Its disadvantages were defined as its unsuitableness for long operations and for operations followed by much pain or smarting, the inconvenience to the operator arising from muscular twitchings (especially during delicate operations), the inconvenience of making, transporting and administering the gas, and its expense. The Committee advised caution with patients affected by disease of the brain, heart, arteries and lungs, etc., and patients of very plethoric habit and short neck.

It also made recommendations on the administration of nitrous oxide among which may be mentioned:

. . . the operator having arranged the head-piece of the chair in a convenient position for the operation, and selected and arranged the instruments to be used, so that no time may be lost when the patient is ready for operation (These directions, *mutatis mutandis*, will apply to the preparation for any surgical operation to be performed under the use of this gas), a gag should be placed between the jaws to keep them apart.

The gag should have a string attached to it . . . it is generally best to place it between the second and the first molars. . . .

The gag may be placed between the incisors, when a molar on both sides is condemned; but, as a caution,

it may be stated that a patient, with projecting incisors, is reported to have bitten so firmly against a gag placed between them, that two of them were forced out . . .

The pulse and breathing should be watched carefully. . . .

In hospital practice there are fewer cases requiring the removal of a large number of teeth, at a sitting, than happens often in private practice, where frequently several have to make way for artificial teeth. The number which may be removed after one inhalation of this gas is limited, *necessarily*, only by the recovery of the patient from the state of anaesthesia. But the sockets from which loose teeth have been removed often bleed so freely, and the accumulation of a large quantity of blood in the pharynx would add so much to the danger of any exceptional case of faintness, or interrupted breathing that the Committee would recommend that the extraction should not be continued beyond a limited number. . . .

Finally, if alarming symptoms come on, in spite of precautions . . . artificial respiration should be resorted to.

At the end of its Report, the Committee mentioned that the nitrous oxide was said to have been administered upwards of 200,000 times in America, with but one death—in a patient suffering from extensive disease of both lungs; and that very favourable statements regarding the efficiency and safety of nitrous oxide as an anaesthesia had been received from both America and the Continent of Europe, from which it concluded that ". . . this gas must . . . be regarded as a very safe anaesthetic".

In an Appendix the Committee noted that: "As a general rule, at the same sitting a patient gets more quickly under the action of the gas at the second administration than under the first, and sooner again at the third than the second." Out of 1,380 administrations, "in 100 protracted and difficult operations it was necessary to give the gas more than once at the same sitting. It was administered a second time to 100 patients . . . a third to 36 patients . . . a fourth to 11 patients . . . a fifth to 2 patients and a sixth to one patient." No attempt was made to explain this in terms of the nitrous oxide retained by the patient, or in terms of his altered state as a result of anaesthesia. It continued: "The lividity and pallor which takes place have been much objected to: but to those accustomed to administer this gas, these symptoms (which, however, do not *always* occur) give no alarm." It mentioned that a species of epileptic seizure may take place and that:

This occurred rather severely in five cases at the Hospital as the patients were recovering after the operation. The spasmodic struggling lasted in these cases about eight seconds, and then passed off on the return of the patient to consciousness. . . . Some patients were anaemic in the extreme, and it was noticed that the colour in the cheeks was better after inhalation than before.

This would have been due to increased skin circulation which usually out-lasts anaesthesia. In two cases: "Faintness followed the recovery of the patient . . . one was supposed to arise from tight lacing to conceal pregnancy." Vomiting was recorded in five cases.

The year 1868.

The record of anaesthetic events in the year 1868 makes fascinating reading. In it one can detect the beginnings of anaesthetic topics which are now—or were until recently—commonplace.

In Clover's (1868a) paper on chloroform and the ensuing discussion, we find mention of the need to control accurately the strength of inhalation anaesthetics. The use of valves made of thin discs "of ivory or vulcanite, made to move in one plane by means of a spindle passing through them, and supported by a spiral spring of fine wire" is described. Taking hold of the tongue with artery forceps is criticized. "He merely raises the chin from the sternum to give effect to the muscles between the chin and the hyoid bone." Mixed vapours were tried. Various types of gags were discussed. Many of them were no more than mouth props, but "Mr. Coleman has invented an excellent gag consisting of a pair of forceps of which the blades do *not* cross, so that pressing the handles together the short blades are separated". Clover's modification of this consisted of inserting a screw between the blades. The question of posture in relation to anaesthesia, syncope and dental operations was also raised.

There is something familiar, even contemporary, about much of the controversy and about the pattern of the professional response to the sudden introduction of the new anaesthetic. There were those who wasted no time in trying it out on their patients for a variety of operations, those who paused to watch and consider and those who first experimented with animals. New devices were invented such as Cattlin's (1868b) reservoir bag and Coleman's carbon dioxide absorber, and Clover's nasal inhaler was adapted for nitrous oxide. Nitrous oxide analgesia, the limitations of hypoxia for producing analgesia or anaesthesia, and the use of air and nitrous oxide mixtures were

also mentioned. Some of the clinical observations will doubtlessly be embarrassingly familiar to many anaesthetists today.

Evans was in London barely a week—as was Colton two months later—but the impact of his demonstrations was considerable. The reasons for this have been expressed ably by Bourne (1960, pp. 2-6)

. . . the phenomena seen with this method of anaesthesia were then new and keenly observed. . . . Today, it may seem remarkable that a method that produced in patients such alarming appearances and had such unsatisfactory features should have so quickly gained favour and passed into general use. . . . There were three reasons for the popularity of the method. First, the Chloroform Committee (1864) four years before Evans' demonstration, had published a report in which the danger of that agent . . . was amply confirmed. . . . Next, there was the American experience . . . "now said to amount to upwards of 200,000 (administrations) with the occurrence of but one death". . . . Finally, the rapid induction of anaesthesia with nitrous oxide, and the rapid recovery from it, appealed to the practical man.

ACKNOWLEDGEMENTS

The idea of allowing the main characters to speak for themselves whenever possible was inspired by Duncum (1947). Mr. Bowdler Henry and Mrs. J. E. H. Fairpo kindly gave assistance in tracing details of some of the members of the Odontological Society of Great Britain.

REFERENCES

Beddoes, T., and Watt, J. (1794). *Considerations on the Medicinal Use of Factitious Airs, and on the manner of obtaining them in large quantities*, 1st ed., Part II, p. 26. Bristol: Bulgin and Rosser.

Bourne, J. G. (1960). *Nitrous Oxide in Dentistry: its Danger and Alternatives*. London: Lloyd-Luke.

British Journal of Dental Science (1868), **11**, 189. Editorial.

British Medical Journal (1868a), **1**, 332. Editorial: A new anaesthetic.

—— (1868b), **1**, 410. Editorial: The protoxide of nitrogen as an anaesthetic.

—— (1868c), **1**, 593. Editorial: The protoxide of nitrogen as an anaesthetic; The administration of nitrogen as an anaesthetic at the Middlesex Hospital.

—— (1868d), **1**, 594. Dr. Colton on protoxide of nitrogen.

Cattlin, W. A. N. (1868a). *Brit. J. dent. Sci.*, **11**, 131.

—— (1868b). *Brit. J. dent. Sci.*, **11**, 208.

—— (1868c). Has protoxide of nitrogen anaesthetic properties, and can it be solely administered to man and the lower animals? *Med. Times and Gazette*, **1**, 618.

—— (1868d). Nitrous oxide as an anaesthetic. *Med. Times and Gazette*, **2**, 78.

Clover, J. T. (1868a). On the administration of chloroform in dental operations. *Brit. J. dent. Sci.*, **11**, 123.

—— (1868b). *Brit. J. dent. Sci.*, **11**, 212.

—— (1868c). Anaesthesia in dentistry by protoxide of nitrogen. *Brit. med. J.*, **1**, 338.

—— (1868d). Letter. *Brit. med. J.*, **1**, 392.

—— (1868e). The protoxide of nitrogen as an anaesthetic. *Brit. med. J.*, **1**, 437.

—— (1868f). The administration of nitrous oxide as an anaesthetic. *Brit. med. J.*, **2**, 201.

—— (1868g). On the administration of nitrous oxide. *Brit. med. J.*, **2**, 491.

Coleman, A. (1862). An instrument for administering the vapour of chloroform through the nose. *Lancet*, **1**, 42.

—— (1868a). *Brit. J. dent. Sci.*, **11**, 204.

—— (1868b). Action of nitrous oxide. *Brit. med. J.*, **1**, 410.

—— (1868c). Re-inhalation of nitrous oxide. *Brit. med. J.*, **2**, 114 (reprinted in *Brit. J. dent. Sci.*, **11**, 442).

Colton, G. Q. (1868). Letter. *Brit. J. dent. Sci.*, **11**, 253.

—— (1888). *Shakspeare and the Bible. Parallel Passages and passages suggested by the Bible with the Religious Sentiments of Shakspeare.* New York: Thomas R. Knox.

Davy, H. (1800). *Researches, Chemical and Philosophical; chiefly concerning nitrous oxide, or dephlogisticated nitrous air, and its respiration.* London: J. Johnson.

Duncum, B. M. (1947). *The Development of Inhalation Anaesthesia: with special reference to the years 1846–1900.* London: Oxford University Press.

Evans, T. W. (1868a). *Sanitary Institutions during the Austro-Prussian-Italian Conflict. Conference of the International Societies of Relief for Wounded Soldiers. An essay on ambulance waggons. Universal Exhibition records and letters. Catalogue of the author's sanitary collection,* 3rd ed. Paris: Raçon.

—— (1868b). *Report upon Dental Surgery and the material which it employs.* Paris Universal Exhibition, 1867. Class XI, Group II.

—— (1868c). Letter to President of the Odontological Society of Great Britain. *Brit. J. dent. Sci.*, **11**, 196.

—— (1869). Physiological action of nitrous oxide gas. *Dental Cosmos*, **11**, 449 (reprinted in *Brit. J. dent. Sci.* (1869), **12**, 337).

—— (1905). *The Memoirs of Thomas W. Evans. Recollections of the Second French Empire.* Edited by Crane, A. Vol. I. London: Fisher Unwin.

Fox, C. J. (1868a). *Brit. J. dent. Sci.*, **11**, 138.

—— (1868b). On nitrous oxide. *Brit. J. dent. Sci.*, **11**, 519.

—— (1868c). On the manufacture of nitrous oxide. *Brit. med. J.*, **2**, 201.

—— (1868d). On nitrous oxide in general surgery. *Brit. J. dent. Sci.*, **11**, 601.

—— (1869a). Letter. *Lancet*, **1**, 32.

Fox, C. J. (1869b). Forms for the registration of nitrous oxide cases. *Brit. J. dent. Sci.*, **12**, 440.

Hepburn, R. (1868). *Brit. J. dent. Sci.*, **11**, 202.

Hill, A. (1877). *The History of the Reform Movement in the Dental Profession in Great Britain during the last twenty years.* London: Trübner.

Kidd, C. (1868). *Brit. J. dent. Sci.*, **11**, 132.

Lancet (1868a), **1**, 481. Protoxide of nitrogen as an anaesthetic.

—— (1868b), **1**, 507. Medical annotation. A new anaesthetic (?).

Lindsay, L. (1955a). Personalities of the past. *Brit. dent. J.*, **48**, 405.

—— (1955b). Personalities of the past. *Brit. dent. J.*, **48**, 455.

Med-chir. Trans. (1864), **47**, 442. Report of the Committee appointed by the Royal Medical and Chirurgical Society to inquire into the uses and physiological therapeutical and toxical effects of chloroform, as well as into the best mode of administering it, and of observing any ill consequences resulting from its administration.

Parkinson, J. (1868). Protoxide of nitrogen as an anaesthetic. *Trans. odont. Soc.* (N.S.), **1**, 31.

Rymer, S. L. (1864). Remarks upon the use of nitrous oxide in dental operations. *Dent. Rev.* (N.S.), **1**, 1.

Sanderson, J. (1869). Protoxide of nitrogen as an anaesthetic. *Trans. odont. Soc.* (N.S.), **1**, 54.

Schoenbein, C. F. (1842). *Mittheilungen aus dem reisetagebuche eines deutshen naturforschers.* Basel.

Sibson, F. (1848). On death from chloroform. *Lond. med. Gaz.*, **42**, 108.

Smith, G. (1869). Protoxide of nitrogen as an anaesthetic. *Trans. odont. Soc.* (N.S.), **1**, 55.

Smith, W. D. A. (1965). A history of nitrous oxide and oxygen anaesthesia. Part II: Davy's researches in relation to inhalation anaesthesia. *Brit. J. Anaesth.*, **37**, 871.

—— (1966). A history of nitrous oxide and oxygen anaesthesia. Part V: The crucial experiment, its eclipse, and its revival. *Brit. J. Anaesth.*, **38**, 143.

Transactions of the Odontological Society of Great Britain (1868) (N.S.), **1**, 31. First Report of the Joint Committee to inquire into the "Value and advantages of the protoxide of nitrogen as an anaesthetic in surgical operations".

Underwood, J. (1868). *Brit. J. dent. Sci.*, **11**, 198.

Vasey, C. (1868). *Brit. J. dent. Sci.*, **11**, 207.

Walton, H. (1868a). *Brit. J. dent. Sci.*, **11**, 209.

—— (1868b). The use of protoxide of nitrogen gas. *Lancet*, **1**, 483.

9

T. W. EVANS—BEFORE AND AFTER*

ON March 2nd, 1868, Clover read a paper before the Odontological Society of Great Britain, entitled 'On the Administration of Chloroform in Dental Operations.' This sets the scene.

The 'Inconvenience and Danger' of Chloroform

Clover began his paper by commenting: 'The experience of Dentists caused them to hail with gladness the introduction of anæsthetics, but they were soon found to be attended with inconvenience and danger. . . . Those practitioners, who, in order to cut short the stage of excitement, gave the anæsthetic in strong doses, not unfrequently found their patients become so prostrate as to cause anxiety, and in a few cases death was produced.'

Clover's solution was to administer a known concentration of chloroform vapour from a large bag which was connected to a valved face mask. For the times the apparatus was well engineered and used with good effect, but none-the-less Clover cautioned: 'no amount of confidence in an instrument should cause us to relax our attention to the pulse for the commencement of faintness.'

Discussing nose-inhalers, Clover again stressed the importance of feeling the pulse: 'For my part, I merely exchange the face piece of my inhaler for a nose-cap provided with valves and apply it over the nose. It is retained *in situ* by a strap . . . and thus the chloroformist has his hands at liberty to watch the pulse.' He added 'it is necessary, if the patient is sitting in the chair, to watch the pulse a few minutes after the operation is over.' Clover claimed to have used his 'instrument in 1,802 cases, not only without any fatal result, but with uniform success in the induction of complete anæsthesia.'

In the discussion that followed this paper, however, Mr. Cattlin got up to say that 'he had no doubt there was less danger when the chloroform was administered according to Mr. Clover's method. Still, no one could have listened to his candid history of cases without observing that even under the most favourable circumstances it could not be given without danger. The chief questions for the Society to consider were, whether there was any antidote against the poisonous effects of chloroform, and if not, whether any means could be devised to lessen the danger of administering it.' These sentiments were echoed by Dr. Kidd, who drew particular attention to a contributory hazard: 'There was a danger in Dental operations', he said,

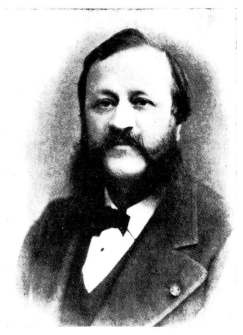

FIG. 1. — Thomas Wiltberger Evans (1823-1897). *By courtesy of the Wellcome Trustees.*

'from the patient's sitting up in the chair; the chair should be reclining. He had investigated the subject, and had collected no less than fifteen cases of death from chloroform in newspapers and journals in Dentists cases. . . .'

The last member to join in the discussion was Charles James Fox, who said that 'he would never consent to a medical man's giving chloroform to a patient at his (Mr. Fox's) house, unless Mr. Clover's apparatus was used. If patients wished their own medical men to administer it, he always expressed his readiness to attend at the patient's house or at the medical man's house, for . . . if an accident should happen, the medical man was not blamed, but it stuck to the dentist if the operation took place in his house. He had felt that so keenly, that he might say he had almost run the risk of offending his medical friends, but generally found a little explanation prevented so undesirable a result.' He added: 'Chloroform was always administered to his patients while they were lying down on a sofa.'

The President, Mr. James Parkinson, then tendered his very best thanks to Mr. Clover for his interesting and practical paper, and adjourned the Society 'until Monday, the 6th of April, when a

*Paper delivered at a meeting of the Lindsay Club on May 7, 1968. This article has been reproduced by kind permission of the Editor of the *British Dental Journal.*

paper will be read by Mr. Harrison, "On a case of Osseus Union of the Upper and Lower Maxillæ".' But events took another course. It was a discussion of a very different topic that took place on April 6 and the change of programme was the direct result of a visit to London, lasting barely a week, of Thomas Wiltberger Evans.

Thomas Wiltberger Evans

Dr. Evans (fig. 1) trained in Philadelphia and, in 1847, he joined a fellow American in Paris. Soon, he opened his own office and built up a successful high-class practice, including Napoleon III and several royal families among his patients. Although he is described in the 'Dictionary of American Biography' as having developed boundless conceit, his professional standards were high and he made significant contributions to advances in his speciality. He was also said to be generous and charitable. The bulk of his fortune went towards the establishment of the Thomas W. Evans Museum and Dental Institute which became the Dental School of Pennsylvania.

Evans Demonstrates Nitrous Oxide Anæsthesia in London

Evans came to London, in 1868, for the specific purpose of introducing his fellow-practitioners in England to the use of nitrous oxide as an anæsthetic agent. He had been instructed in its use by none other than Gardner Quincy Colton whom he had met in Paris in connexion with the Universal Exhibition held there in 1867. Evans soon became enthusiastic about the use of nitrous oxide and in a report upon the dental exhibits at the Paris Exhibition he wrote 'Dr. Colton has re-established by thousands of experiments the superiority of the protoxyde of nitrogen gas over other anæsthetics in Dental Surgery, particularly in operations which may be promptly effected.' He continued 'The gas has recently been even employed with success in Paris under my own direction in the gravest surgical operations. . . . Much and ingenious apparatus has been constructed in America for the preparation and inhalation of this valuable anæsthetic substance.'

The point has been made that Evans arrived in London at a time when there was anxiety about the use of chloroform for dental operations. This undoubtedly contributed to the outcome of his visit. But concern about chloroform anæsthesia was not new. Mortality figures had previously led the Royal Medical and Chirurgical Society to appoint a committee to look into the matter. Reporting in 1864, it gave details of animal experiments which confirmed that cardiac syncope was easily produced by high concentrations of chloroform, and that 'at times, even with every care, and with the most exact

dilution of the vapour, the state of insensibility may in a few moments pass into one of imminent death.'

By 1864, however, Colton was already achieving considerable success in America with the use of nitrous oxide for dental extractions. Why then was it necessary to wait until Colton visited Paris in 1867 and instructed Evans and until Evans had visited London in 1868, before nitrous oxide anæsthesia caught on in this country? The answer may be that practitioners in Britain were influenced by the indecisive attempts of Samuel Lee Rymer to emulate Colton in 1864.

Previous Experiments in London by Samuel Lee Rymer

In the previous year, 1863, Rymer noticed a brief account, in the *Dental Cosmos*, of two nitrous oxide anæsthetics administered by Colton. Soon afterwards the *Dental Cosmos* carried an advertisement which announced that Dr. Colton had 'associated himself with two eminent dentists . . . who devoted their exclusive attention to the extraction of teeth by the use of the gas.'

The advantages of the gas were summed up as follows: 'First—It *is perfectly harmless* and there is no danger of giving too much. Second—The insensibility induced is perfect and complete in *all cases* where a sufficient quantity is given. Third—The effects all pass off within three minutes from the commencement of the inhalation, leaving the patient feeling as well as before. Fourth—The danger and disagreeableness of inhaling ether and chloroform are all avoided.' It was added that 'to accomplish these results the gas must be made *very pure*, and be properly administered, and that Dr. Colton has already exhibited it for the extraction of more than 4,000 teeth, and with very decided success.'

At the meeting of the Odontological Society held in December 1863 Rymer rose to 'call the attention of the Society to a statement in the *Dental Cosmos* that the nitrous-oxide gas is being employed in America to produce anæsthesia' . . . and he said 'I merely call the attention of the Society to what is going on in America with regard to this nitrous oxide, because there may be value in it.' Mr. Coleman replied 'There is no novelty in the employment of nitrous oxide gas as an anæsthetic. Sir Humphry Davy first suggested it, and from his suggestion it was tried, and with some success; its failure on some occasions led to the introduction of ether. It is only the revival of an old idea.' Coleman may have made some trials of this 'old idea', on his own account, around that time, because in 1868 he mentioned that 'From experiments conducted by himself several years ago he did not consider that there was any very great difficulty in preparing the gas pure from nitrate of ammonia.'

Samuel Lee Rymer none-the-less went ahead with some preliminary experiments which were published early in 1864. He described his method thus: 'The usual method of inhaling nitrous oxide is from a bladder filled with the gas, and to which is attached a tube of wood. The mouth-piece is held by the right hand of the person inhaling the gas, the nostrils being held with the left. The tube is placed in the mouth, and the gas breathed from and into the bladder.

'For a practical purpose, such as the extraction of a tooth, the orifice of the tube must be much larger than for common experiments—in other respects, the inhalation is conducted after the same manner, except that it ought to be under the direction of a professional man, and it is desirable that two persons should be left in attendance on the patient—one to administer the gas, and the other to extract the tooth.'

His first subject was a lady of about twenty years, who inhaled the gas for two minutes, 'at the expiration of which period she bore pretty severe pinching without feeling, but she was not unconscious . . . the same patient inhaled the gas again (two days after the above trial), a more convenient mouthpiece having been adjusted to the bag. In less than two minutes, and with no excitement, complete unconsciousness ensued, from which she soon recovered (in about two minutes), and experienced no inconvenience. The sensation was described as remarkably pleasant. The eyes were closed, pupils fixed, and the pulse was considerably augmented.'

Mr. Hopgood then inhaled the gas and 'He scarcely felt some very sharp pinches administered to him during the experiment, although their effects were visible for two or three days afterwards upon his flesh.' The next subject was a young woman who behaved in much the same way as the first did at her second inhalation, from a bag.

Rymer considered the fifth and last experiment to be the most important. 'The patient (was) sixteen years of age . . . without the smallest excitement, (she) became unconscious, and appeared in a calm but profound sleep. An upper bicuspid tooth, considerably decayed, and requiring care in its removal, was then deliberately extracted by Mr. Perkins. Entire consciousness returned in two minutes. No unpleasant effect was experienced, but the reverse. . . . There could be no two opinions about this experiment. We who observed it, agreed that it was a complete success. The patient upon returning consciousness was surprised to learn the tooth had been extracted as she knew nothing at all about it.'

Rymer's final comment was 'I have only to add that the *uniform* success claimed by Dr. Colton is

to me a matter of perplexity. . . . Whether more complete knowledge will result in giving the operator a generally reliable agent in nitrous oxide gas remains to be proved or disproved.'

Rymer reported neither cyanosis nor lividity, although four years later he did admit that the experiments were discontinued because, apart from the inconvenience of manufacturing the gas, 'Dr. Odling advised them, if they proceeded at all, to do so with the utmost possible caution, because he considered its exhibition was attended with the greatest possible danger.' He mentioned that a vulcanised india-rubber bag and a bladder were used alternately, but he did not state the capacity of the bag. Recent experiments with ox bladders suggest that they are unlikely to have held more than about 4 litres.

Importance of the Size of Rebreathing Bag

Rymer described five administrations. He said that a *bag* was used for the second, so it should also have been used for the fourth. Consciousness was lost at the second and fourth administrations, and also at the fifth. Consciousness was not lost at the first administration and it does not appear to have been lost at the third. It is tempting to make the tentative suggestion that the bag was larger than the bladder and that it was used instead of the bladder for the fifth administration, perhaps in the light of the greater success achieved with the second and fourth administrations.

Horace Wells did not state the size of the bag he used at his unsuccessful attempt to demonstrate nitrous oxide anæsthesia at the Massachusetts General Hospital in 1845. If the bag was small this would help to explain his failure. We do know, however, that by 1868 Colton was using 8 gallon, or 30 litre bags. (He also mentioned that 2 to 3 gallon bags were then used for entertainment.) The significance of bag size has been demonstrated by the following simple laboratory experiments (Smith, 1967).

Illustrative Experiments

In the first experiment (fig. 2) a subject rebreathed about 5 litres of 80 per cent nitrous oxide from a spirometer, for one and a half minutes. There were subjective sensations but no loss of consciousness. The contents of the spirometer were reduced by about 1·2 litres and this can be accounted for mainly by the uptake of nitrous oxide from the lungs by the pulmonary circulation. He then rebreathed from a second spirometer which was filled initially with air. Note that the volume contents of this spirometer remained the same, suggesting that none of the nitrous oxide taken up during the first part of the experiment escaped from the body during the

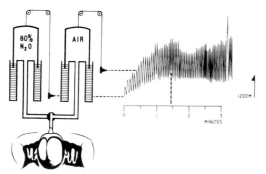

Fig. 2.—First Experiment: spirograms obtained while rebreathing first 5 litres of 80 per cent nitrous oxide, and then 5 litres of air, each for one and a half minutes.

second half. The reason for this will be made clear by the second experiment.

The second experiment (fig. 3) was a repetition of the first, but this time the gases passing into and

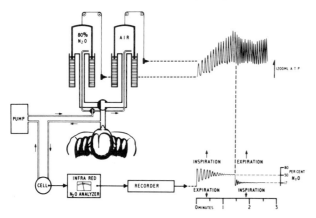

Fig. 3.—Second Experiment: repetition of the first experiment (fig. 2) while analysing the gases respired for nitrous oxide.

out of the mouth were analysed continuously for nitrous oxide. Although the concentration of nitrous oxide inhaled at the first breath was 80 per cent, the concentration inhaled at subsequent breaths fell to about 50 per cent, due to the gases initially in the lungs diluting the nitrous oxide initially in the spirometer. It is not surprising that the subject remained conscious. During the second half of the experiment, the nitrous oxide in the lungs at the end of the first part of the experiment contaminated the air in the second spirometer, so that the concentration of nitrous oxide inspired rose from nothing to about 17 per cent.

It so happens that if 1·2 litres of nitrous oxide taken up had been redistributed rapidly throughout the body's extracellular fluid, (a wider distribution might be expected) it would have been in equilibrium with 17 per cent nitrous oxide in the gaseous phase

in the lungs. This explains why no nitrous oxide was eliminated from the pulmonary circulation back into the lungs. The partial pressure of nitrous oxide was about the same in the pulmonary arterial blood and the alveoli. This effect was made use of in the third experiment.

In the third experiment (fig. 4) the amount of nitrous oxide mixture rebreathed was increased to about 12 litres—about half that used by Colton.

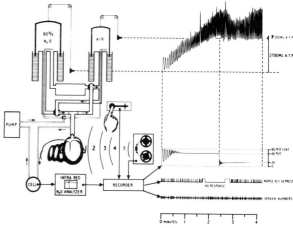

Fig. 4.—Third Experiment: similar to the first and second experiments, except that a larger volume of nitrous oxide was rebreathed and consciousness was lost. Non-return valves were arranged so that the subject inspired directly from the left hand spirometer, and breathed back into it through a rigid reservoir. While conscious, the subject responded to numbers broadcast from a tape recorder by pressing a Morse key.

The inspired concentration did not fall below about 60 per cent and the subject lost consciousness. In order to record the onset and duration of unconsciousness, numbers were spoken from a tape recorder, to which the subject responded by pressing a Morse key. Both the stimuli and the responses were recorded, as indicated. Consciousness was lost after about one and a half minutes Even though, as in the second experiment, no nitrous oxide was eliminated on rebreathing air from the second spirometer, the subject regained consciousness about half a minute after the change-over. The nitrous oxide which had been taken up was distributed throughout the body fluids. Its partial pressure in the body fell to levels less than that required to maintain narcosis.

These experiments make the point that the nitrous oxide rebreathed from a small bag would be too diluted by the gases already in the lungs to be able to produce anæsthesia, whereas unconsciousness can be produced by using a larger bag. The last experiment also demonstrates that two factors combine to hasten recovery after a brief anæsthetic; nitrous oxide is eliminated from the body and it is redistributed within the body.

Evans' Measurement of Nitrous Oxide Uptake

The volume of nitrous oxide taken up during the third experiment was just under three litres. Evans also measured the uptake of nitrous oxide and he obtained about the same result. He wrote: '. . . it is to be observed that when the condition of anæsthesia has been produced by the inhalation of nitrous oxide, the blood is by no means fully saturated with the gas.

'I have endeavoured to ascertain about how much nitrous oxide it is necessary to introduce into the blood to develop the anæsthetic state—to produce insensibility. In practice, five or six gallons are required, on the average, to put to sleep an adult. Some of this is wasted—nearly the whole quantity is expired during administration. How much really remains in the system . . . when the inhalation is suspended?

'Placing a large bell-glass in a pneumatic trough, after filling it with a given quantity of gas, I have caused the gas to be inspired in such a way as that the products of expiration should be received into another glass over the same trough . . . the difference between the volumes of gas in the two jars will show very nearly the actual amount of gas absorbed by the blood at the moment the inhalation is suspended. I have found this difference rarely to exceed *three quarts*.'—in other words, about three litres.

In this instance, Evans measured the uptake from a non-breathing system and it was a non-rebreathing system, using inspiratory and expiratory valves, which he demonstrated during his brief visit to London in 1868. The events of that week are revealed in the proceedings of the meeting of the Odontological Society of Great Britain which did take place on April 6, 1868.

Evans' Demonstrations Discussed by the Odontological Society of Great Britain

The President, Mr. Parkinson, opened the meeting by saying that 'They were no doubt aware that during the past week several operations in Dental Surgery had been performed, both at the Hospital and the residence of their zealous friend Mr. Hepburn, under the influence of nitrous oxide gas as an anæsthetic, brought under their notice by Dr. Evans of Paris. . . .' He then read out a letter written by Evans, addressed from Paris and dated April 5. Here are two extracts: 'Constantly occupying myself with the means of mitigating human sufferings, and being much impressed both with the advantages and the inconveniences which attend the employment of ether and chloroform, I interested myself with anæsthetical researches made in Europe and in America, and more especially with those experiments made in the United States in view of rendering practicable the employment of nitrous oxide gas for surgical operations. . . . I made arrangements with Dr. Colton, in order that, utilising his large experience and adding my own observations and my conscientious investigations, I might surely and effectually introduce the employment of this anæsthetic in Europe.'

'The results that I made in Paris were so satisfactory that I felt it my duty to make them known to my fellow-practitioners of England, and the generous and unanimous approbation they have given to my demonstrations have proved to me that I was right to rely upon their collaboration.

'. . . desirous that the largest possible number, and especially the poor of London, should benefit by the advantages which result from the employment of this agent when administered by skilful hands and competent men, I beg to offer to the Dental Hospital of London "One Hundred Pounds", to be used for the purchase of apparatus and materials to manufacture the nitrous oxide gas.'

Evans apparently appreciated that nitrous oxide might not provide the final answer, for he continued: 'However, if, after more experience, our common hope should not be entirely realised, and the officers of the Hospital should decide to discontinue its use, they would be authorised to employ the remaining sum for the employment of any other anæsthetic that in their judgement would better fulfil the object in view.'

Offer to Administer Nitrous Oxide at the Dental Hospital

Mr. Underwood then described how, on Monday, March 30, 1868, he had been approached by Dr. Evans who had offered to administer nitrous oxide on the following day at the Dental Hospital. Underwood reported that 'Dr. Evans laid special stress that the gas should be made at least twenty-four hours before it was used and that it should be washed thoroughly four times.' He said that 'Evans told him that inhalation took an exceedingly short time; that it was necessary that the operator should be as rapid as possible, as the patient would recover in the course of a very few seconds after the operation was concluded. The gas was contained in a very large bag with a gutta-percha tube having attached to it a bone or ebony mouth piece . . . and and ordinary stop cock which contained an inspiring and expiring valve.' He continued: 'Dr. Evans told him that the signs of unconsciousness were pallidity of the face, snoring, extreme dilation of the pupil and fixedness of the eye. . . . Dr. Evans, in commencing, introduced into the mouth a wooden gag on the opposite side to that on which they were about to operate.'

Underwood went on to describe the first eleven

cases anæsthetised at the Dental Hospital. All but three were females. Ages ranged from 11 to 34 years, averaging 22. Duration of administration was not stated in one case and was uncertain for another, but with the remainder it lasted from 47 seconds to one minute and 54 seconds, averaging 67 seconds. No patient felt pain, although one, a very nervous woman of 34, who had an excessively tender abscess, felt the tooth coming out. He remarked upon the decided blue cast of the face and that there were symptoms 'which in the case of chloroform he should have looked upon as alarming, and should have discontinued its use. . . . He believed that the agent was an exceedingly valuable one, but it must be used . . . with excessive care, especially in the hands of practitioners who had not given their attention to the subject of anæsthetics . . . it appeared to him that the patient was brought apparently to the verge of dissolution, and that instantly the gas was removed a reaction took place.'

Mr. Hepburn, after commenting that Dr. Evans had fitted up a room at the Langham Hotel[1] for the purpose of preparing the nitrous oxide, went on to say that the experiments he had witnessed 'were thoroughly successful. . . . In fact the results were perfectly marvellous.' He thought that the gas 'would do away with a great deal of the time occupied, to say the least of it, in chloroform cases, and that it was a boon and a blessing to humanity.'

Mr. Coleman maintained that: 'Nitrous oxide gas appeared to offer advantages which neither chloroform nor ether procured.' These he detailed as: rapidity of effect; rapidity of recovery; fewer disagreeable side effects and the agreeable taste of the gas. Although he commented that 'None of the patients complained of sickness, giddiness or headache' he was cautious about this point, for he went on to say 'Still, they had at present too little data to go upon, and it might be remembered that some of the celebrated chemists of the last century had suffered from sickness and fainting, which effects did not pass off for some days after inhaling the gas.'

He considered that 'the gas resembled air in a state of effervescence.'

Two Disadvantages Named

He named two disadvantages. The first was the same as the second advantage—rapidity of recovery. The second was 'the greater difficulty of obtaining this agent over chloroform or ether.' He agreed with Underwood that the appearance of patients during nitrous oxide anæsthesia 'certainly would, in a patient under chloroform, appear very alarming. But, perhaps, the great ground for safety in this

agent might be considered to be . . . that the inhalations occupied so short a time, that the moment the agent was removed, the individual was able to inspire pure air, and very soon threw off the effects of the anæsthetic. . . . The real condition here rather more approached that of asphyxia than narcotism. . . . The question of safety could only be decided by long experience, and though Dr. Evans spoke very confidently, and said they would soon get accustomed to those symptoms, and even disregard them, yet he hoped it would be a long time before operators would disregard such symptoms as those, and it was evident from the cautious way in which Dr. Evans administered this gas, that he himself was aware that it was a thing not to be trifled with.'

Mr. Vasey reinforced Mr. Underwood's remarks, saying that: 'The appearance of the patient whilst under the influence of nitrous oxide was most appalling. There was a general asphyxiated condition, the whole countenance and lips presented a most fearfully livid appearance, and one of the gentlemen who was watching the pulse, said it was depressed. . . . It seemed to him as if Dr. Evans, from great experience, was able to tell the precise moment when the inhalation should cease and the operator perform the operation. He thoroughly supported that a committee should be appointed, so that the whole subject should be carefully investigated. It would be well that experiments should be performed on some of the lower animals.'

Mr. Coleman, however, thought that 'a question like this should not be confined to a small committee but could only be answered by a very large number of experimenters entering the field with a view of discovering whether they were really a great boon to humanity, or whether it were too dangerous an agent for them to operate with.' Mr. Cattlin, on the other hand, 'thought the Society should suspend its sanction to the use of nitrous oxide until its action as an anæsthetic had been thoroughly investigated by a committee of the Society.'

Clover then 'contrasted the effects of laughing gas in use in former times, and the effects experienced with protoxyde of nitrogen lately' and he made the point that 'it used to be inhaled by means of a bladder . . . the result of which was he would never at any time breathe so pure a nitrous oxide as he did in the present plan, by which expired air at once escaped by valves. There would not be such a complete arrest of oxidation in the former method as there was now.' He 'thought that the instrument he exhibited at the last meeting would be of great service, having a contrivance for completely covering the mouth and nose, and for regulating the admission of air. He also exhibited a nose-piece which would be very useful in dental operations

---

[1]Situated opposite Broadcasting House, now called 'The Langham' and used by the British Broadcasting Corporation for office accommodation.

where the mouth was required to be open.' He concluded with the following words of comfort: 'As long as the gas was given pure, the results would be exceedingly uniform, and would be very much a mixture of faintness and asphyxia. In all cases where the effects were fully produced, there would be a great failing of the pulse, and in some instances, it would be found to be arrested. But it was likely to be a much less serious affair to have the heart stopped as the result of an agent of this kind than when chloroform had been administered for some considerable time.'

The Nitrous Oxide Committee

After some further discussion, Mr. Cattlin proposed that 'Mr. Tomes, Mr. Coleman, Mr. Hepburn, Mr. Underwood, with the President, Treasurer, and Secretaries be a committee to investigate the anæsthetic properties of nitrous oxide gas with power to call in any scientific aid, and to report the results of such investigation at some future meeting.' This was agreed to and the President then adjourned the Society until Monday, May 4, when it was arranged that Mr. Harrison would read his paper on a 'Remarkable Case of Deformity of the Mouth remedied by Treatment.'

The Brevity and Impact of Evans' Visit

Evans gave his first demonstration in London on Tuesday, March 31, he returned to Paris on Saturday and he wrote a letter on Sunday which was read out at the meeting of the Odontological Society on Monday, April 6. The decision to change the subject of that meeting must have been taken within this short period. Underwood's opening remarks read as if he had known nothing of Evans before Monday, March 30, yet, one would have expected Evans to have taken some steps to pave the way for his visit. Evidence of this appears to be lacking. The immediate impact of his visit is astonishing. It is not obvious how much this was due to his personal qualities and how much to the nagging anxieties about chloroform.

Subsequent Developments

Coleman's wish was granted. A large number of practical experimenters did enter the field—even if their experiments were not particularly scientific—and their evidence was collected by the committee. But the committee's preliminary report, made at the end of 1868 and its final report made in 1872, made no startling contributions. Conclusions drawn from animal experiments had little to add to those made by Davy in 1800. Caution was advised in the use of nitrous oxide with patients with disease of the brain, heart, arteries and lungs, and patients of very plethoric habit and short neck. It con-

sidered the gas unsuitable for long operations. The significance of lividity and pallor was played down with these words 'to those accustomed to administer this gas, these symptoms give no alarm.'

The final report drew the conclusion that nitrous oxide 'induced anæsthesia by preventing oxidation.' The use of mixtures of nitrous oxide and oxygen was tried, but with unsatisfactory results and the experiments were dropped. By 1872 the committee had collected 58,000 cases of administration of the gas.

The year 1868 saw the beginnings of other facets of nitrous oxide anæsthesia with which we are familiar, such as the use of gas and air by Clover and Fox; the absorption of carbon dioxide by Coleman; Cattlin's reservoir bag; the importance of avoiding leaks due to flow resistance in the anæsthetic apparatus which Clover tackled by placing a supplemental bag near the face and so on.

In 1868, Evans' visit was followed by one from Colton, and it was observed that 'Dr. Colton pushes the gas much further than we have been in the habit of doing; he looks upon a sound approaching to stertorous breathing, and on the twitching of fingers, as indications that the patient is in profound sleep.' Once the gas was accepted as expedient, however, subsequent progress was slow. Sixteen years later Buxton expostulated: 'All, at present, is more or less tentative; our evidence is fragmentary; our deductions open to cavil. Of one thing there is no uncertainty—that our present methods are clumsy and unscientific; that in their adoption we

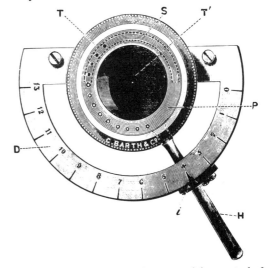

FIG. 5.—The nitrous oxide and oxygen mixing control of Hewitt's original gas and oxygen apparatus as made by Messrs. Barth & Co. The central tube T conducted nitrous oxide. Oxygen was conducted from the outer concentric tube T' through small holes, the number uncovered depending upon the position of the lever H.

risk the welfare of our patient, and by shutting our eyes to their imperfection we close the door to useful research.' The previous year he had drawn attention to Paul Bert's classic experiments with gas and oxygen, yet it was another nine years before Hewitt introduced the first practical apparatus for administering reasonably controlled mixtures containing up to 10 per cent oxygen (fig. 5). (No example of this apparatus appears to have survived.)

It was not until very late in the last century that interest in the nasal administration of nitrous oxide was revived and its adaptation for use with mixtures of gas and oxygen had to wait for Bellamy Gardner early in this century. Its adoption was slow, however, even in teaching hospitals.

There is a familiarity about many of these early discussions surrounding dental anæsthesia. It would be salutary to know the verdict of an historian of anæsthesia, writing in 2068, on present practice and controversies—assuming that our civilization is extant.

ACKNOWLEDGMENTS

Assistance from the Wellcome Trust is gratefully acknowledged. Figures 2, 3 and 4 are reproduced by permission of the *British Journal of Anæsthesia*.

BIBLIOGRAPHY

Buxton, D. W. (1883) *Brit. J. dent. Sci.*, 26, 1141.
—— (1884) *Brit. J. dent. Sci.*, 27, 147.
Chloroform Committee (1864) *Med.-Chir. Trans.*, 47, 442.
Clover, J. T. (1868) *Brit. J. dent. Sci.*, 11, 123.
Coleman, A. (1868) *Brit. J. dent. Sci.*, 11, 205.
Colton, G. Q. (1868) *Brit. J. dent. Sci.*, 11, 253.
Davy, H. (1800) Researches, Chemical and Philosophical: chiefly concerning nitrous oxide, or dephlogisticated nitrous air, and its respiration. J. Johnson, London.
Evans, T. W. (1868) Report upon Dental Surgery and the material which it employs. Paris Universal Exhibition, 1867. Class XI, Group II.
—— (1869) *Dent. Cosmos*, 11, 449.
Gardner, H. B. (1907) Prolonged Anæsthesia under Nitrous Oxide and Oxygen for Dental Operations. John Bale, Sons and Danielsson, London.
Hewitt, F. W. (1892) *Trans. odont. Soc.*, N.S., 24, 194.
Nitrous Oxide Committee, First Report. (1868) *Trans. odont. Soc.*, N.S., 1, 31.
——, Second Report (1872) *Trans. odont. Soc.*, N.S., 5, 11.
Rymer, S. L. (1863) *Brit. J. dent. Sci.*, 11, 543.
—— (1864) *Dent. Rev.*, N.S., 1, 1.
—— (1868) *Brit. J. dent. Sci.*, 11, 202.
Smith, W. D. A. (1967) *Brit. J. Anæsth.*, 39, 464.

10

TWENTY YEARS OF NITROUS OXIDE ANAESTHESIA IN GREAT BRITAIN

But the necessity for a means of prolonging the anaesthesia became vastly more important when nitrous oxide came into use, and here it was that our friends of now quite a past generation were sadly perplexed. They spoke of the agent in no very complimentary terms, and their patients were in much the same condition of mind as the Irish gentleman who described his experience of a ride in a Sedan chair. "If it had not been for the honour of the thing he would rather have walked." The unfortunate gentleman had been put into one without bottom or seat.

(Coleman, 1898)

Almost as soon as it became known in Great Britain that the use of nitrous oxide as an inhalation anaesthetic was a practical proposition a Committee was formed to investigate its anaesthetic properties. This presented a Preliminary Report within the year (*Trans. odont. Soc.,* 1868), and its conclusions were outlined in Part VII (Smith, 1966). Its Final Report was not presented until 1872 (*Trans. odont. Soc.,* 1872).

The Final Report had nothing to contribute towards an understanding of the physiological action of nitrous oxide, other than to draw the general conclusion, from experiments carried out on animals and humans, that nitrous oxide induced anaesthesia by preventing oxidation. In Great Britain, it was not until fourteen years later that Buxton (1886) reintroduced the idea ". . . that nitrous oxide produced narcosis by virtue of other than asphyxiating properties".

With regard to ". . . prolonging the anaesthetic effect of the gas, so as to make it more available for operations on the mouth requiring time, or for surgical operations generally", the Committee reported that

. . . this has been accomplished in a number of ways; viz., when the operation is in the mouth, by continuing the inhalation of the gas through the nose during the operation, by means of a nose-piece adjusted to the gas tube, the supply of gas being regulated according to circumstances; or by throwing a jet of gas into the mouth at each inspiration while the operation is proceeding, the nose, in the latter case, being closed by a spring clip; and when the operation is on any other part of the body, by checking and re-supplying the gas through the face-piece from time to time, as circumstances may require.

The Committee reported that with the improvement in the making and in the administration of the gas, the occurrence of anomalous symptoms had become less frequent; and it regretted that the gas was not used more often in many minor operations of surgery. The members of the Committee closed their Report by

. . . recording their opinion of the comparative safety of this anaesthetic as contrasted with any other yet discovered, seeing that out of the 58,000 cases of its administration in this country of which they have records, and the thousands of its known administration both in this and other countries of which no special records have reached them, not a single case of death fairly referable to the action of this gas has occurred; but while they have great pleasure in recording this fact, they feel it to be an imperative duty to repeat here the caution for proper care in its administration, given in their former Report, as it is clear, from its effects on animals when carried beyond a certain point, that death may be produced by it in the human being, if carelessly or recklessly used, or if used by persons not properly trained to its administration.

The Final Report of the Nitrous Oxide Committee added little to its Preliminary Report of 1868: indeed, there were no radical changes in the practice of anaesthesia for the ambulant patient in Great Britain during the next twenty years, apart, perhaps, from an increasing use of nitrous oxide instead of chloroform for short operations, and apart from the early introduction of ether as a means of prolonging nitrous oxide anaesthesia. As late as 1895, however, Buxton wrote:

Even in Great Britain the employment of nitrous oxide is not very common except in the larger towns of England. In the country districts, and in Scotland, chloroform still reigns supreme, and not a few medical men are almost ignorant of the practical points involved in the administration of laughing gas. . . . Whether every hospital possessing say, fifty beds, owns an apparatus for giving the gas at present is, we think, very doubtful. Thus it would appear that either nitrous oxide is an unsatisfactory anaesthetic, or its uses are restricted within too narrow a compass.

Although the actual practice of anaesthesia may not have changed significantly, there were signs of a changing attitude to the subject and of an awareness of developments taking place on the Continent. These crystallized in the publication of three textbooks on anaesthesia which were published in 1888 (Buxton; Hewitt; Silk), and in Hewitt's preliminary communication on nitrous oxide and oxygen anaesthesia published in 1889.

By 1874, Clover claimed to have used nitrous oxide in 6960 cases. He did not indicate how many of these were for dental extractions, but he mentioned its use for a variety of operations.

It is by far the best anaesthetic for many short operations, such as the extraction of teeth, opening abscesses or boils. It answers very well in operating for strabismus. Removal of the eyeball was performed lately by Mr. Bowman for a lady, who said she had no consciousness of the operation. It is well suited for examining hysterical cases, wrenching stiff joints and reducing luxations of recent date. I do not think that it is suitable for cases where it is necessary to

keep the patient quiet for more than three or four minutes; but, if the patient be allowed to recover consciousness after one inhalation before another is commenced, the anaesthesia may be kept up tolerably well for half an hour. I have never kept a patient unconscious for more than between six and seven minutes; but if quietude is not important, I have no doubt that a patient could be prevented from feeling pain for an hour. But although this is possible, I am sure the recovery afterwards would not be satisfactory.

Prophetically, Clover (1874) wrote: "If nitrous oxide should prove fatal, I think it will happen from the occurrence of syncope, from some other cause, during the inhalation." He continued: "Arrested breathing would soon be remedied by artificial respiration, if the heart were still beating. I have, on three occasions, been obliged to resort to this means, and the recovery in all these cases was satisfactory in less than three minutes."

Clover (1874) used nitrous oxide to prepare the way for giving ether in two ways:

(1) By means of a bag of gas, I make the patient unconscious, and then give ether as usual; but the patients sometimes wake up enough to struggle against the ether. . . . (2) By using a small bag which

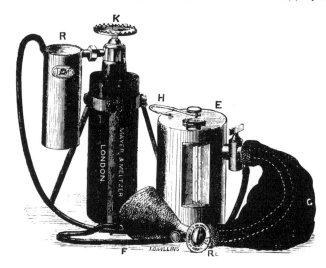

FIG. 1

Clover's apparatus for administering nitrous oxide gas and ether singly or combined.

F face-piece; Re regulator; G indiarubber bag; E ether vessel; H hook to attach the latter to a strap passing round the neck; K foot key; R gas rarifier.

By adjusting the regulator the patient could be made to breathe either directly into the bag or indirectly through the tube and the ether vessel.

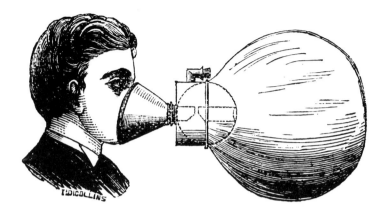

FIG. 2
Clover's portable regulating ether-inhaler.

is supplied with gas during the inhalation, and by diverting the current of gas and making the supply of gas pass over ether, as soon as the patient loses consciousness, enough ether can be got into the system in this way to keep up anaesthesia for three minutes with the mouth open. It is, therefore, well suited for small operations in the mouth, such as the extraction of difficult teeth.

Two years later Clover (1876) introduced a machine designed specifically for administering nitrous oxide and ether, singly or combined (fig. 1). Later (Clover, 1877) he commented:

Experience in more than three thousand cases in which I have used it convinces me that the administration of ether may be made far less unpleasant to the patient, and equally effective and safe, by first giving enough gas to render the patient unconscious to its taste. . . . The apparatus, however, requires a little more attention to temperature and other details, and is rather too complicated for general use.

He overcame the difficulty (Clover, 1877) by "having the ether-vessel placed close against the face-piece, so as to receive more warmth from the patient's breath and from the hand of the administrator". The new apparatus was called the "portable regulating ether-inhaler" (fig. 2). It consisted essentially of a face-piece, a vaporizer and a bag connected in series. There were no valves and the patient rebreathed through the vaporizer into the bag. One half of the ether vessel was surrounded by a water jacket, and the proportion of respired air passing through the ether vessel could be adjusted by rotating the

vaporizing unit on the facepiece. It was intended for giving ether without gas, "but, by connecting the bag with a supply of nitrous oxide, it forms a tolerably efficient substitute for the gas and ether-inhaler above mentioned". Later he wrote: "My experience with this portable inhaler is limited, simply because I prefer my original Gas and Ether Inhaler" (Duncum, 1947, p. 344).

Meanwhile Coleman was also active in the field of dental anaesthesia. In 1869 he introduced his economizing apparatus for reinhaling the gas (fig. 3), in which a canister containing lime was interposed between the mask and two reservoir bags. The reservoir bags were connected in series but separated by a non-return valve. Fresh gas was supplied to the distal bag as required, and rebreathing into the proximal bag was controlled by manipulating the expiratory valve. The apparatus was "used by Mr. Coleman at the Dental Hospital of London every Thursday morning", but it did not come into general use.

In 1871 he demonstrated to members of the Odontological Society

. . . a very simple contrivance for always enabling them to have the pads of their face-pieces tense. Both air and water, they were aware, found their way after a time through india-rubber tube. To the pad, then, he had connected a small india-rubber tube, through which, at any time, air or water could be introduced.

Coleman (1875) presented his own apparatus for administering nitrous oxide with ether (fig. 4).

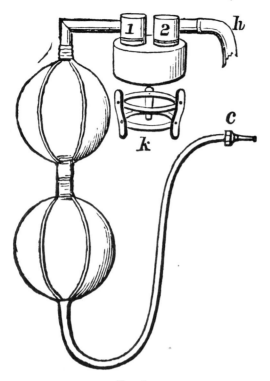

FIG. 3

Coleman's economizing apparatus.

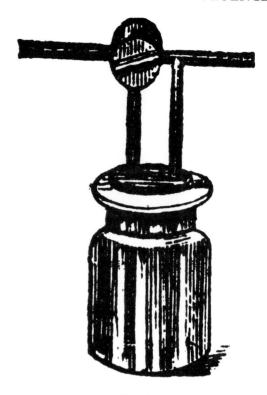

FIG. 4

Coleman's apparatus for administering nitrous oxide with ether.

In bringing the apparatus into notice he was especially anxious

... that it should not be forgotten that to Mr. Clover is due the great credit for first employing these two anaesthetics in combination, thereby doing away with the great drawbacks of each, viz., the short period of insensibility afforded by nitrous oxide, and the pungent irritating effects of ether.

The apparatus was "not offered to compete with the very perfect instrument which has been introduced by Mr. Clover", but it was "simply a much less costly and complex arrangement". He described his method of using it.

When employed for a short operation pure gas alone is permitted to enter the bag, and the patient so anaesthetised; when, however, it is desired to prolong anaesthesia, about a gallon of gas is allowed to enter the bag, and when this has been respired about a gallon more is permitted to enter the bag, but in so doing is made, by turning the two-way stopcock, to first pass through the ether, and so take up a considerable quantity of that fluid. By closing the expira-tory valve (there being no inspiratory valve) the mixture of gas and ether is respired over and over again. The results, after a considerable experience, are said to be most satisfactory.

Marsh (1880) gave some indication of the variety in techniques of nitrous oxide anaesthesia used at the time.

Gas administration is conducted in so many ways, that what with Clover's supplemental bag, Cattlin's bag, Coleman's economizer, Barth's apparatus, and various gasometers now in use, all of which have their special advantages and supporters, one is liable to fix upon a way of giving gas and fancying *this method* the *best of all*. For the sake, then, of discussing this point, pardon my saying, I prefer using a twelve-gallon gasometer fitted up with a hundred-gallon iron bottle of gas underneath. . . .

In the light of present beliefs, some of the practices of that period were not above criticism. For example, Tanner (1892b), describing the routine administration of nitrous oxide, wrote:

No absolute rule can be laid down as to when to cease administration of the gas. Experience alone will teach this. The slow regular respirations which immediately succeed the rapid breathing of the earliest stage, is a sign that anaesthesia is complete; and immediately after a slight tremor or twitching will probably appear; this is soon after followed by signs of laryngeal stertor. A sufficient degree of anaesthesia has now been produced for the commencement of most small operations, as the extraction of one or two teeth or loose roots; should, however, the operation be likely to last longer, a few more inspirations of the gas may be allowed with perfect safety. The respiration now becomes markedly stertorous and distinctly intermittent; convulsive twitchings extend to the arms and legs, amounting almost to jactitations; and if the gas is still pressed tonic spasm sets in. The pulse is distinctly intermittent. Beyond this it is dangerous to proceed and in the majority of cases it is not advisable to proceed further than the development of stertor, as the very trifling prolongation of the anaesthesia obtained is more than counteracted by the trouble in restraining the movements of the spasmodic patient.

Tanner (1892a) advised against the administration of more than two anaesthetics to the same patient on the same day!

Hilliard (1898) described the methods which were used for prolonging anaesthesia:

Anaesthetists are agreed that nitrous oxide would be a perfect anaesthetic for dental anaesthetics but for the brevity, after removal of the face-piece, of the available anaesthesia produced by its inhalation. Hitherto, therefore, only operations of the shortest duration could be attempted where nitrous oxide has been employed, while for those cases requiring an anaesthetic of two or more minutes duration the nitrous oxide has to be in the vast majority of cases supplemented by the use of ether.

After commenting on the unpleasant side effects that are liable to follow the use of ether, Hilliard (1898) continued:

It is obvious, therefore, that if an anaesthesia of several minutes duration, after removal of the face-piece, can be obtained with nitrous oxide, by whatever means, this agent will be used with increasing frequency. . . . Up to the present time the means adopted for prolonging the anaesthetic effect of nitrous oxide have been very imperfect, being based for the most part upon the principle of preventing the elimination of the gas, thereby obtaining merely a slightly prolonged anaesthesia; but by preventing this elimination we must prevent or impede respiration also. Such methods, for instance, as pushing backward the lower jaw together with the tongue, thereby closing the orifice of the larynx, or by passing a sponge upon a holder backwards and downwards into the pharynx, produced very marked congestion and cyanosis with jactitation—in fact, the signs of impending asphyxia. The patient under these circumstances is in a very dangerous condition. . . . In almost every reported case of death occurring during the exhibition of nitrous oxide it has resulted from obstructed respiration and consequent asphyxia.

One might ask why the idea of using a nasal inhaler with nitrous oxide and air (Clover, 1868a, b, c, d; Coleman, 1862) was not followed up, but according to Hilliard (1898) this was abandoned because

. . . the results did not prove sufficiently satisfactory. . . . The apparatus was difficult to keep properly adjusted, so much air was breathed through the mouth that the anaesthesia was uncertain, and finally the gas could not be supplied at sufficient pressure to obviate this evil without being likely to cause damage to the olfactory region, the frontal or even the maxillary sinuses.

Nineteen years after Evans's introduction of nitrous oxide anaesthesia into Great Britain, O'Neill (1887) expressed his dissatisfaction with the lack of subsequent progress in no uncertain terms.

Since the introduction of nitrous oxide as an anaesthetic agent into the realms formerly held in almost absolute sovereignty by chloroform, there is probably no other operative branch of dentistry which has remained so much the same, and which has seen less change about its surrounding requirements as the methods of administering nitrous oxide gas. . . . When the gas had achieved its first success, so as to draw the power and attention of good men to its use, it is undeniable that the verdict among good operators, mostly habituated to rely upon chloroform, was decidedly averse and unpropitious towards it, as being unreliable, of short duration in its anaesthetic action, etc. But this decision has received, at the hands of many eminent and skilful men, great modification. . . . Reviewing the science of dentistry—British or otherwise—as applying to any advancement made in the direction of the administration of the gas and its surrounding concomitants, a mediocrity will be seen in comparison with many other branches of dental art that have effected improvement with rapid and brilliant strides.

O'Neill was not alone. Buxton (1883a) (fig. 5) had already complained about the lack of research in this country.

In spite of the most untoward disabilities under which all research of an experimental nature is prosecuted in England, the solution of many burning questions in the field of anaesthetics may yet be hoped for, and may be, are not too far distant. It is a matter of regret, that most English observers in this department have devoted themselves more exclusively to what we may call the clinical side of research. . . . To satisfy us upon these points we must go outside English laboratories, and seek in France and Germany for those philosophical experiments which, it appears to us, should have originated here.

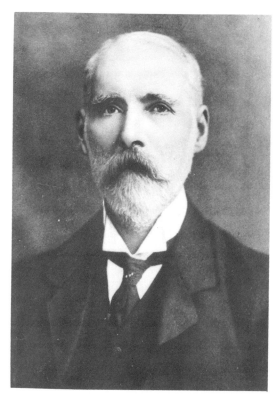

FIG. 5
Dudley Wilmot Buxton (1855–1931).
(By courtesy of the *Lancet*.)

Dealing more specifically with nitrous oxide, Buxton (1883a) said:

The drugs which we now employ have to enter the blood stream, and so exert their deleterious effects to every organ of the body, as in the case with nitrous oxide. . . . To Dentists it is a matter of no small importance that the patient should be absolutely quiet, and his efforts should not be frustrated by a cumbrous mouthpiece or too rapid recovery from anaesthesia. And although nitrous oxide is so largely used by the profession, it cannot be doubted that they would welcome with avidity, either a more perfect method for the administration of nitrous oxide, or its replacement by an agent as safe, but which is capable of prolonging the length of time which anaesthesia endured.

Later (Buxton, 1883b), after condemning the attempts made in America to prolong nitrous oxide anaesthesia by the repeated application and removal of the mask, he drew attention to the work of Paul Bert in France, which had led to the performance of operations lasting up to 26

minutes using nitrous oxide and oxygen mixtures at high pressure, recovery taking place within half a minute and without ill effects.

Buxton (1884) summed up the position at that time, in these words:

All, at present, is more or less tentative; our evidence is fragmentary; our deductions open to cavil. Of one thing there is no uncertainty—that our present methods are clumsy and unscientific; that in their adoption we risk the welfare of our patient, and by shutting our eyes to their imperfection we close the door to useful research and a line of physiological discovery likely to produce vast stores of information such as will prove of immense service to the whole human race.

ACKNOWLEDGEMENTS

I am indebted to the Department of Medical Photography, the University of Leeds and Leeds United Hospitals, for figures 1–4, and to the Department of Illustrations, the Wellcome Historical Medical Library and Museum, for figure 5.

REFERENCES

Buxton, D. W. (1883a). The experimental study of the action of anaesthetics. *Brit. J. dent. Sci.*, **26**, 1093.
—— (1883b). The experimental study of the action of anaesthetics. II: *Brit. J. dent. Sci.*, **26**, 1141.
—— (1884). The experimental study of the action of anaesthetics. IV: *Brit. J. dent. Sci.*, **27**, 147.
—— (1886). On the physiological action of nitrous oxide. *Trans. Odont. Soc.*, N.S. **18**, 133.
—— (1888). *Anaesthetics: their uses and administration.* London: H. K. Lewis.
Clover, J. T. (1868a). On the administration of chloroform in dental operations. *Brit. J. dent. Sci.*, **11**, 123.
—— (1868b). *Brit. J. dent. Sci.*, **11**, 212.
—— (1868c). The administration of nitrous oxide as an anaesthetic. *Brit. med. J.*, **2**, 201.
—— (1868d). On the administration of nitrous oxide. *Brit. med. J.*, **2**, 491.
—— (1874). Remarks on the production of sleep during surgical operations. *Brit. med. J.*, **1**, 200.
—— (1876). On an apparatus for administering nitrous oxide gas and ether, singly or combined. *Brit. med. J.*, **2**, 74.
—— (1877). Portable regulating ether-inhaler. *Brit. med. J.*, **1**, 69.
Coleman, A. (1862). An instrument for administering the vapour of chloroform through the nose. *Lancet*, **1**, 42.
—— (1869). Mr. Coleman's economizing apparatus for re-inhaling the gas. *Brit. J. dent. Sci.*, **12**, 443.
—— (1871). *Trans. odont. Soc.*, N.S. **3**, 236.
—— (1875). Apparatus for administering nitrous oxide with ether. *Brit. J. dent. Sci.*, **18**, 354.
—— (1898). On a method of administering anaesthetics through the nose. *Trans. Soc. Anaesth.*, **1**, 117.
Duncum, B. M. (1947). *The Development of Inhalation Anaesthesia: with special reference to the years 1846–1900.* London: Oxford University Press.

Hewitt, F. (1888). *Select Methods in the Administration of Nitrous Oxide and Ether.* London: Baillière, Tindall & Cox.

—— (1889). On the anaesthesia produced by the administration of mixtures of nitrous oxide and oxygen (preliminary notice). *Lancet*, **1**, 832.

Hilliard, H. (1898). A method of prolonging nitrous oxide anaesthesia in dental practice. *Lancet*, **1**, 1244.

Marsh, H. (1880). Notes on nitrous oxide gas. *Brit. J. dent. Sci.*, **23**, 1015.

O'Neill, T. G. (1887). Concerning nitrous oxide gas. *Brit. J. dent. Sci.*, **30**, 267.

Silk, J. F. (1888). *A Manual of Nitrous Oxide Anaesthesia*, p. 28. London: Churchill.

Smith, W. D. A. (1966). A history of nitrous oxide and oxygen anaesthesia. Part VII: 1868—Nitrous oxide anaesthesia takes root in Great Britain. *Brit. J. Anaesth.*, **38**, 551.

Tanner, F. L. (1892a). General anaesthetics in the dental surgery. *Brit. J. dent. Sci.*, **35**, 97.

—— (1892b). General anaesthetics in the dental surgery. *Brit. J. dent. Sci.*, **35**, 155.

Transactions of the Odontological Society of Great Britain (1868), N.S. **1**, 31. First report of the Joint Committee appointed by the Odontological Society of Great Britain, and the Committee of Management of the Dental Hospital of London, to inquire into the "Value and Advantages of the Protoxide of Nitrogen as an Anaesthetic in Surgical Operations".

Transactions of the Odontological Society of Great Britain (1872), N.S. **5**, 11. Second Report of the Joint Committee appointed by the Odontological Society of Great Britain, and the Committee of Management of the Dental Hospital of London, to inquire into the "Value and Advantages of the Protoxide of Nitrogen as an Anaesthetic in Surgical Operations".

11

THE INTRODUCTION OF NITROUS OXIDE AND OXYGEN ANAESTHESIA

It is to be much regretted that the vast difference between anaesthesia and asphyxia has been almost entirely overlooked by writers on anaesthesia.

(Hayes, 1887)

The inhalation of a mixture of nitrous oxide and oxygen was tried by Hermann as early as 1867:

. . . on two occasions, when he inhaled this gas (nitrous oxide) in a pure state, he was completely asphyxiated. The effect nevertheless was not unpleasant, because the intoxicating effect of the gas overpowered the sensation of dyspnoea, although it was undoubtedly present. This condition of asphyxia, in which the face is pale and the lips blue, differs very much from that produced by inhaling the same gas mixed with oxygen, in the proportion 4 to 1. The experimentalist is intoxicated, but in a less degree, and the face retains its natural colour. M. Hermann remarks that surgeons, not now contented with ordinary anaesthetics, are trying this kind of inhalation; he thinks that, inhaled by itself, the protoxide of nitrogen is dangerous, as it is likely to produce a mortal asphyxia; and if administered mixed with oxygen, it is a very weak anaesthetic of a very short duration. [*Brit. med. J.*, 1867.]

In the following year Edmund Andrews (fig. 1) published a paper on the use of oxygen with nitrous oxide. He wrote:

Every surgeon who has seen the prompt and pleasant anaesthetic action of the nitrous oxide gas, so much used by dentists, has wished that in some way it might be made available in general surgery. The patient usually goes under the influence in 30 or 40 seconds, and wakes with equal promptness, without vomiting or other unpleasant symptoms, all of which is in striking contrast with the slowness, the nausea, and the discomforts of chloroform and ether. [Andrews, 1868, 1869.]

Andrews was not critical of the dentists' use of gas without oxygen, indeed, he went so far as to say that ". . . pure nitrous oxide, when given for brief operations appears to be the safest anaesthetic known". He did mention, however, that "Dr. Rogers, a dentist of this city (Chicago), states that he used a mixture containing one third free oxygen for several years, and that in his opinion it is far pleasanter than unmixed nitrous oxide." If this is true, then Dr. Rogers may have been the first to use gas and oxygen for dental extractions, though one may doubt that he used quite such a high proportion of oxygen.

Andrews' hope was that by adding oxygen, it would be possible to use nitrous oxide anaesthesia for general surgical operations. He experimented with rats, showing that death occurred within 10 minutes when pure nitrous oxide was administered, whereas anaesthesia was obtained, with

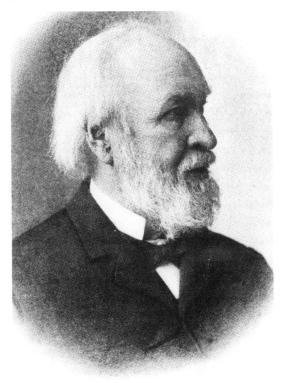

Fig. 1

Edmund Andrews (1824–1904). Chicago surgeon. (By courtesy of "The Wellcome Trustees".)

subsequent complete recovery, when nitrous oxide was administered with 25 per cent oxygen for 30 minutes. Lime-water was used "to absorb the carbonic acid produced by its breathing".

Lichtenstein and Method (1953) reproduced Andrews' case history No. 6064 in which the effects of ether, gas, and gas and oxygen were compared in the same patient:

Oct 3. 1868 Mrs Baber, very nervous temperament. Ingrowing toe nail. 9 months ago took sulph ether for operation on left foot for the nail. Got to sleep slowly felt no pain. Waked up wild and continued so a good while. 6 months ago. Took pure nitrous oxide for extraction went to sleep in about a minute, felt no pain. Face blue, was wild for a long time after waking and felt uncomfortable several days. Today. Oct 3. Took gas mixed with one 3d oxygen for extirpation of other nail. Anaesthetised in $1\frac{3}{4}$ minutes no blueness of lips. Kept inhaling 3 minutes from beginning. Waked up wild after three minutes more. Continued wild some 15 minutes, but recovered quicker & with more comfort than from pure nit ox gas.

His experiments and his clinical trials left Andrews with the "impression that the best proportion of oxygen would be found to be one-fifth by volume, which is the same as in atmospheric air".

Lilly (1869) followed this with the suggestion that only one sixth of the oxygen need be used. "We do not need for practical purposes, during the short time that anaesthesia endures, the full allowance of oxygen . . .", but at that time the idea did not appear to be taken any further in either America or Great Britain.

Mixtures of nitrous oxide and oxygen, in various proportions, had been tried by the Committee of the Odontological Society of Great Britain, but in the discussion following the presentation of its second report, Coleman (1872) said that "they had not been attended with success; they produced much struggling and excitement, with but imperfect anaesthesia".

The next big step forward was taken in France by Paul Bert (fig. 2). He reintroduced the idea of using oxygen with nitrous oxide and he revealed the significance of the partial pressures of inhaled gases.

The fact that nitrous oxide must be administered pure indicates that in order to be absorbed by the organism in sufficient quantity, the tension of the gas must be equal to one atmosphere. In order to achieve this at normal pressure, the gas must be in the proportion of 100 per cent. But let us suppose that the

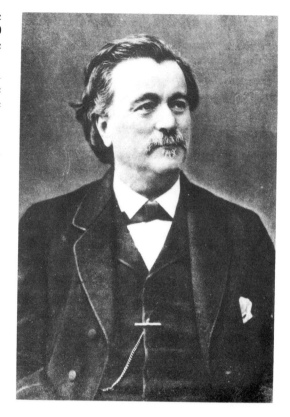

FIG. 2

Paul Bert (1833–1886). French physiologist. (By courtesy of "The Wellcome Trustees".)

patient is placed in an apparatus where the pressure can be increased to two atmospheres; then one could submit him to the desired tension by making him inhale a mixture of 50 per cent nitrous oxide and 50 per cent air. Thus one could achieve anaesthesia while maintaining the normal quantity of oxygen in the blood, and it follows that the normal conditions of respiration would be preserved. That is in fact what has been done; but I must add that up to the present I have experimented only upon animals.

I now feel justified by the results of my experiments on animals, in most strongly recommending to surgeons the use of nitrous oxide under pressure in order to obtain an anaesthesia of long duration. [Bert, 1878; translation taken from Duncum, 1947, p. 357.]

In the following year his suggestion was taken up by two surgeons in Paris, M. Péan of the Hôpital St.-Louis and M. Leon Labbé of Lariboisière, and an ingrowing toenail was successfully removed from a nervous girl of 20 years. The patient and the surgeons were enclosed in a

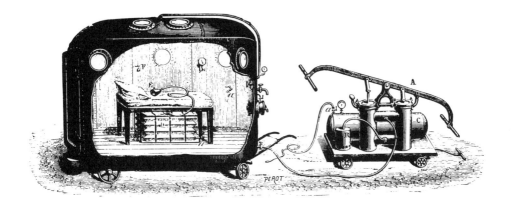

FIG. 3

"La Cloche Mobile" of Dr. Fontaine, for the administration of hyperbaric nitrous oxide and oxygen anaesthetics. It was 2 metres wide, 3.5 metres long and 2.65 metres high, and it was said to hold ten to twelve people. The hand pump was capable of delivering 400–600 litres of air per minute. The air passed through a "réfrigérateur B" to prevent the temperature in the chamber from rising more than one or two degrees above ambient temperature. The container C contained 350 litres of anaesthetic gas mixture compressed to a pressure of 10 atmospheres (3.5 cubic metres at atmospheric pressure). (From Rottenstein, 1880.)

sheet-iron chamber (of Dr. Daupley's aerotherapeutic establishment), in which the pressure was raised to 920 mm Hg, while a mixture of 85 per cent nitrous oxide with 15 per cent oxygen was administered to the patient through a face-piece (Bert, 1879). A number of operations were performed in this way by M. Péan at Dr. Fontaine's therapeutic establishment (Rottenstein, 1880, p. 312) and Fontaine designed a mobile pressure chamber on wheels (fig. 3) which was transported from hospital to hospital (Rottenstein, 1880; Allinson, 1881), but the method did not survive for routine anaesthesia (Buxton, 1887). According to Brille (1936), Ambard and de Martel took over the original anaesthetic chamber and obtained excellent results with it in 1913, but the First World War put an end to their experiments.

Bert was conscious of the practical disadvantages of using nitrous oxide under pressure, and in 1883 he wrote:

I have no hesitation in saying that this method of anaesthesia as nearly as possible approaches perfection. . . . Unfortunately, the necessity for employing complicated and costly mechanical apparatus—cast iron chambers to withstand the pressure, pumps, steam engines—makes it possible for large hospitals only to use this valuable method. In Paris a very fine installation has been made at Hôpital Saint-Louis; and I know of others, at Lyons, at Geneva, in Brussels and in some German cities. [Translation taken from Duncum, 1947, p. 362.]

This communication (Bert, 1883) also contains the surprising sentence, "En Allemagne, on a même ainsi pratiqué des accouchments."

It is possible that the installation in Geneva was operated by a private practitioner. Inglis (1965) has published recently an illustration of a compressed air "cloche" for dental anaesthesia, which was found among the advertisements in an old guide book to Spain dated 1880 (Publicité des Guides Joanne, 1881). The complete advertisement, which was discovered quite by chance (Raeburn, M., 1965, personal communication), is reproduced in figure 4.* It acknowledges the contribution of Paul Bert and draws attention to the use of nitrous oxide under pressure for anaesthesia during dental operations by Docteur Guillermin, of Geneva.

Dr. Guillermin (fig. 5) set up in practice in 1870, a full decade before bringing his pressure chamber into use. It is not known how many

---

* There appears to be some doubt as to the present whereabouts of the particular copy of the guide book to Spain in which this advertisement was discovered, but the advertisement can also be seen in a guide book to Mediterranean Winter Resorts which was published in the same year (Joanne, 1880).

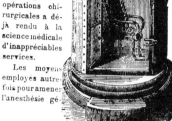

CLOCHE A AIR COMPRIMÉ
(Système **PAUL BERT**)
POUR LES OPÉRATIONS DENTAIRES

Le Nouvel appareil à AIR COMPRIMÉ de M. Paul Bert, employé dans les hôpitaux de Paris pour produire le sommeil et l'insensibilité pendant les grandes opérations chirurgicales a déjà rendu à la science médicale d'inappréciables services.

Les moyens employés autrefois pour amener l'anesthésie générale, surtout par le protoxyde d'azote, ne laissaient pas que d'offrir dans certains cas, un véritable danger, tandis qu'avec la méthode de M. Paul Bert on peut saturer le patient du mélange gazeux avec la sécurité la plus absolue, pendant tout le temps nécessaire pour les opérations les plus compliquées.

CLOCHE A AIR COMPRIME
Employée par le docteur GUILLERMIN, dentiste à Genève.

En appliquant la merveilleuse découverte du professeur Bert aux opérations dentaires, le **Docteur Guillermin**, de GENÈVE, a rendu un réel service à la nombreuse classe des personnes qui souffrent des dents. En effet, si le nombre des grandes opérations chirurgicales est nécessairement limité, il n'en est pas de même de l'extraction des dents, cautérisation ou arrachement des nerfs, etc., toutes opérations fort douloureuses et qui s'effectuent sans douleur et avec une sécurité parfaite, dans les cloches à air comprimé.

FIG. 4

Advertisement from Publicité des Guides Joannes, 1881. (By courtesy of the Courtauld Institute of Art and Messrs. Weidenfeld and Nicolson.)

patients were anaesthetized in it, or when it was abandoned, but I have been unable to trace a reference to it in the Publicité des Guides Joanne of any year other than 1881 (Joanne 1880), and it had disappeared by February 1905, when his son joined him in practice. His son, Professor Paul Guillermin, has confirmed that the chamber was used much. This is supported (although not conclusively) by a surviving appointment form (fig. 6), which is decorated with a small picture of the "Cloche Anesthésique", similar to that in the advertisement but differing from it in minor details. The form was printed in the 1880s. A footnote states that the "Cloche" had been used for dental operations by Dr. Guillermin for several years with absolute safety, and Professor Guillermin

feels sure that his father would not have continued to use the chamber if he had encountered any ill effects. The appointment form also gives the name of Dr. Guillermin's assistant, but no descendants have been traced. The chamber was heavy and strongly reinforced, and was just big enough for the patient, the dentist and his assistant. Dr. Guillermin allowed it to be advertised in the guide book in order to please his father-in-law, Achille Faure, who was one of the founders of the guide. The advertisement was printed in the same year that the Institut de Médecine Dentaire was founded in Geneva, but no details of the "Cloche" have been found in the archives of that Institute (Malherbe, J. H., 1966, personal communication).

It is not known how Dr. Guillermin came to apply Paul Bert's methods to dental anaesthesia.

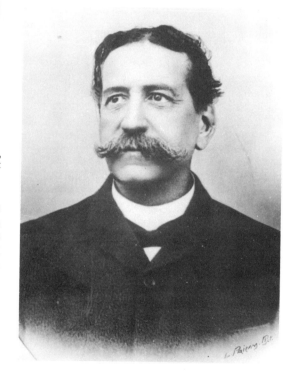

FIG. 5

Dr. Guillermin, Médecin dentiste (died 1924). (By kind permission of Professor Paul Guillermin.)

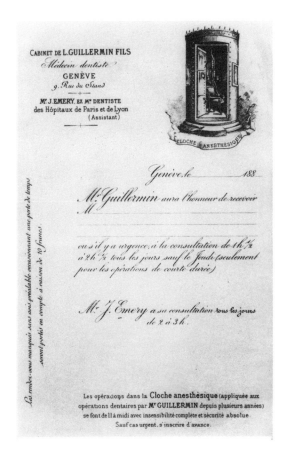

over such a pre-existing chamber in Geneva. Technical details of the pressurization and decompression of the chamber, and of the method of administering nitrous oxide and oxygen, are unknown. The appointment form, however, does provide one clue about the economics of the system. Failure to keep an appointment cost the patient 10 francs!

Rendell-Baker and Jacobson (1965) have published an illustration of a chamber designed by Howland in the United States in 1883, which was described as an "inhaling air chamber for dental and surgical operations". This, however, was taken from Howland's patent application, and the chamber may never have been built (Rendell-Baker, L., 1966, personal communication).

Until the early work of Guillermin came to light it was assumed that the first application of hyperbaric nitrous oxide and oxygen anaesthesia for dental extractions was that made by Tindal in 1941 (see figure 8). His account of this (Tindal, 1941) probably remains the earliest known clinical description:

On 11th January, 1941, a male human subject permitted himself to be anaesthetised in the pressure chamber. Operation. Removal of right lower wisdom tooth. Patient and self compressed to 15 lbs in tank, patient in sitting position. Nose mask applied delivering mixture O_2 10% N_2O 90% measured by Coxeter's flow meters (at atmospheric pressure), and filled into

FIG. 6

An appointment form used in Dr. Guillermin's practice in the 1880s. (By kind permission of Professor Paul Guillermin.)

It may or may not be relevant that his assistant came from Paris and Lyons where pressure chambers had been used for anaesthesia. Dr. Guillermin's "Cloche Anesthésique" looks like some of the chambers used for compressed-air therapy earlier in the century, such as Bertin's chamber of 1868 (see Rendell-Baker and Jacobson, 1965). An illustration of a similar chamber from Dr. Fontaine's aerotherapeutic establishment was published by Rottenstein (1880). It is reproduced in figure 7. Just as pre-existing pressure chambers in aerotherapeutic establishments in Paris were adapted for the first hyperbaric nitrous oxide and oxygen anaesthetics, in response to Paul Bert's suggestion, so may Dr. Guillermin have taken

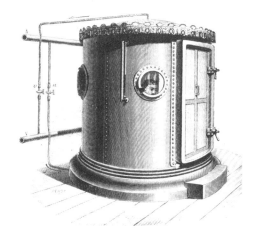

FIG. 7

A compressed "Cloche" used in Dr. Fontaine's "Etablissement Aérotherapique". (From Rottenstein, 1880.)

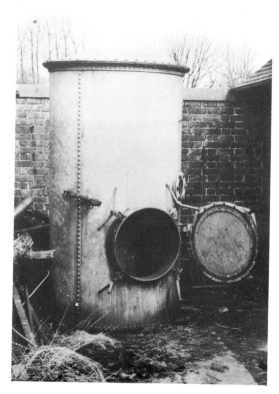

FIG. 8

The pressure tank used by Dr. Andrew Tindal. (By kind permission of Dr. Andrew Tindal.)

pheric pressure and then maintaining anaesthesia using a nitrous oxide and oxygen mixture, the proportion of oxygen being about the same as in air. If anaesthesia became too light, a deeper plane was re-established by giving nitrous oxide for a breath or two. He recommended the method to surgeons, and the idea was taken up in Austria by Hillischer, a Viennese dentist, who published a report of the trial of the method for dental anaesthesia in 1886, but many of his cases were imperfectly anaesthetized (Hewitt, 1889).*

In Hillischer's apparatus nitrous oxide and

a Douglas bag beforehand. Patient very rapidly lost consciousness, and snored after about 6 breaths. Colour was bright pink. About 6 breaths later the whole muscular system suddenly relaxed. Eyeballs were fixed centrally. Corneal reflex almost abolished. Light reflex very sluggish. Mouth opened with gag, but gag was unnecessary. Jaw was depressed with the fingers of the left hand (no spasm). Throat was packed, no reflexes, no swallowing. No reaction to removal of the tooth. Patient recovered consciousness in about 30 secs. The tank was then decompressed. Patient vomited, and for some time was very nauseated, having had some breakfast about ½ hour before compression started. At no time was there any hint of cyanosis, the lips all through being brick red. There was no doubt about the deep anaesthesia in this case, but this case should have been anaesthetised with the patient lying down, as the muscular relaxation was so complete that it must have caused considerable vascular upset, which probably was the principal cause of nausea and vomiting. This frequently occurs when a patient has been deeply anaesthetised for exodentia in an upright position in the dental chair.

In 1883 Bert tried inducing anaesthesia in animals using 100 per cent nitrous oxide at atmos-

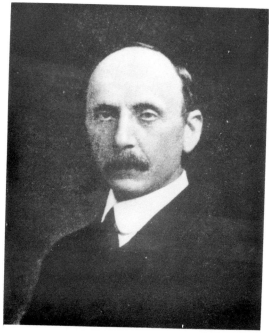

FIG. 9

Sir Frederick William Hewitt (1857–1916). (By courtesy of Elliot and Fry Studios and the *Lancet*.)

* Hewitt (1889) stated that Kreutzmann of San Francisco also used mixtures of the two gases, quoting Lyman (1889). Lyman (1889) did indeed state that "Kreutzmann, of San Francisco, has tried a mixture of nitrous oxide and oxygen gas 10–20 per cent. For this he claims rapid effects, less nausea, and a speedy recovery." The source quoted by Lyman, however, (Kreutzmann, 1887) mentions only mixtures of chloroform and oxygen.

oxygen were supplied separately, from individual Chinese silk reservoir bags, through the two sides of a double compartment tube, to a mouthpiece. An assistant kept the reservoir bags filled from cylinders. Rotation of a revolving semicircular plate, which was interposed between the end of the double tube and the mouthpiece, adjusted the proportions of nitrous oxide and oxygen delivered. Hillischer started his administrations using 10 per cent oxygen (Hewitt, 1893, p. 120).

Hillischer's work was drawn to the attention of Frederick William Hewitt (fig. 9) who began his own experiments with nitrous oxide and oxygen in the same year. His first report on the subject (Hewitt, 1889) confirmed that there had been no advance in nitrous oxide anaesthesia during the previous twenty years. He wrote:

. . . certain phenomena occur to which I would direct special notice—phenomena which necessitate the withdrawal of the anaesthetic and the admission of air to the lungs. Amongst these phenomena may be mentioned lividity or actual cyanosis (varying with the previous colour of the patient's face), true stertor, jerky and irregular respiration, clonic movements in the extremities and elsewhere, dilatation of the pupils, and considerable acceleration of the pulse rate. Most, if not all, of these symptoms occur whenever the gas is administered to full surgical anaesthesia, and they are I believe, asphyxial in origin.

He demonstrated their asphyxial nature later (Hewitt, 1892):

At the instigation of Sir George Johnson, Mr. Braine and I administered nitrogen, not only practically free of oxygen but with known and small percentages of this gas, to several patients at the Dental Hospital of London; and the phenomena were to the by-standers indistinguishable from those of an ordinary nitrous oxide administration. No one can, I think, deny that the "stertor", "jactitation" and lividity produced by nitrogen are of asphyxial origin.

At the same time he pointed out that "The unsuitability of atmospheric air as an oxygenating agent (during nitrous oxide anaesthesia) is due to its useless nitrogen."

Details of the administration of nitrogen were given by Johnson (1891a, b; see also Hewitt, 1893, p. 267):

Mr. Braine was good enough to administer this gas (compressed nitrogen containing 0.5 per cent by volume of oxygen and 0.3 per cent of carbon dioxide) in five instances to members of the staff of King's College, who volunteered to submit to the experiments. . . . Encouraged by these results Mr. Braine felt justified in administering the gas to patients at the Dental Hospital for anaesthetic purposes. The only difference, in the opinion of some of those present,

being that the anaesthesia was less rapidly produced, and somewhat less durable, than that from nitrous oxide, although in each case the tooth was extracted without pain. . . . On a subsequent occasion the same gas was administered by Dr. Frederick Hewitt at the Dental Hospital. As before nine patients took the gas. The maximum period required to produce anaesthesia was 70 seconds, the minimum 50 seconds, and the mean time 58.3 seconds. . . . In the case of 3 per cent gas (3 per cent of oxygen with nitrous oxide), which was given to five patients, the time required to produce anaesthesia varied from 60 to 75 seconds, the average time being 67.5 seconds. In each case the tooth was extracted without pain, the duration of anaesthesia being somewhat longer than with pure nitrogen. In each case there was lividity, dilatation of the pupils, and more or less jactitation. On the same day Dr. Hewitt gave nitrogen with 5 per cent oxygen to four patients. With this mixture the time required for the production of anaesthesia ranged from 75 to 95 seconds, the average being 87.5 seconds. . . . In all four cases there was slight lividity before the face piece was removed, but in only one case was there jactitation of the limbs.

Hewitt (1889) experimented with a number of ways of mixing nitrous oxide and oxygen but most of his early attempts at producing surgical anaesthesia with these mixtures were unsatisfactory. For his fifth series of cases his patients inhaled from a gasometer filled at different times with known but different mixtures. A reservoir bag was interposed near to the mask. When he tried using $12\frac{3}{4}$ per cent oxygen in the mixture he met with success in eleven consecutive cases. His reaction to this was almost as revealing as his description of nitrous oxide anaesthesia without oxygen:

The anaesthesia which was produced astonished me. There was no excitement; the respiration was regularly and quietly performed; the colour of the face and lips remained unimpaired or was even increased; and there was no stertor; the available period of narcosis was longer than that of nitrous oxide narcosis; and the recovery was perfect.

When trying to repeat this result in his sixth series, however, he failed to obtain surgical anaesthesia with this mixture in four out of fourteen subjects, and he came to realize that individual requirements varied.

Hewitt's next step was to charge the gasometer with one-eighth, by volume, of oxygen and seven-eighths of nitrous oxide, but to leave the supplies of oxygen and nitrous oxide connected so that either could be turned on quickly in order to alter the mixture delivered to the patient according to the moment-to-moment clinical requirements. Hewitt gave 78 anaesthetics in this way and detailed records were kept of 59 of them. "With one or two exceptions every patient was readily anaesthetised . . . and in those instances in which excitement occurred, it either subsided spontaneously as the administration proceeded, or was controlled by freely supplying nitrous oxide to the gasometer." The average period of administration was 126 seconds and the average duration of subsequent anaesthesia was 44 seconds. A further revealing comment which Hewitt made was: "It was often difficult to decide when to discontinue the administration and to allow the operator to commence, for nearly all the usual phenomena of full nitrous oxide anaesthesia were absent."

Encouraged by this experiment, Hewitt then attempted to devise portable apparatus.

Messrs. Barth and Co., therefore made for me two small india rubber bags having respectively the capacities of ten gallons and a half and one gallon and a half, and connected together by a wide metal tube and stop-cock. The large bag was fed from a pair of bottles containing nitrous oxide; the small one from a pair of bottles containing oxygen. From the large bag there passed a wide tube to the face-piece. The large bag was filled with nitrous oxide, and the small bag with oxygen; the stop-cock between them was opened, and their contents allowed to diffuse.

The idea of increasing the pressure at which gas and oxygen mixtures are delivered to the patient may have originated from his early experiments with this apparatus, for he wrote:

I had never fully appreciated the part played by pressure when using a gasometer. It soon became obvious, however, when comparing the results obtained by the use of the bags with those observed when employing a gasometer, that the pressure at which the mixture had been inhaled when using a gasometer was a most important element in the administration. I found, when administering the mixture from the bags described, that unless the bags were compressed during the inhalation the anaesthesia was liable to be imperfect and transitory; whereas, if by the aid of an assistant pressure was brought to bear upon the bags, the anaesthesia was similar in its main features to that obtained by the gasometer. I purposely conducted a few administrations without employing pressure, and waited until signs of excitement and imperfect narcosis commenced to appear; I then asked my assistant to compress the bags, and the result was that the symptoms mentioned subsided and full anaesthesia became established.

Hewitt's conclusion was unjustified in the absence of measurements of the gas mixtures actually delivered to the patients under the three sets of conditions. Subsequently he tried deliberately

controlling the free action of the expiratory valve, by weighting it, in a series of twenty-nine cases. "The results, however, were negative in character" (Hewitt, 1892).

In the previous year Buxton (1888), Silk (1888) and Hewitt (1888) published textbooks of anaesthesia. Buxton (1888) referred to Bert's work (p. 44) but explained that: "In England the method has not been employed, as nitrous oxide and ether are practically as safe, and the large and expensive chamber and apparatus render its use, save in hospitals, almost impossible." Silk (1888) wrote:

While admitting that a very marked dissimilarity may exist between the phenomena observed during the two sets of conditions (asphyxia and inhalation of nitrous oxide), it would be perfectly compatible with all we know of either state to attempt to explain the symptoms following nitrous oxide administration on the first supposition, that they are due partly, and in the first instance to the specific action of the gas, and partly, in the later stages, to the absence of oxygen.

After a description of Paul Bert's work he continued:

Without being so sanguine as to expect that the time will ever arrive when it may be possible, for the sake

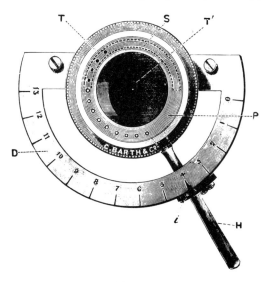

FIG. 10

The nitrous oxide and oxygen mixing control of Hewitt's original gas and oxygen apparatus as made by Messrs. Barth & Co. The central tube T' conducted nitrous oxide. Oxygen was conducted from the outer concentric tube T through small holes, the number uncovered depending upon the position of the lever H. (From Hewitt, 1892.)

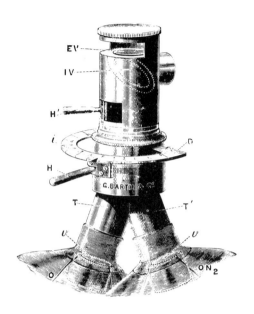

oxygen. He tried them out on a total of 805 patients, the last 162 of whom were anaesthetized using his final apparatus (Hewitt, 1892).

His main criticism of Hillischer's apparatus was that a small movement of the mixture control made a big change to the mixture inhaled. In order to overcome this, oxygen was admitted to the mixture chamber of Hewitt's apparatus through small holes, the number of holes in use being controlled by moving a lever (fig. 10). Nitrous oxide and oxygen were supplied through individual reservoir bags (figs. 11 and 12). Hewitt appreciated that one of the limitations of this arrangement was the fact that the mixture delivered varied with the pressure in the reservoir bags as well as with the number of holes in use.

He gave an analysis of 153 dental anaesthetics administered using this apparatus (Hewitt, 1892) and a summary of it is given in the appendix. In making comparisons with present and recent

Fig. 11

The mounting of the oxygen and nitrous oxide reservoir bags, the mixture control, the stopcock and the non-return valves of Hewitt's original gas and oxygen apparatus. (From Hewitt, 1892.)

of anaesthesia alone, to conduct all operations in specially constructed chambers, either in hospitals, or movable from house to house on wheels as his followers would suggest, but at the same time bearing in mind the ridicule showered upon, and the arguments urged against the now almost universal system of antiseptic surgery, it may not be altogether absurd to look forward to a practical development of the plan above mentioned. Subsequently the same investigator proposed to prolong the anaesthetic action by means of a mixture of oxygen and nitrous oxide in definite proportions under normal pressure. Experimentally this plan was found to be of some value, but it does not seem to have been carried beyond this stage.

Meanwhile Hewitt was experimenting along these very lines, but there was no hint of the possible use of oxygen with nitrous oxide in his book (Hewitt, 1888).

Hewitt continued these researches for another three years by the end of which time he had experimented with thirteen different schemes for mixing and administering nitrous oxide and

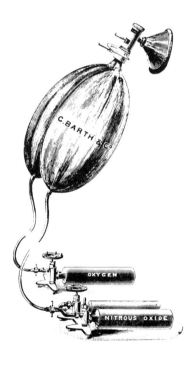

Fig. 12

The complete assembly of Hewitt's gas and oxygen apparatus. (From Hewitt, 1892.)

dental anaesthetic techniques, however, it must be borne in mind that Hewitt did not use a nose-piece such as used by Clover (1868) and Coleman (1898). His dental patients were operated on while recovering from anaesthesia induced using gas and oxygen delivered from a facemask.

At the meeting of the Odontological Society at which this method was first discussed, Hewitt (1892) concluded:

So far as my experience has gone, I am inclined to regard the use of oxygen with nitrous oxide as of distinct advantage in the majority of cases in dental practice. But we cannot shut our eyes to the fact that the administration of the mixed gases involves more time, more attention to detail, and more skill than are essential for the employment of nitrous oxide; whilst the risks of unpleasant side effects are a trifle greater. . . . I need hardly remind you that it is not always an easy matter to prophesy the duration of an operation.

During the discussion which followed Hewitt's paper introducing nitrous oxide and oxygen anaes-thesia for dental operations, the main criticism came from Bailey, who had claimed previously (Bailey, 1887) that "As a practical man he could positively state that all symptoms met with during the administration of nitrous oxide were not due to asphyxia", and who later affirmed (Bailey, 1890) that "Jactitation . . . is the only reliable symptom of anaesthesia". Bailey's (1892) contribution was reported as follows:

Mr. G. H. Bailey very warmly eulogised the enthus-iasm, ability and energy which Dr. Hewitt's paper displayed. He had not had the experience of Dr. Hewitt with nitrous oxide and oxygen combined, but he thought from Dr. Hewitt's figures the average of "going off" was over two minutes, the average anaes-thesia seemed to be thirty-four to forty seconds, but curiously enough the number of teeth got out did not appear to be so many as with ordinary nitrous oxide —2.7 did not seem to him to be a large number; he could not help thinking that with ordinary gas it would be more. The patient certainly had no loss of colour, no jactitation, no "phonation"—although he saw no objection in this—there was no rigidity; these were advantages. At the hospital they had an excellent nurse, and he had asked her, "What difference do you find between the days we have pure nitrous oxide and the days we have the mixture—have you less noise but more sickness?" And she said, "Certainly." This was in favour of the mixture. But he had observed in conversation with Dr. Hewitt, that the complication of the apparatus and the uncertainty of the amount to be given were objections. Now as to the change of colour under the gas, he did not think there was very much change of colour with nitrous oxide; his custom was to use the expiratory valve only, and to keep a gentle pressure with the hand upon the bag, and practically

one obtained good anaesthesia lasting at least twenty seconds. Now he would just take the list of cases he had had that day:
1. Pure nitrous oxide and a little ether administered. The eye of the patient was taken out in two minutes. Now with Dr. Hewitt's apparatus the patient would be "going under" during this two minutes.
2. A boy aged 10; a lower molar removed, no change of colour, no jactitation, nitrous oxide being given alone.
3. Nitrous oxide and a little ether: ten teeth re-moved in one minute and a half.
4. A gentleman of large build, very muscular, tooth removed without noise in one minute and a half. Nitrous oxide.
5. A boy, who had just come in from cricket, said that ether disagreed with him; had pure gas, tooth out in fifteen seconds.
6. Five teeth removed from a very ruddy full-blooded man; no unpleasantness. Nitrous oxide only.
7. A young fellow of the bull-dog sort, very bad teeth, had gas only; the tooth broke, but afterwards came out; no change of colour, no jactitation, barring a little kicking.
That was his experience of the day. If he had given the mixture in these cases he thought that they would have said he had had a good result. . . . Dr. Hewitt thought the recovery was not so good with the mixture as with nitrous oxide. If that were the case, surely, with the complication and other disadvantages, it was not so valuable. As to length of time "going off", Dr. Hewitt very kindly gave him (Mr. Bailey) gas on two occasions, and the last time he said "shall I give you a mixture with oxygen?" But he (Mr. Bailey) said, no, he would rather not, as he took the gas so very well. However, he was a long time getting under the influence of the gas. He thought the length of time getting into a state of anaesthesia was a very serious objection, as it was very trying to the friends of the patient. . . . He could not help thinking that Dr. Hewitt troubled himself unnecessarily about the change of colour. When nitrous oxide first began to be given the leading physicians, Gull, Jenner, and others objected to it, owing to the change of colour which it produced, but what happened? After they had seen it given for a little time, they all said they saw no harm whatever in this symptom, and that, Mr. Bailey thought, was at present the general concensus of opinion. The jactitation might be, certainly, a bad thing, but that would vary enormously and very seldom proved troublesome. . . . With regard to the apparatus, it seemed to him to be all but perfect, except for its somewhat ungainly bulk, but the question was if it was desirable to have so complicated an apparatus. In conclusion he begged to thank Dr. Hewitt most heartily for the manner in which he had carried out his investigations.

In his reply

Dr. Hewitt thought that 2.7 was a very good average for students. Perhaps in private practice it was possible to get more teeth out. . . . Mr. Bailey said that there was very little change in colour; Dr. Hewitt would not contradict this. It was possible that one did not always recognise the change of colour; he usually got others to notice the lividity under nitrous oxide, and want of change of colour in oxygen cases. He should say no more on the subject, but he maintained that there was no change—or very much less with the mixture than with the nitrous oxide alone. Dr. Hewitt did not claim that the combination was best for all cases, but he looked upon it as a good alternative to nitrous oxide, and better than it for many cases. . . . He had said very little about the actual safety of the mixture, but if it could be said that anything was safer than nitrous oxide, he thought it might be said of nitrous oxide and oxygen.

Hewitt's ideas were also criticized by Edgelow (1893) who wrote:

With the mixture of oxygen and nitrous oxide, the period of consciousness preceding anaesthesia is undoubtedly lengthened. . . . Lastly, the after effects are more pronounced. A feeling of drowsiness and desire to remain still are manifest. Nausea, retching and vomiting are more likely to occur than with nitrous oxide alone. Thus although this mixture gives an advantage in point of time to the operator, and is on that account of much service in cases demanding an increased duration of insensibility, as well as in such cases as Hewitt has specially designated, yet in the ordinary run of patients, nitrous oxide has such undoubted advantages over the mixture, that there is little likelihood of the latter displacing the pure gas. And I may add that the results Hewitt claims for the combination are to be readily obtained by the method of giving a whiff or two of air with the ordinary apparatus.

Wolfenden (1895), on the other hand, confirmed Hewitt's findings: ". . . after a considerable experience with the use of the mixed gases, I fully and confidently bear testimony to all the advantages claimed by him for this method of producing anaesthesia . . . sooner or later the old system will have to give way to the new". Buxton (1895) added his emphatic support:

If, as is submitted, nitrous oxide can be given without any cyanosis, jactitations (clonic or tonic spasms) or other signs of oxygen starvation, it may be employed with safety and convenience for practically all persons and ages. To effect this it becomes necessary to adopt a procedure somewhat different from that formerly taught in text books and practised by most persons. . . . It is not denied that a mixture narcosis of air or oxygen and nitrous oxide is less simple to manage, and possibly requires more skill to bring it to a successful termination, but certainly the important aid it renders us in dealing with difficult and dangerous cases outweighs any disadvantages it may possess in this respect.

Later he went further and wrote (Buxton, 1896): "All methods involving asphyxial symptoms are open to grave censure."

Further details of this work and arguments in favour of using oxygen were contained in two textbooks written later by Hewitt (1893, 1897). The first of these went into five editions, the last being published posthumously in 1922, and there can be little doubt about Hewitt's influence in introducing nitrous oxide and oxygen anaesthesia. By the time of the publication of the first edition of his *Anaesthetics and their Administration* in 1893, Hewitt was able to report that he had records of over 2000 administrations of nitrous oxide and oxygen.

Referring back to his original experiments in which fixed percentages of oxygen were administered to patients he wrote:

. . . the best results have been secured with those [mixtures] containing 5, 6, 7 or 8 per cent oxygen, according to the type of patient . . . percentages of oxygen above those administered, are, as a general rule, unnecessary. That cases arise in which lower or higher percentages should be given is beyond doubt; but such cases can only be successfully met when a regulating apparatus is used. . . . I have found (when using the gasometer) that the chief objection to higher percentages is the liability to excitement. It must be remembered, too, that with 5 per cent of oxygen one is very near asphyxial borderland. Indeed, when administering a mixture containing this percentage of oxygen, cases will occasionally be met with in which minor degrees of stertor, jactitation and lividity are present.

Of the relative proportions of nitrous oxide and oxygen which his apparatus was capable of furnishing, Hewitt (1897, p. 33) wrote: ". . . much will depend upon the state of the bags during the inhalation, and especially upon whether they are kept of equal size throughout . . .", and ". . . each apparatus possesses slight peculiarities of its own. . . . The result is that the anaesthetist must observe what his particular apparatus is capable of doing." Hewitt (1897, p. 45) recommended inducing anaesthesia with the control lever set to position 2 at which ". . . roughly about 2, 3 or 4 per cent oxygen will be breathed." Then (p. 48):

. . . the anaesthetist must regulate the admission of oxygen in accordance with the type of his patient, and the symptoms that the patient displays. There is, unfortunately, no rule which will apply to every case. . . . Generally speaking, a gradual and progressive increase in the percentage of oxygen is advisable . . . starting the inhalation, as already mentioned with 2 to 4 per cent of oxygen, and then progressively increasing this proportion to 8 or 9 per cent. It seems to me that it is a mistake to adopt the plan which is customary in Germany, and to begin with 10 per cent of oxygen. It is surely more rational to make an allowance for the oxygen present in the lungs when the administration begins, and we should therefore commence with a very small percentage of this gas. As the lungs lose the air they contained, so the percentage of oxygen in the mixture may be increased, provided that no symptoms of excitement arise. If a 10 per cent mixture be used from the commencement, excitement is liable to ensue from the undue proportion of oxygen [p. 49].

Hewitt also remarked (p. 54) that the anaesthetist ". . . must bear in mind that a little interval must necessarily elapse before the effects of an increase or decrease in oxygen admission will become manifest".

Hewitt's "gas and oxygen" technique was a great advance on the previous "straight gas" and "gas and air" administrations, but by present-day standards it would still come under the heading of a "hypoxic" technique. On the other hand, it must be remembered that anaesthesia was not then prolonged by using a nasal inhaler during the operation.

Hewitt (1897, p. 53) claimed that:

The small, feeble and exceedingly rapid pulse which not infrequently may be felt at the acme of an ordinary nitrous oxide inhalation, is not met with when oxygen is present with the nitrous oxide in sufficient quantities. I have never, in fact, come across any indications of circulatory failure during the administration of the mixed gases. The tongue and adjacent structures are less engorged than when nitrous oxide is administered free from oxygen.

He considered (p. 81) that:

When sufficient oxygen is administered with nitrous oxide to prevent asphyxial complications there is every reason to believe that the anaesthesia produced is free from risk to life. A careful study of every fatality which has been recorded in connection with the use of nitrous oxide gas shows that in most, and in probably all cases in which this agent has caused death, absence of oxygen has been primarily responsible for the occurrence. The same may also be said of those reported cases in which alarming symptoms have taken place during the administration of nitrous oxide by the customary method.

APPENDIX

SUMMARY OF 153 DENTAL ANAESTHETICS ADMINISTERED BY HEWITT (1892) USING HIS NITROUS OXIDE AND OXYGEN APPARATUS

Sex. 123 females; 29 males; 1 not stated.

Age. 7–61 years.

Typical cases (good colour, no jactitation, no stertor, more or less complete muscular relaxation and quietude during the operation) 117 cases (76.4 per cent).

Atypical cases.
20 variable degrees of lividity (otherwise typical).
10 rigid (otherwise typical).
1   livid with rigidity.

1   livid with very slight clonus.
2   ordinary symptoms of nitrous oxide anaesthesia accidentally allowed to appear.
2   intentionally terminated by nitrous oxide free from oxygen.
——
36 Total.

Signs of readiness for operation (from notes on 137 cases).
104 conjunctival reflex absent.
9   conjunctival reflex not abolished, but slight softly snoring breathing or muscular relaxation.
24   conjunctival reflex not noted but other signs relied upon.

Phonation. 29 cases (usually not excessive, but violent screaming in 2 cases).

Muscular excitement, struggling or kicking (rigidity not included) 8 cases.

4 *cases terminated by nitrous oxide,* 3 because too much oxygen given at first and one because patient became excited.

Period of inhalation.
Average for 67 cases, 110.5 seconds.
Range, 66 to 186 seconds.

Available period of resulting anaesthesia.
Average for 69 cases, 44 seconds.
Range, 21 to 90 seconds.

Number of teeth extracted. Average for 129 cases, 2.7 teeth.

Pain. All except three cases denied feeling pain. One of these probably felt no pain, one felt pain towards the end of operation lasting 66 seconds and one felt pain at the end of a difficult extraction of a wisdom tooth.

After effects. Recovery was not quite so speedy as after nitrous oxide. One case, retching; and 1 case, transient nausea.

ACKNOWLEDGEMENTS

It gives me pleasure to thank Professor Paul Guillermin for his good-natured and helpful letters outlining the part played by his father in the history of nitrous oxide and oxygen anaesthesia. It was Mr. O. M. Ashford who kindly made local enquiries in Geneva and provided his address. I am indebted to Mr. Michael Raeburn of Messrs. Weidenfeld and Nicolson Ltd. for providing me with a full-page reproduction of Dr. Guillermin's advertisement of 1881 (only the illustration of the "cloche" appeared in Inglis (1965)). Miss J. H. Malherbe was good enough to search the archives of the Institut de Médecine Dentaire, Geneva, and to draw my attention to Brille (1936). Dr. L. Rendell-Baker went out of his way to furnish me, among other things, with references and literature on pressure chambers. I am delighted that Dr. Andrew Tindal has provided a photograph of the pressure tank used by him in 1941. As in previous instalments, wherever possible, the presumption of trying to speak for others has been avoided by allowing the main characters to speak for themselves. This method of presentation has been taken from Duncum (1947). I am indebted to the Department of Medical Photography of the University of Leeds and United Leeds Hospitals for figures 3, 7, 9, 10 and 11.

REFERENCES

Allinson, T. R. (1881). Letter. An anaesthetic car. *Brit. med. J.*, **2**, 110.

Andrews, E. (1868); see Andrews (1869).

—— (1869). Oxygen mixture, a new anaesthetic combination. (Reprinted from *Chicago med. Exam.* (1868), **9**, 656.) *Brit. J. dent. Sci.*, **12**, 22.

Bailey, G. H. (1887). On the physiological action of nitrous oxide (discussion). *Trans. odont. Soc. N.S.*, **19**, 122.

—— (1890). An analysis of a series of one thousand nitrous oxide administrations recorded systematically (discussion). *Trans. odont. Soc. N.S.*, **22**, 263.

—— (1892). On the anaesthetic effects of nitrous oxide when administered with oxygen at ordinary atmospheric pressures (discussion). *Trans. odont. Soc. N.S.*, **24**, 240.

Bert, P. (1878). Sur la possibilité d'obtenir, à l'aide du protoxyde d'azote, une insensibilité de longue durée, et sur l'innocuité de cet anesthésique. *C.R. Acad. Sci. (Paris)*, **87**, 728.

—— (1879). Anesthésie par le protoxyde d'azote mélangé d'oxygène et employe sous pression. *C.R. Acad. Sci. (Paris)*, **89**, 132.

—— (1883). Anesthésie prolongée obtenue par le protoxyde d'azote à la pression normale. *C.R. Acad. Sci. (Paris)*, **96**, 1271.

Brille, J. M. (1936). *Analgésie et Anesthésie en chirurgie dentaire*, p. 95. Paris: Les Archives Hospitaliere.

Brit. med. J. (1867). Progress of Medical Science. Protoxide of nitrogen as an anaesthetic. **1**, 482.

Buxton, D. W. (1887). On the physiological action of nitrous oxide. *Trans. odont. Soc. N.S.*, **19**, 90.

—— (1888). *Anaesthetics: their uses and administration*. London: H. K. Lewis.

—— (1895). Nitrous oxide anaesthesia. *Brit. J. dent. Sci.*, **38**, 865.

—— (1896). The nature of anaesthesia. *Brit. J. dent. Sci.*, **39**, 104.

Clover, J. T. (1868). On the administration of chloroform in dental operations. *Brit. J. dent. Sci.*, **11**, 123.

Coleman, A. (1872). Second Report of the Joint Committee to inquire into the value and advantages of the Protoxide of Nitrogen as an Anaesthetic in Surgical Operations (discussion). *Trans. odont. Soc. N.S.*, **5**, 50.

—— (1898). On a method of administering anaesthetics through the nose. *Trans. Soc. Anaesth.*, **1**, 117.

Duncum, B. M. (1947). *The Development of Inhalation Anaesthesia: with special reference to the years 1846–1900*. London: Oxford University Press.

Edgelow, P. (1893). Anaesthetics. *Brit. J. dent. Sci.*, **36**, 304.

Hayes, S. J. (1887). Anaesthesia versus asphyxia. *Brit. J. dent. Sci.*, **30**, 44.

Hewitt, F. W. (1888). *Select Methods in the Administration of Nitrous Oxide and Ether*. London: Baillière, Tindall & Cox.

—— (1889). On the anaesthesia produced by the administration of mixtures of nitrous oxide and oxygen (preliminary notice). *Lancet*, **1**, 832.

—— (1892). On the anaesthetic effects of nitrous oxide when administered with oxygen at ordinary atmospheric pressures: with remarks upon 800 cases. *Trans. odont. Soc. N.S.*, **24**, 194.

Hewitt, F. W. (1893). *Anaesthetics and their Administration. A manual for medical and dental practitioners and students*. London: Charles Griffin.

—— (1897). *The Administration of Nitrous Oxide and Oxygen for Dental Operations*. London: Claudius Ash.

Inglis, B. (1965). *A History of Medicine*. London: Weidenfeld and Nicolson.

Joanne, P. (1880). *Les Stations d'hivers de la Méditerranée*. Paris: Librairie Hachette.

Johnson, G. (1891a). On the physiology of asphyxia and on the action of pure nitrogen. *Proc. roy. Soc.*, **49**, 144.

—— (1891b). On the physiology of asphyxia and on the action of pure nitrogen. *Lancet*, **1**, 814.

Kreutzmann, H. (1887). Anaesthesia by chloroform and oxygen combined. *Pacific M. & S. J.*, **30**, 462.

Lichtenstein, M. E., and Method, H. (1953). Edmund Andrews, M.D., a biographical sketch with historical notes concerning nitrous oxide-oxygen anaesthesia. *Northwest. Univ. med. sch. Quart. Bull.*, **27**, 337.

Lilly, H. M. (1869). Oxygen and nitrous oxide mixture (reprinted from *Medical and Surgical Reporter*). *Brit. J. dent. Sci.*, **12**, 99.

Lyman, H. M. (1889). Anaesthetics. *Annual of the med. Sci.*, **2**, 511.

Publicité des Guides Joanne (1881). Appendice 1881–1882. V. Supplement, p. 79. Paris (see Joanne. 1880).

Rendell-Baker, L., and Jacobson, J. H. (1965). Hyperbaric oxygenation: international anesthesiology clinics. *Ventilation*, **3**, 319.

Rottenstein, J. B. (1880). *Traite d'anesthesie chirurgicale contenant la description et les applications de la methode anesthesique de M. Paul Bert*. Paris: Librairie Garmer Baillier.

Silk, J. F. (1888). *A Manual of Nitrous Oxide Anaesthesia*. London: Churchill.

Tindal, A. (1941). The perfect anaesthetic: anaesthesia by the method of Paul Bert. *Surgo. Glasgow Univ. med. J.*, **7**, 33.

Wolfenden, A. B. (1895). Nitrous oxide and oxygen. *Brit. J. dent. Sci.*, **38**, 625.

12

THE EARLY MANUFACTURE, STORAGE AND PURITY OF NITROUS OXIDE

A considerable time elapsed before I was able to procure the gas in a state of purity, and my first experiments were made on the mixtures of nitrous oxide, nitrogene and nitrous gas (Nitric oxide), which are produced during metallic solutions. [Davy, 1800b, p. 454.]

. . . the gas must be made very pure. [Colton, 1863; cited Rymer, 1864.]

Parsimony, which tampers with life and health by employing a corrupt article of nitrate of ammonia, a half-washed gas, and unsuitable appliances for administering this, should charge the fault where it belongs—on the user, not on the thing used. . . . Chemically pure nitrous oxide, rightly and liberally administered, we believe the most harmless anaesthetic yet discovered. [Sprague, 1864.]

. . . the ordinary gas of dentists . . . never makes the least approach to purity, containing always from 10 to 25 per cent free nitrogen and oxygen. As it is impossible to separate free nitrogen without apparatus for reducing the gas to liquid form, I suspended experiments until this deficiency could be supplied. [Andrews, 1872, cited Lichtenstein and Method, 1953.]

BEFORE 1863

In the early days of nitrous oxide anaesthesia the gas had to be made on the spot, and nitrous oxide generators soon became available commercially. These followed the general plan of the apparatus originally designed by James Watt (fig. 1) and advertised for the production of "factitious airs" in 1796 (Beddoes and Watt, 1796).

ADVERTISEMENT

LEST the difficulty of constructing and procuring the apparatus should prove an obstacle to the extension of its use, BOULTON & WATT undertook to manufacture them. The difficulties of this new branch are so far overcome as to enable them to supply orders without delay. A list of the parts furnished by them, both of the larger and smaller apparatus, is subjoined, but they can only state the price by approximation, as the business is too new yet to enable them to determine the positive cost at which they shall be able to construct them in future.

	£	s.	d.
A PNEUMATIC APPARATUS, large size, comprehending Furnace, Fire-tube, and End Pieces, Water-pipe, conducting pipe, Circulating Refrigeratory, and Hydraulic Bellows, fitted up as described in the preceding pages, will come to about . .	8	8	0
The AUXILIARY ARTICLES necessary to make the Apparatus quite complete, viz. two Fire-pots, two spare Fire-tubes, a large and a small Air-holder, a Close Refrigeratory, a cast iron pan to fit the Furnace for a Sand Heat, &c., &c., will come to between 4l. and	5	0	0
A PNEUMATIC APPARATUS, small size, comprehending Articles as above for the large one, will come to about	5	15	6
The AUXILIARY ARTICLES, no Fire-pots included, about	3	0	0
N.B. If the small Furnace is combined with the large Bellows and Refrigeratories, which is recommended for private Practitioners, with all the extra Articles, it will come to between 10l. and . . .	11	0	0

It was this apparatus that Humphry Davy used for making nitrous oxide by heating ammonium nitrate, but for his preliminary experiments he used another method:

In the beginning of March, I prepared a large quantity of impure nitrous oxide from the solution of zinc. Of this I often breathed quantities of a quart and two quarts generally mingled with more than equal parts of oxygene or common air. In the most decisive of those trials, its effects appeared to be depressing, and I imagined that it produced a tendency to fainting: the pulse was certainly rendered slower under its operation.

At this time, Mr. Southey respired it in an highly diluted state; it occasioned a slight degree of giddiness, and considerably diminished the quickness of his pulse.

Mr. C. Coates likewise respired it highly diluted, with similar effects. [Davy, 1800b, p. 454.]

There can be no doubt that Davy was concerned about the effects of the impurities that may be found with nitrous oxide, because he followed up his first jubilant announcement of the respirability of nitrous oxide with a hasty warning:

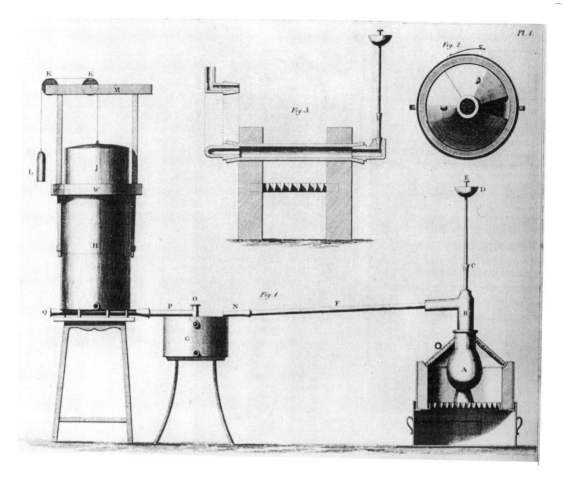

FIG. 1

"Fig. 1, Elavation of the Large Pneumatic Apparatus, with the Alembic. Fig. 2, Bird's Eye View of the Furnace, with its Covers. Fig. 3, Section of the Fire-tube and Furnace, according to the first construction." From Beddoes and Watt (1796). The Alembic is the pot A. G is the Refrigeratory. HJ is the Hydraulic Bellows "to receive and measure the air as it comes cooled from the Refrigeratory through the Communicating-pipe P". The Hydraulic Bellows was normally connected to an air-holder at Q (see Part I; Smith, 1965, fig. 1). Another drawing in Beddoes and Watt (1796) shows the Hydraulic Bellows and the Circulating Refrigeratory in section (Plate 2, fig. 1). The Spirometer of today has the same basic design as the Hydraulic Bellows: "To avoid the incumbrance of a great weight of water, the outer vessel H is made double, so that only an interstice of about half an inch is left between its two cylinders for the vessel J to move up and down in." The Refrigeratory was "made in three different ways, according to the nature of the airs to be cooled". The spiral ether chamber in Snow's (1847) vaporizer was reminiscent of the Circulating Refrigeratory, which "is used for airs which require washing as well as cooling, to make them deposit any extraneous matters which they would otherwise carry over with them." This consisted of an outer cylindrical vessel which was flushed continuously with water, cold fresh water entering at the lower aperture shown in the diagram above, and waste water leaving at the top. Projecting into the surface of the water from above was an "inner vessel; it is open at the bottom, but its cover is convex, and has a spiral chamber winding along the underside, which being likewise opened below, the air coming from the Alembic or Fire-tube, by the pipe N, at the circumference, passes through the whole of it in constant contact with the water in the Refrigeratory, until it arrives at pipe O, fixed near the centre, which delivers it to the Hydraulic Bellows." (By courtesy of the Royal Society of Medicine.)

In a subsequent communication Mr. Davy expresses his apprehension, lest a general notice of the respirability of gaseous oxyd of azote should induce anyone to make injurious experiments on himself, and therefore wishes it should be added, that the circumstances of safety and of hazard should be speedily pointed out to the public. A train of experiments, by which he hopes to clear up this perplexed subject, are in progress . . . [Davy, 1799.]

In a further note to *Nicholson's Journal*, Davy (1800a) added:

Since my discovery of the respirability, and extraordinary effects of the gaseous oxide of azote in April, 1799, a great portion of my time has been devoted to experiments on its properties, composition, and mode of action on living beings. These experiments are nearly compleated: but as at least two months will elapse before they can be published, and as some of the facts to which they relate have been made known to the world in Dr. Beddoe's Notice, to prevent dangerous and inconclusive experiments, I beg leave to communicate to the public, by means of your Journal, a short account of the mode in which it is usually prepared for experiments on respiration. Nitrate of ammoniac perfectly neutralised, and rendered as dry as possible, must be exposed to a heat not below 310° (154°C), or above 400° of Fahrenheit (204°C). (This decomposition was discovered by the illustrious Berthollet. I have found that at a temperature of 500° (260°C), nitrous gas (nitric oxide) and nitrogene are evolved as well as nitrous oxide. Whenever there is a luminous appearance in the retort, more or less of the two substances will be produced.) At this temperature it is decomposed into water and gaseous oxide of azote, or as I would rather call it, nitrous oxide.

The gas must be passed through water and suffered to remain in contact with it at least an hour and a half before it is respired.

This letter was amplified in his *Researches, Chemical and Philosophical; chiefly concerning nitrous oxide, or dephlogisticated nitrous air, and its respiration* (Davy, 1800b, p. 108 et seq.). He concluded that at high temperatures "nitrate of ammoniac is wholly resolved into water, nitrous acid, nitrous gas (nitric oxide), and nitrogene; whilst a vivid luminous appearance is produced" (p. 112): and that "From the rapidity with which the deflagration of nitrate of ammoniac proceeds (at high temperatures), and from the immense quantity of light produced, it is reasonable to suppose that a very great increase of temperature takes place. The tube in which the decomposition has been effected, is always ignited after the process" (p. 113). For the production of large quantities of nitrous oxide, Davy recommended the use of "fibrous nitrate of ammoniac. . . . This salt undergoes no decomposition till the greater

part of its water is evaporated, and in consequence at the commencement of that process, is uniformly heated" (p. 118).

Davy again emphasized that the gas produced "must be suffered to rest at least for an hour after its generation. At the end of this time it is generally fit for respiration. If examined before, it will be found to contain more or less of a white vapour, which has a disagreeable acidulous taste, and strongly irritates the fauces and lungs" (p. 118). Further experiments demonstrated "that solutions of green sulphate of iron dissolve nitrous gas (nitric oxide) in quantities proportional to their concentrations" (p. 175); and "that the solution of green muriate (chloride) of iron absorbs nitrous gas" (p. 186): so, Davy was able to advise that "For separating nitrous gas from gases absorbable to no great extent by water, a well boiled solution of muriate of iron should be employed" (p. 193). Apparently, however, he did not use wash-bottles containing these solutions for routine purification of nitrous oxide prepared for respiration, although this was recommended when nitrous oxide was later prepared for anaesthesia (figs. 5, 7, 8, 9, 10).

The cost of raw material was also considered. Davy (1800b, p. 121) mentioned in a footnote that: "A pound of nitrate of ammoniac costs about 5s. 10d. This pound, properly decomposed, produces rather more than 34 moderate doses of air; so that the expense of a dose is about 2d. What fluid stimulus can be procured at so cheap a rate?" (p. 121). He also noted that:

A mode of producing ammoniac at little expense has been proposed by Mr. Watt. Condensed in the Sulphuric Acid, it can be easily made to combine with nitric acid, from the decomposition of nitre by double affinity. And thus if the hopes which the experiments at the end of those researches induce us to indulge, do not prove fallacious, a substance which has been heretofore almost exclusively appropriated to the destruction of mankind, may become, in the hands of philosophy, a means of producing health and pleasurable sensation [p. 232].

The air-holders in which Davy stored nitrous oxide were enclosed tanks filled, initially, with water. As the water was drained from the bottom of a tank, nitrous oxide was aspirated into the top from the hydraulic bellows, and: "The water thrown out of the airholders in consequence of the introduction of the gas, is preserved in a vessel

The combustion and deflagration of inflammable substances, metals, and various compounds in oxygen gas, form some of the most beautiful and interesting experiments in modern chemistry. The intense splendour of the liberated light and the variety of its colours astonish the spectator, and become a pleasing addition to our national amusements, while the experiments serve at the same time to elucidate some of the great laws of nature.

Many people, however, have complained that, notwithstanding the simplicity to which apparatus for such experiments has been reduced, something was still desirable to enable those who have not had many opportunities of acquiring habits of experimenting to enjoy this interesting science without the inconvenience of being obliged to use a pneumatic cistern for the purpose of transferring the gas. To accommodate some friends of this description, I contrived a gas-holder, which not only obviates the above inconvenience, but it is capable of being employed to transport the gas from place to place, and to preserve it from being contaminated, and of being used for experiments with the blow pipe [fig. 2].

It is such an air-holder that is illustrated on the title-page of the song "Laughing Gas" which was sung by Mr W. Smith around 1830 (see Part II; Smith, 1965b). Similar air-holders were used well into the second half of the century. They were described by Wylde (1872) who also referred to a way of preparing oxygen in a cylinder:

When oxygen is required in large quantities, ... the most common [arrangement] is that of a mercury bottle, into which a bent iron tube is screwed. The bottle is then charged with the oxygen mixture (two parts of chlorate of potassium and one part of black oxide of manganese), and heat is applied from a common fire. ... To receive the gas, gasometers of various shapes and sizes are constructed. Our diagrams [fig. 3], will give you an idea of both the mercury bottle and a very convenient form of gasometer or gas holder.

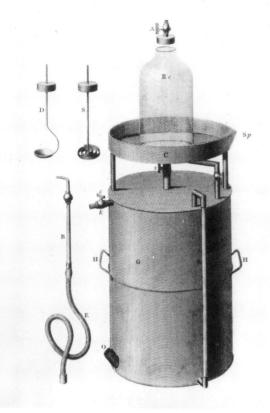

FIG. 2

Pepys's (1802) gas-holder. The gas-holder G had a capacity from 2 to 10 gallons. "Bladders mounted with cocks may be filled with gas by first emptying them of atmospheric air, then screwing them to cock *ck*, filling the cistern (C) with water and opening the cock 2 ... the quantity used may be ascertained from [the water level in] the register (R) which has a scale of pints or cubic inches attached to it." (By courtesy of the Brotherton Library, University of Leeds.)

adapted for the purpose, and employed to fill them again; for if common water is employed in every experiment, a great loss of gas would be produced from absorption" (p. 120). Davy also appreciated that if he used common water, the nitrous oxide would be diluted by "air previously contained in the water, (which in no case can be perfectly freed from it by ebulliation) ..." (p. 93).

A popular version of Watt's air-holder was designed by Pepys (1802) for more general use, and in particular for oxygen:

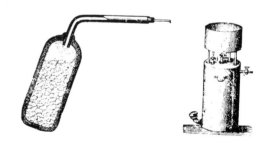

FIG. 3

On the left: a mercury bottle containing "two parts of chlorate of potassium and one part of black oxide of manganese" for generation of oxygen. On the right: a version of Pepys's gas-holder, illustrated as late as 1872. (By courtesy of the Regent Street Polytechnic; Dept. of Medical Photography, University of Leeds and United Leeds Hospitals.)

That these were in fairly common use at the time is evident from their casual presence on the floor of a laboratory illustrated above one of the chapter headings in Wylde's book (fig. 4).

Despite the precautions that he took to prevent anyone making "injurious experiments upon himself", Davy (1800b, p. 479), ". . . during a fit of enthusiasm produced by the respiration of nitrous oxide . . . resolved to endeavour to breathe nitrous gas (nitric oxide)."

"114 cubic inches (1870 ml.) of nitrous gas were introduced into the large mercurial airholder; two small silk bags of the capacity of seven quarts were filled with nitrous oxide.

After a forced exhaustion of my lungs, my nose being accurately closed, I made three inspirations and expirations of nitrous oxide in one of the bags, to free my lungs as much as possible from atmospheric oxygen; then, after a full expiration of nitrous oxide, I transferred my mouth from the mouth-piece of the bag to that of the airholder, and turning the stop-cock, attempted to inspire the nitrous gas. In passing through my mouth and fauces, it tasted astringent and highly disagreeable; it occasioned a sense of burning in the throat, and produced a spasm of the epiglottis so painful as to oblige me to desist instantly from attempts to inspire it. After moving my lips from the mouth-piece, when I opened them to inspire common air, aeriform nitrous acid was instantly formed in my mouth, which burnt the tongue and palate, injured the teeth, and produced an inflammation of the mucous membrane which lasted some hours. . . . I never design again to attempt so rash an experiment.

It is likely that Davy inhaled lower concentrations of the higher oxides of nitrogen unintentionally on a number of occasions. That the nitrous oxide inhaled was not always pure was implied by his statement that: "Whenever the gas was in a high state of purity, it tasted distinctly sweet to the tongue and palate, and had an agreeable odour" (Davy, 1800b, p. 460). He also described incidents when impurities were undoubtedly present, for example:

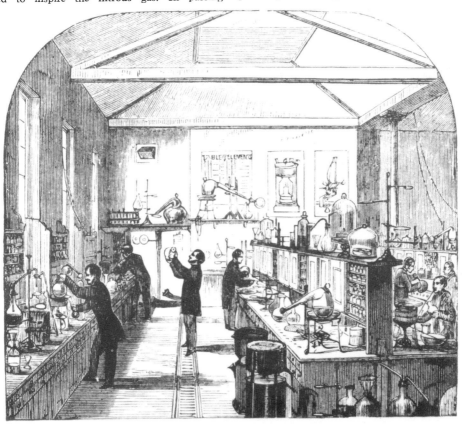

FIG. 4

An illustration of a chemical laboratory published in 1872, indicating that Pepys's gas-holders (centre floor) were still in common use. (By courtesy of the Regent Street Polytechnic; Dept. of Medical Photography, University of Leeds and United Leeds Hospitals.)

On May 3rd. To ascertain whether the gas would accelerate or retard the progress of sleep, I breathed at about 8 o'clock in the evening, 25 quarts of nitrous oxide, in quantities of six at a time, allowing short intervals between each dose. The feelings were much less pleasurable than usual, and during the consumption of the last two doses, almost indifferent; indeed the gas was breathed rather too soon after its production and contained some suspended acid vapour which stimulated the lungs so as to induce coughing.

After the experiments, for the first time I was somewhat depressed and debilitated; my propensity to sleep, however, came on at the usual hour, and as usual was indulged in, my repose was sound and unbroken.

Between May and July, Davy "habitually breathed the gas, occasionally three or four times a day for a week together; at other periods, four or five times a week only". But it is impossible to assess how carefully the nitrous oxide was prepared, and to what extent the subjective consequences of breathing it were due to the inhalations, or to his general mental and physical activity at the time. In his own words:

The doses were generally from six to nine quarts; their effects appeared undiminished by habit, and were hardly ever exactly similar. Sometimes I had feelings of intense intoxication, attended with but little pleasure; at other times, sublime emotions connected with highly vivid ideas. . . .

The general effects of its operation upon my health and state of mind, are extremely difficult of description. . . .

I slept much less than usual, my mind was long occupied by visible imagery. I had a constant desire of action, a restlessness, and an uneasy feeling about the praecordium analogous to the sickness of hope.

But perhaps these phaenomena in some measure depended on the interest and labour connected with the experimental investigations relating to the production of nitrous oxide, by which I was at this time incessantly occupied.

My appetite was as usual, and my pulse not materially altered. . . .

During the last week in which I breathed it uniformly, I imagined that I had increased sensibility of touch. . . . I was certainly more irritable, and felt more anxiety from trifling circumstances. My bodily strength was rather diminished than increased. . . .

Between September and the end of October, I made but few experiments on respiration; almost the whole of my time being devoted to chemical experiments on the production and analysis of nitrous oxide.

At this period my health being somewhat injured by the constant labour of experimenting, and the perpetual inhalation of the acid vapours of the laboratory, I went to Cornwall; where new associations of ideas and feelings, common exercise, a pure atmosphere, luxurious diet and moderate indulgence in wine, in a month restored me to health and vigour.

So long as nitrous oxide was rebreathed from a bag, its effectiveness was reduced due to its

mixture with the air already in the lungs (Clover, 1868; see Part VII, Smith, 1966b). The same argument can be applied to the inhalation of impurities, but this is not to say that they can be rebreathed with impunity, as was pointed out in a contribution to the *Journal of Science and the Arts*, by Michael Faraday* (M. F., 1819; Jeffreys, 1960). Oddly, the higher oxides of nitrogen were not mentioned:

Instances have occurred where the respiration of this gas (nitrous oxide) has been said to produce, in place of pleasant sensations, very injurious and alarming effects on the health of the body and state of the spirits; but it is probable that many of these have been occasioned by impurities in the gas. There are two or three products very frequently obtained in small quantities, by the distillation of common nitrate of ammonia, which, if not removed from the nitrous oxide, must have injurious effects: these are chlorine, the vapour of azotane or chloride of nitrogen, and perhaps may be mentioned also nitrogen.

When muriate of ammonia is present with the nitrate of ammonia, these substances are always disengaged: if the quantity of muriate is small they may be removed by standing over water, but when occurring in large proportions, they may remain for some time in the gas. When a mixture of nitrate and muriate of ammonia are heated together, there is an action between the elements much more violent than if the nitrate were pure, a great proportion of the muriate is decomposed, and but little distils over unaltered. It would seem that the nitrous oxide in the nascent state acted upon both ammonia and the muriatic acid, for the products of a distillation of this kind are nitrogen, chlorine, muriatic acid, and a portion of the chloride of azote in vapour, and scarcely any nitrous oxide is obtained.

It is evident that a gas containing the above substances in mixture must be very deleterious when respired; and I have rarely found the nitrate of

---

* Faraday liquefied nitrous oxide a few years later (Faraday, 1823). Two fluids were obtained, one was a "heavier fluid found to be water, with a little acid and nitrous oxide in solution; the other was nitrous oxide". He also observed: "A gauge being introduced into a tube in which liquid nitrous oxide was afterwards produced, gave the pressure of its vapour as equal to 50 atmospheres at 45° (F)". Later (Faraday, 1845), using two mechanical pumps in series, and cooling the gas, solidified nitrous oxide which "appeared as a beautiful clear crystalline body. The temperature required for this effect must have been very nearly the lowest, perhaps 150° (F) below 0°." At this time he found that the liquid nitrous oxide "gave very uncertain results at different times as to the pressure of its vapour; results which can only be accounted for by supposing that there are two different bodies present, soluble in each other, but differing in the elasticity of their vapours". He thought that the second gas was probably nitrogen. He also acknowledged that M. Natterer had obtained liquid nitrous oxide in "considerable" quantities "by the use of pumps only". Faraday died in 1867, the year before Evans re-introduced nitrous oxide anaesthesia to Great Britain.

ammonia of commerce that did not produce them.*
It is, however, easy to guard against their ill effects,
by testing the first portions of gas that come over.
When a nitrate containing muriate is distilled, the first
effect is a mutual decomposition of the salts, and a
resolution of them into substances mentioned, and this
goes on until all the muriate is destroyed (supposing
the nitrate to be in excess); the nitrate is then left
pure and gives excellent gas, though before scarcely
any nitrous oxide could be obtained from it. The odour
from the gas is sufficient, even without any reference
to the usual tests of the purity of nitrous oxide, to tell
the presence of chlorine and chloride of nitrogen in
the first portion; and when the gas obtained by a
moderate distillation, is free from the peculiar odours
of these bodies, it may always be breathed with safety,
except by the few who experience effects apparently
anomalous to those which belong to the gas.

It was probably because he had witnessed the
consequences of breathing impurities in imperfectly prepared nitrous oxide that Brande (1827)
warned that he had "seen ill effects from having
inhaled it". Stanley (1842) also revealed an
awareness of the dangers of overheating ammonium nitrate (see Part II; Smith, 1965b).

There is evidence that gases may have been
compressed into bottles for medical use even
before Colton revived the use of nitrous oxide for
dental anaesthesia in 1862–63 (see Part V; Smith
1966a). Davison (1954) came across an anonymous
booklet entitled *Pneuma-Therapeia* which was

---

* This is not true today. Ammonium nitrate was first
manufactured by Imperial Chemical Industries Ltd. in
1926, primarily for explosives and "nitro-chalk" fer-
tilizer, but it was not sold to manufacturers of nitrous
oxide until 1936. The principal impurities that made
ammonium nitrate unsuitable for this purpose before
1936 were iron and chlorine. Iron, derived from
materials of construction of the plant, would have been
present in concentrations of about 60 p.p.m. Chlorine,
introduced at Tees Valley water, then used in the
manufacture of weak nitric acid, would have been in
concentrations of about 50 p.p.m. Improved materials
of plant construction and the use of a condensate
source of water have reduced these impurities to well
within the specification of not more than 10 p.p.m. of
iron, and not more than 15 p.p.m. of chlorine (Peacock,
J. M., I.C.I. Ltd., personal communication). Coxeter
& Son Ltd. purchased ammonium nitrate from I.C.I.
Ltd. in 1939. Between 1931 and 1939 it was imported
from Belgium, and before that from Norway (Edmundson, W., personal communication). Silk (1888) recommended testing a solution of the ammonium nitrate
with "solutions of chloride of barium, and nitrate of
silver . . . the formation of even a faint cloudiness or
precipitate . . . should lead to the rejection of the salt".
He added: "It [N₂O] is now, however, very seldom
prepared at home." Fox (1868b) obtained his granu-
lated ammonium nitrate from Hopkins and Williams,
New Cavendish Street; and from Messrs. Evans and
Lescher, of Bartholomew Close.

published by the Medical Pneumatic Company,
Piccadilly, as early as 1856. At the bottom of
the title-page was the signature "G. Barth" in
pencil. The booklet advertised oxygen and other
gases compressed in wrought iron bottles of
"little more than five pints fluid measure
capacity".* It stated:

The Medical Pneumatic Apparatus Company is ready
to execute orders and supply gas. A prospectus and
description of their apparatus, with charges for sale
or hire, and all other information, will be forwarded
gratis by post, or furnished personally by applying to
the Manager, Medical Pneumatic Apparatus Company,
46, Regent Circus, Piccadilly, London.

It had this to say about nitrous oxide:

The inhalation of the protoxide of nitrogen (laughing gas of Sir Humphry Davy) is well known as a
curious and amusing lecture room experiment. If used
diluted with air in properly regulated doses, the customary effect of large doses undiluted is never produced; it has then a most beneficial influence in many
deranged functional conditions; rapid cures of defective
vision, deafness,† and certain forms of paralysis have
been accomplished by it. It has also a remarkable effect
on the animal spirits, and causes a happy tone of feeling which is not succeeded by depression as is customary after the use of alcoholic stimulants. A single
dose is often sufficient to avert an approaching fit of
melancholy or hypochondriasis. As it powerfully in-
creases muscular strength it certainly deserves to be
tried in cases of lingering and difficult parturition
where the expulsive uterine efforts are nearly exhausted.

This company, however, was not mentioned in
the anaesthetic literature of the period, and it is
not known whether it ever thrived. Davison (1954)
suggested that the commercial supply of bottled
gases was at least ready to be launched.

THE PREPARATION OF NITROUS OXIDE AFTER THE
REVIVAL OF ITS USE FOR ANAESTHESIA

Colton (1868) and Fox (1868a) recommended the
Sprague model of nitrous oxide generator which
was made in America, complete with retort, wash
bottles and gasometer. Particular claims for this
apparatus were that it provided for automatic
control of the production of nitrous oxide, and
that it avoided rebreathing by the use of valves.
To quote Sprague (1864):

---

* The Viennese fire brigade used a "rescue apparatus"
that consisted of a large tin bottle filled with compressed air, in 1833. The first regeneration apparatus
containing chemicals and compressed oxygen was
constructed by Schwann of Liege in 1854 (Teleky,
1948).

† See Addendum Chapter 4.

With apparatus where the heat shall be accurately
and uniformly regulated by the flow of nitrous oxide
itself, precluding the possibility of overheating the
nitrate of ammonia, a pure gas, unwatched, may be
prepared at a trifling cost. This has recently been
effected.

In defence of the use of nitrous oxide for
anaesthesia he wrote:

Attempts have been made, by interested parties, to
prejudice the public against the use of nitrous oxide,
by representing the ordinary mode of inhaling it as
"filthy and disgusting". Such a puerile objection we
deem unworthy a reply, and should pass it, but for
the fact that it is not without its influence with morbid
and unreflecting minds. That there are slatterns in
dentistry as in culinary offices, is not a question of
doubt. Who is so simple as to decry all catering, because the dishes of certain hotels have been found in
some cases improperly rinsed? The same idea holds
true in the use of nitrous oxide. But admitting, if you
please, the return of the breath to the bag as neither
safe nor cleanly (which we deny where the quantity of
the gas is sufficient), the objection may be readily met
by a use of the valved breathing tube attached to the
cock of the bag, allowing no return of the breath to
this. Such we have tried with the best of results—
producing perfect anaesthesia, with a moderate
quantity of gas.

Duncum (1947, p. 275) illustrates the type of
apparatus designed by Sprague c.1863 for generating, purifying and collecting nitrous oxide gas,
but this does not provide for the passage of
nitrous oxide through a "regulator" for controlling the amount of heat applied to the retort.
Similar apparatus (fig. 5) was illustrated by
Thomas (1870), whose book was published by
S. S. White of Philadelphia. Samuel S. White also
advertised this apparatus in the back of the book.
A complete apparatus of 40 gallons capacity cost
$71.50. The 50-gallon size cost $75 and boxing
was an additional $2.50. Retorts were advertised
at $1.50, and, fused nitrate of ammonia cost 60
cents per lb. for quantities less than 25 lb., or
50 cents per lb. for 25-lb. or 50-lb. boxes. For
those unable to afford a gasometer, Thomas suggested the adaptation of a barrel to serve for the
washing, collection and storage of nitrous oxide
(fig. 6). The barrel was first filled with water
from the top. Nitrous oxide was then aspirated
from the retort by letting water run out at the
bottom. The bubbling of the gas through the
remaining water was considered sufficient for
washing and purifying it. Nitrous oxide was displaced from the barrel when required by letting
more water run in at the top.

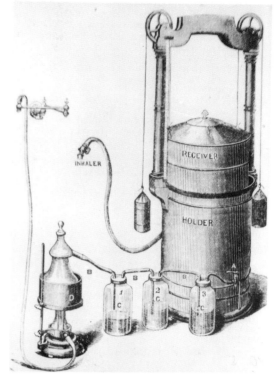

FIG. 5

S. S. White's apparatus for generating, washing, purifying and storing nitrous oxide (Thomas, 1870). A solution of sulphate of iron was used in one bottle and
water in the other two. (By courtesy of the Royal
Society of Medicine.)

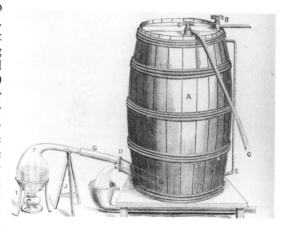

FIG. 6

A barrel used for the washing and storing of nitrous
oxide generated in a retort (Thomas, 1870). (By
courtesy of the Royal Society of Medicine.)

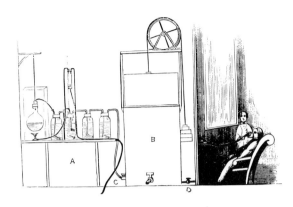

FIG. 7

Sketch showing the Sprague apparatus in use (Fox, 1868b) (Dept. of Medical Photography, University of Leeds and the United Leeds Hospitals).

Fox (1868b), in considering the manufacture of nitrous oxide, was enthusiastically in favour of the Sprague apparatus. His sketch of the layout he used is shown in figure 7.

. . . there are many plans, all, with one or two exceptions, based upon the same principle. The most easy proceeding for those who do not wish to be at the trouble of making their own apparatus is to order Sprague's or White's apparatus from one of the Dental depots. My only objection to White's [fig. 5] is that the connecting tubes are metallic, and liable, therefore, to oxydise and clog, and there is no regulator attached. If you order one of Sprague's apparatus with his regulator you will have, in my opinion, the very best apparatus that has yet been contrived for making the gas. It is the only one I have found after every trial to act with uniform comfort and regularity.

He continued:

If you desire to fit up your own apparatus, all you need is a flask or retort, connected with glass tubing, of about one quarter of an inch to one half of an inch in the bore, to a set of three Woulfe's bottles, holding about four pints each, stoppered with perforated corks to receive the tubes, which should be connected with india rubber tubing (in the wash bottles should be placed—in the first, pure water; in the second, a solution of caustic potash, half a pound of potash to one gallon of water to take up any nitrous acid that may be found; and in the next a solution of protosulphate of iron, one half pound to one gallon of water to purify the gas from any nitric oxide. This is a precautionary measure only, as, if the gas is made with proper care, none of these products should be evolved).* All these matters can be obtained at Griffin's, Garrick Street, Covent Garden, or any manufacturing chemist. This was the plan I adopted first, and is the one still used at Messrs. Bell & Co.'s, the eminent chemists in Oxford

* See also Sculley (1871).

Street, who make all the gas supplied to the Dental Hospital. Mr. Porter, the gentleman who has the especial charge of this department, takes particular pride in the purity of his gas, and the completeness of his apparatus, and he has certainly contrived one of the most complete, and, I may almost say, automatic gas making arrangements that I have ever seen, by which not only the amount of coal gas turned on is regulated, thereby controlling the heat, but, in case of any accident causing the nitrous oxide to be evolved too rapidly, a whistle sounding calls attention to the danger.

A drawing of Mr. Porter's (1868) apparatus is shown in figure 8. The pressure generated in the nitrous oxide supply line was used to control the amount of coal gas supplied to the burner. Messrs. Crapper & Co. (*Brit. J. dent. Sci.*, 1871a) supplied similar apparatus (fig. 9) but they acknowledged the regulator as Sprague's. This type of apparatus was apparently still in vogue when Silk's *Manual of Nitrous Oxide Anaesthesia* was published in 1888 (fig. 10). Mr. Ash's regulator was also described in 1869 (*Brit. J. dent. Sci.*):

. . . it has one great advantage over Sprague's, and that is, that in the event of the coal gas going quite out perfect safety is insured by a little valve which admits the external air into the flask, thereby preventing the formation of that disastrous vacuum which has caused the fracture of so many flasks.

Various designs of gasometer were marketed. Fox (1868b) mentioned the name of a man making them in London: "Jordon, of Wells Street, Oxford Street, is now an experienced hand at making these gasometers, and I can strongly recommend him." The following are illustrated here: S. S. White's, figure 5; Crapper's, figure 9; a decorated gasometer illustrated in Rottenstein (1880), figure 11; and one from Ash & Sons (Silk, 1888), figure 12. Other examples have been illustrated by Cohen (1941) and by Macintosh, Mushin and Epstein (1958). (See figure 0.15 on page xxiv for a gasometer which has survived in Sheffield.)

The firms of Barth and of Coxeter & Son were both manufacturing nitrous oxide in 1868 (*Brit. J. dent. Sci.*, 1868a), and they wasted little time in changing from supplying it in bladders and bags, to supplying it in iron bottles (fig. 13). (See footnote, p. 364, Fox (1869).) In the same year there was also a notice in the *British Journal of Dental Science* (1868c) to say that: "C. Ash & Sons have set aside one of their show rooms at Broad Street, Golden Square . . . for the occasional

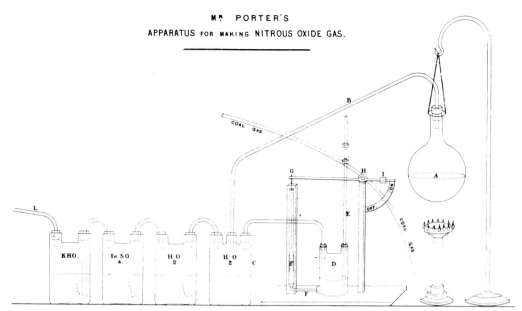

FIG. 8

Mr. Porter's apparatus. The flask A is connected to a three-necked Woulfe's bottle C; one neck leads to the wash-bottles, and the other is connected to another bottle D. This is partly filled with water into which dips tube E which is connected to a whistle. Another tube F connects bottle D, below the water level, to another bottle containing a float f, and this is connected to a lever G-H which is counterpoised by the weight I, the fulcrum being the plug of a gas tap. (Dept. of Medical Photography, University of Leeds and United Leeds Hospitals.)

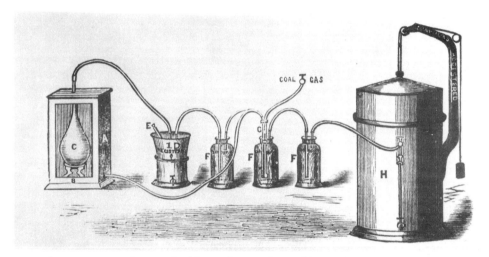

A. Iron retort case, improved with ventilator and portable top for the ready adjustment of flask. Height 1 ft. 10 inches.

B. Bunsen burner.

C. Retort fixed on sand-bath and Bunsen burner.

D. Porcelain condenser, divided into two chambers (see sectional view), the upper, No. 1, water bath for cooling the connections; No. 2, lower reservoir for collecting the condensed moisture given off during the boiling of the nitrate of ammonia. No. 3 is made of porous body, causing the gas to cool rapidly. Height 1 ft. 1 inch.

E. Cork to be drawn to prevent vacuum immediately upon ceasing making the gas.

F.F.F. Wash bottles, with porcelain mounts and stands. Height 12 inches.

G. Sprague's coal gas regulator.

H. Eighty-gallon gasometer. Height 6 ft. 7 inches.

FIG. 9

Messrs. Crapper & Co.'s apparatus for manufacturing nitrous oxide. (Department of Medical Photography, University of Leeds and the United Leeds Hospitals.)

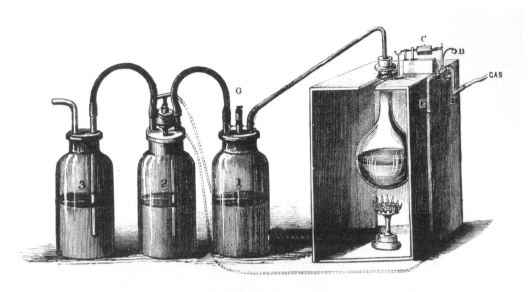

—Apparatus for the preparation of Nitrous Oxide. The Ammonium Nitrate is placed in
the flask and heated by the burner below. A, B, C, arrangement for regulating the
supply of coal gas; D, E, pipe supplying coal gas to the burner. 1, 2, 3, wash bottles.

FIG. 10
Apparatus for the manufacture of nitrous oxide supplied by Ash & Son and illustrated in Silk
(1888). "When the flask and its contents fall below a weight regulated by the counterpoise C,
the catch B is released, and presses at A upon the pipe E.D, supplying burner F, and at the
same time the flask itself is raised." (Dept. of Medical Photography, University of Leeds and
the United Leeds Hospitals.)

manufacture of nitrous oxide, in order that those
Dentists intending to make it themselves may be
instructed in the best way of doing so."

George Barth, and Coxeter & Son, did not
succeed in liquefying the gas until 1870 (*Brit J.
dent. Sci.*, 1870; *Brit. med. J.*, 1870) (fig. 14)
despite the suggestion having been made by Mr.
Ernest Hart in 1868 (*Brit. med. J.*, 1868), and
despite Evans (1868) having brought over a bottle
of liquid gas in the same year. A later nitrous
oxide bottle, taken from Rottenstein (1880) is
shown in figure 15.

The signature of G. Barth on the title-page of
the booklet *Pneuma-Therapaeia* discovered by
Davison (1954) is tantalizing, but it is not certain
whether Barth had any direct connection with the
Medical Pneumatic Apparatus Company. It may
be relevant to note that in 1868 it was reported
that: "Mr. Barth tells us he has bottles in use now

which were made fifteen years ago" (*Brit. J.
dent. Sci.*, 1868a). Those bottles, therefore, would
have been made in 1853. Shuter (1912) provided
further evidence, although he did not quote his
sources. He wrote:

As patients increased in numbers it became inconvenient for surgeons and dentists to make their own
gas, consequently a demand quickly grew for reliable
sources of supply.

At first gas was sold by Bell and other chemists in
large rubber bags, which were so bulky and cumbrous
that the need of a more portable container was keenly
felt. As soon as the demand was sufficient to make
the business pay, Mr. George Barth solved the difficulty. He was already selling compressed oxygen for
medical purposes,* and it was a short step to treat

* When a death following nitrous oxide anaesthesia
occurred in Exeter, in 1873 (see below), Barth was
quick off the mark in writing to the *British Journal of
Dental Science* suggesting the use of oxygen for restoring animation in cases where respiration ceases before
the action of the heart: "It has been suggested to us

nitrous oxide in the same fashion. He used old puddled iron mercury bottles which he tapped and fitted with a valve, but these were so big and heavy that he substituted brazed copper cylinders, each of a quart size containing fifteen gallons of gas,* so the pressure in them was really below the limits of safety and in more than one instance the end blew off.

Soon afterwards Mr. Orchard was enabled by ingenious improvements in the machinery to supply liquefied gas under much safer conditions, and from that time forward nitrous oxide has been stored and used in the liquid state except in inaccessible districts where the original method of retorting and storing in a gasometer is still in vogue.

Up to that time the "Dental Hospital" was still making its own nitrous oxide. At a meeting of the Odontological Society of Great Britain held in December 1870, Mr. Braine revealed that:

. . . since the 1st of April last year, nitrous oxide gas had been administered more than 2,100 times in the Dental Hospital; some of the gas used having been supplied by Messrs. Bell, and some having come from Messrs. Coxeter, both in the compressed and in the liquid form; but by far the largest quantity had been made in the building by their late excellent house surgeon, Mr. Milward Harding.

The main reason for compressing nitrous oxide into bottles was to facilitate its distribution and use. An added advantage of liquefying it was thought to be that a purer product could be obtained. This possibility was appreciated by Andrews when he was experimenting with mixtures of nitrous oxide and oxygen (see Lichtenstein and Method, 1953). In 1868 he wrote:

Dr. Evans, the well-known American dentist in Paris, asserts that the ordinary nitrous oxide is very far from pure, even when well made. He states that he has been in the habit of purifying his gas by mechanically condensing it into a liquid under high pressure. This liquid being absolutely pure nitrous oxide, is then allowed to reassume the gaseous form in a bag or gasometer. He finds that the gas thus purified, only requires about half the usual quantity to anaesthetise a patient.

that the anaesthesia produced by nitrous oxide is generally supposed to arise from deprivation of oxygen . . ., a ready means of inflating the lungs with that gas in its pure state in combination with the ordinary method of producing artificial respiration would be very desirable. We have therefore prepared iron bottles containing oxygen gas in a highly compressed state with connections to fit the apparatus ordinarily in use for administering the nitrous oxide gas."

* If this had been so, the pressure in the cylinder would have been 60 atmospheres and the gas would have liquefied (cf. fig. 13).

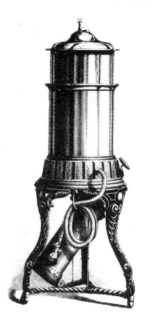

Fig. 11

A gasometer illustrated in Rottenstein (1880). (Department of Medical Photography, University of Leeds and the United Leeds Hospitals.)

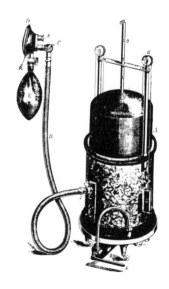

Fig. 12

A gasometer made by Ash & Sons and illustrated in Silk (1888). (Department of Medical Photography, University of Leeds and the United Leeds Hospitals.)

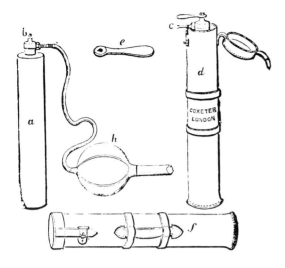

FIG. 13

Coxeter's vessels for compressed gas. "*a*, represents one of these iron vessels holding 36 gallons of compressed gas; it is 28½ inches long and 4½ inches in diameter, weighing 23 lbs. . . . The gas issues with great force from the tap, *b*, which is turned by the handle, *e*. . . . To allow the force with which the gas, owing to its compressed state, issues from the bottle, to be expanded, it is first received into what is known as Cattlin's bag, from which it is inhaled by the patient with as much ease and comfort as from an ordinary gasometer. The tube connecting the Cattlin's bag to the bottle is of small calibre, but the one at the other end of the bag to which the usual stopcock and facepiece is attached is of the usual size. The bag and small tube is attached to the bottle by a screw union at *c* and can be readily detached" (Fox, 1869). These data suggest that the gas was compressed to about 28 ats. (Dept. of Medical Photography, University of Leeds and United Leeds Hospitals.)

It was not until 1872 that he was able to write:

Many months ago I made experiments on the use of nitrous oxide pure, and nitrous oxide mixed with oxygen, with the view of adapting them to the purpose of anaesthesia in general surgery. These experiments . . . showed that there were several difficulties in the way of using, for prolonged operations, the ordinary gas of dentists—one of which was that the gas never makes the least approach to purity, containing always from 10 to 25 per cent free nitrogen and oxygen. As it is almost impossible to separate the free nitrogen without apparatus for reducing this gas to the liquid form, I suspended the experiments until this deficiency could be supplied. Three weeks ago I received from Johnston Brothers' Dental Depot, New York, an apparatus and a supply of liquid nitrous oxide equal to 100 gallons of the gas.* . . . The liquid was contained in a strong iron flask

about four inches wide and twelve inches long. When it is desired to use the anaesthetic a faucet is turned slightly, allowing the gas to escape into a rubber tube leading to a small sack, and then to an ordinary inhaler, so contrived, with valves, that the inspirations are drawn from the sack, and the expirations pass into the open air. . . . The intention is to have the flasks kept ready filled at drug stores and dental depots, where the surgeon can return his empty flasks and procure filled ones.

FIG. 14

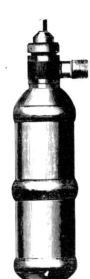

Barth's liquid nitrous oxide. "The 25-gallon copper bottles of liquid gas . . . measure exactly 8¾ inches (including the valve) by 2 inches diameter, and weigh when full 2 lb. 1 oz. only . . . they may be easily carried in the pocket if desired" (*Brit. J. dent. Sci.*, 1871c). The account finished on a cautious note. "But we should first like to be quite assured as to the safety of these slight-looking vessels. We cannot forget the alarm that was once raised about Coxeter's much more solid-looking vessels. But we have no doubt Mr. Barth could give us equal strong proofs of the safety of his arrangement. We remember that when Mr. Coxeter first introduced liquid nitrous oxide, he supplied 25-gallon bottles, 6 inches long and 2 inches in diameter, but those holding 50 gallons were so portable that no demand arose for the 25-gallon bottles." (Dept. of Medical Photography, University of Leeds and United Leeds Hospitals.)

Although Andrews received at least one bottle of the liquefied gas, he does not appear to have left any record of having resumed experiments with oxygen and "pure" nitrous oxide mixtures.

A vivid account of the beginnings of the manufacture and distribution of nitrous oxide in this country has been given by H. S. Coxeter (quoted by Boyle, 1934), a great-grandson of the original Coxeter:

---

* James Coxeter & Son (1873) drew attention to the fact that "Messrs. Johnston obtained the complete nitrous oxide apparatus from us, including Mr. Clover's facepiece, supplemental bag, stop-cock, and two-way stopcock, Mr. Catlin's Reservoir bag, and the iron vessel containing 100 gallons of liquid nitrous oxide designed by ourselves, and after careful examination decided to copy it, as they considered it would be difficult to improve upon the arrangement. . . ."

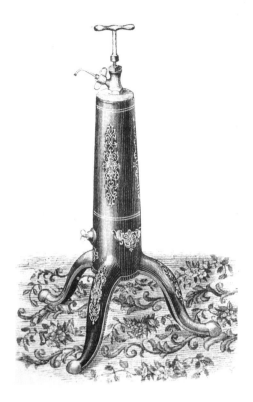

FIG. 15

An ornate nitrous oxide bottle illustrated in Rotten-stein (1880). (Dept. of Medical Photography, University of Leeds and United Leeds Hospitals.)

For some of the earliest cases of nitrous oxide anaesthesia, both in the laboratory and in private dental practice, the gas was supplied in ox bladders, the patient inhaling the gas through the outlet tap, while his nose was pinched by one assistant and the bladder was squeezed by another. It is true that these early cases were mostly of an experimental nature, although slight operations were often performed under a sufficiently deep, but often unexpectedly short anaesthesia. These bladders* of nitrous oxide were regularly supplied by J. Coxeter & Son for use at the old University Hospital opposite their premises. The gas was made by heating ammonium nitrate in glass laboratory retorts over a bunsen burner and collecting it under water, no further washing being considered necessary. The interest taken by the surgeons in the new anaesthesia, and its immense popularity among the students, due largely to the amusement caused by the hilarious

---

* S. S. White, in America (Thomas, 1870), advertised "Rubber Gasometers, Square". They ranged in size from 18×24 inches at $6 to 30×40 inches at $12. They also advertised six sizes of "Rubber Gas Bags, Oval" from the 5-gallon size at $4.25 to the 10-gallon size at $9.50.

excitement exhibited by the patient under this crude method of administration, pointed to a great future for "laughing gas".

Delivery by messengers carrying bundles of bladders like a toy balloon seller was obviously impracticable, and Mr. Coxeter quickly had some cylinders made of wrought iron tubes with welded tops, bottoms and seams.* Into these the gas was pumped by hand, with great expenditure of time and energy, and the gas sold according to the varying amount it had been reasonably possible to pump in. As the demand increased it became obvious that a more rapid method of manufacture and filling was necessary, and a factory was started in a covered yard, in which a gas-engine-driven compressor was installed. The heating of the ammonium nitrate was now done in cast iron retorts, into which melted ammonium nitrate was poured through a funnel and the orifice plugged securely. The retort was then heated over a gas ring, and the nitrous oxide bubbled through into a Woulfe's bottle containing a solution of caustic potash, entering a small gasometer, from which it was pumped into cylinders.

For a time there was considerable tension in the workshop, as no-one quite knew what might or might not happen either during the manufacture of the gas or the filling of the cylinders; the latter, although extremely heavy, had a nasty habit of developing a sudden and alarming leak at one end of the seams. Also the ammonium nitrate, not having the same high degree of purity obtained later, was somewhat erratic in its behaviour, and upon the appearance of white fumes in the Woulfe's bottles, hose pipes were turned on to the retort with all speed. Sometimes even this was ineffective, and as the gas came off with ever increasing force and fury, it was left in sole possession of the workshop, and the workmen anxiously awaited events outside. Improved methods of manufacture have been in use for some years, and the gas is now delivered in a very pure state. The unsatisfactory iron bottles were replaced by drawn seamless cylinders. Cast brass valves were replaced by those of tougher alloy, stamped or drop-forged.

Nowadays cylinders of liquefied gas are taken for granted, but when they were first introduced this was far from the case, as illustrated by the following exchange between Fox (1870b) and Coleman (1870a) in 1870 at a meeting of the Odontological Society of Great Britain.

Fox. The next matter he desired to bring before the notice of the Society was by this time, perhaps, rather an old story; namely the liquid nitrous oxide. After the last meeting of the Society several gentlemen ex-

---

* Fox (1869) described iron vessels $28\frac{1}{2}$ inches long and $4\frac{1}{2}$ inches in diameter holding 36 gallons of compressed gas and weighing 23 lb. (fig. 13). Larger vessels containing 72–90 gallons weighed about 35 lb. Later (Fox, 1870a) Messrs. Coxeter supplied the liquid gas in iron vessels of the same make and form, but of different size. The 100-gallon size was 12 inches long, $3\frac{1}{4}$ inches in diameter and weighed 9 lb. 1 oz. The 50-gallon size was $8\frac{1}{2}$ inches long, 3 inches in diameter and weighed 5 lb. 11 oz. The 25-gallon size was 6 inches long, 2 inches in diameter and weighed 3 lb. 5 oz. (cf. fig. 14).

pressed to him their great disappointment at not having seen some exhibition of it. He has therefore induced Mr. Coxeter to send a bottle this evening, which, though containing a hundred gallons, measured only 12 inches in length, $3\frac{1}{2}$ inches in diameter and 9 lb. in weight.

Coleman. . . . earnestly entreated it should not be handed about by warm hands in a warm room: there was great peril in so doing, and if an accident *should* occur, it would put an end to the Odontological Society as there represented.

Fox. After the remarks made by Mr. Coleman he must add that Mr. Coxeter had recently made very careful experiments on this subject, and it was only after one of these bottles had been subjected to a pressure of 6000 lb. on the square inch that it had actually burst. They might remember to their comfort that at present it was exposed to a pressure of 750 lb. to the square inch. When on the occasion of Mr. Coxeter's experiments the bottle did at last give way, it did not explode scattering itself into fragments, dealing destruction around, but it simply rent to an extent of about four inches, making a noise like the discharge of a rifle. He might add that one of these bottles had stood for the last two months in his own house, directly opposite a large fire in a warm room, and had been pretty considerably handled by his friends from the country.

Coleman (1870b) was not entirely reassured:

He (Mr. Coleman), with regard to the confidence expressed by Mr. Fox at the last meeting, might ask the Society to accept his statements with reservation, and for the gentleman's own safety he must urge him not to presume too much upon his calculations, which, being erroneous, might suddenly deprive the Odontological Society of his services . . . a bottle burst by hydraulic pressure, though a proper means of testing its actual strength, ought not be regarded as an example of what would occur to one burst by an elastic fluid.

Apparently not everyone heeded the warning, because Silk (1888) was later to write:

Keep the bottles as far as possible at an equable temperature, recollecting its susceptibility to changes; do not at any rate place them in hot water, or near or in the fire, as it is recorded has been done by more than one ingenious individual, with astonishing and sometimes fatal results.

Ritson (1871) told of another cause of "explosions":

The frequent bursting of Cattlin's bags during the exhibition of nitrous oxide, especially when the vessel is fully charged, may be prevented by fixing the vessel upright, valve end uppermost. The gas can then be made to flow gently or quickly as required. Since adopting this plan I have had no trouble, but in one case before I adopted this plan the sudden burst of gas from a fully charged vessel startled a patient when just anaesthetised, so that he leapt from the chair, and was violent for about three minutes. On recovery, said he thought he was drowning. I always have an assistant to regulate the supply of gas.

The firms of J. Bell & Co., George Barth & Co., and Coxeter & Son have been mentioned. Messrs. Ash & Son, of London, supplied the nitrous oxide which was administered to a patient who died in Exeter in 1873 (*Brit. J. dent. Sci.*; Willett, 1901). Another firm that supplied nitrous oxide during the last century was the Condensed Gas Co. Ltd., Manchester. This was founded by Mr. J. F. Blennerhassett, and in 1883 he entered into an agreement with a Manchester dentist, Mr. J. H. Parkinson, for the sale and delivery of nitrous oxide gas, and appliances for delivering and administering it, within the London area (Oscroft, 1934).* Cock (1934) added further details:

In 1887 my old fellow-student, Dr. Dudley Buxton, the anaesthetist, introduced me to J. F. Blennerhassett, who fitted me out with anaesthetic apparatus for a good many years. The N$_2$O bottles were of steel, with flat bottoms welded in. "J.F.B." was a quaint old bird, clever, ingenious, and perfervid, even to making interruptions at the local vestry or similar meetings: longhaired, with much tangled beard, and withal a very likeable chap. After he died, or gave up, I was supplied by Barth & Co. for many years. Somewhere in the early 'nineties I attended an old gentleman named Orchard, who claimed to be the first to condense oxygen in cylinders.† . . . The early cylinders were a great nuisance by reason of the freezing of water vapour in the neck.

Early doubts about the purity of nitrous oxide.

The first recorded death in this country following a dental extraction under nitrous oxide occurred in 1873 (*Brit. J. dent. Sci.*). Although this fatality appeared to be unrelated to the inhalation of impurities, the possibility was in the dentist's mind, and he made a point of saying:

I obtained my gas from Messrs. Ash and Son, of London. I am satisfied the gas was pure. I had used the very same flask for two patients before, and everything on these occasions went well. They are the first makers in London, and the gas comes to us in short iron jars. Six gallons is the quantity I generally use.

---

* According to an Army Council Instruction of 1920, the supplies of nitrous oxide for military hospitals in the Home Commands were to be obtained from this company—except for those situated in Middlesex, Kent, Surrey, Berkshire, Buckinghamshire, Dorsetshire, Wiltshire and Hampshire which were to be supplied from the Army Medical Store, Woolwich (*Lancet*, 1920).

† An early hand pump used for the purpose in America is illustrated by Sykes (1960, p. 8).

The apparatus I use is Clover's patent, manufactured by Coxeter, of London.*

Roberts (1884) was openly dubious about the purity of commercially liquefied gas. He mentioned no specific chemical tests, but he gave reasons to support his doubts:

I find from personal experience the gas is much safer and pleasanter to inhale, after being in contact with water for a few hours. This to my mind clearly proves that the purity of the gas . . . is very questionable, . . . instead of being passed through several purifying solutions . . . it appears to be purified upon the theory, that, notwithstanding any impure gases which may pass over the flask . . . only nitrous oxide becomes condensed and liquefied. . . .

For some years I have used both the liquid gas and the diffused gas from the gas holder—I mean chemically purified gas from the gas holder—and have noticed a marked difference, in fact such a difference that where medical men have taken the diffused gas themselves or their patients, they decidedly objected to the liquid gas afterwards. . . .

The compressed gas has a sweet taste and frequently produces a sense of suffocation. . . . Now with the diffused gas, if perfectly pure, there is not any recognisable taste. . . .

This, Sir, I think, clearly proves the theoretical purity of nitrous oxide gas to be very faulty, and although both liquid and condensed answer the chemical test, that test is also very unreliable.

Silk (1888) gave no indication of any serious trouble having arisen from the inhalation of impurities, in fact he implied that the gas was usually pretty pure, but he left little doubt that from time to time it could be grossly contaminated. Under the heading "Adulterations and Impurities" he wrote:

The simplicity of its manufacture, and the cheapness of the drugs employed in its preparation, render it less liable to adulteration or impurity than might otherwise be the case. It may, however, occasionally present traces of nitric oxide, and other oxides of nitrogen, owing to the distillation of the ammonium nitrate having been allowed to proceed too rapidly or to be conducted at too high a temperature; or it may contain traces of chlorine. . . . The presence of these impurities may be suspected if the gas has an irritating or suffocating taste and smell or causes undue coughing on inhalation, and if the gas thus suspected be passed by

means of a glass tube through a solution of nitrate of silver, a precipitate will indicate that a chloride is present, and inasmuch as the other gaseous oxides of nitrogen usually yield yellow or orange fumes upon being brought into contact with air, their presence is easily ascertained.

The gas may also occasionally have a rancid, disagreeable odour, due to the decomposition of the oils used to lubricate the condensing machinery and taps.

It is perhaps needless to remark that any of these impurities, even if only suspected, should lead us to reject the use of the particular bottle or sample.

Hewitt (1893, 1907) was impressed by the usual purity of nitrous oxide but acknowledged the possibility of contamination:

The nitrous oxide supplied for anaesthetic purposes is usually free from impurities. It is stated, however, that the gas has sometimes been found to contain other oxides of nitrogen and chlorine. These gases would give the nitrous oxide an irritating odour and would induce coughing. The former impurities would be best detected by passing a slow stream of nitrous oxide through a cold solution of ferrous sulphate, acidulated with sulphuric acid; should the solution darken, the presence of other oxides of nitrogen would be indicated. . . .*

TWENTIETH CENTURY

A fatality possibly related to nitrous oxide impurities.

Buxton (1907) suggested that the inhalation of impurities with nitrous oxide might have contributed to a fatal outcome in one case, although from the details given this is not entirely convincing.

Spasm of the larynx has been reported and its possible supervention, even without the mechanical irritation caused by fragments of teeth, &c., must be remembered, as death has resulted from impaction of foreign bodies in the larynx when the patient was under nitrous oxide. This spasmodic closure probably was the cause of one of the deaths and followed inhaling impure and irritating gas. Cough and difficulty of respiration should always suggest this possible complication and the gas should be tested before the patient is allowed to inhale it, if the first attempt causes severe laryngeal irritation. The administrator can easily determine whether the gas is impure by himself after inhaling a few breaths of it.

Standard of purity considered in America.

Because the "increasing use of nitrous oxide gas, not only as the sole anaesthetic in minor

---

* i.e., about 27 litres from a non-rebreathing system would have been inhaled before the mask was removed and the tooth extracted. This dentist found that "Generally speaking patients are perfectly insensible in about forty-five seconds. I have known cases where patients have taken a minute and a half to become insensible, which is the extreme of my experience." Using such a technique, even if impurities had been present, the total quantity inhaled should have been small.

* In the 5th edition of Hewitt's textbook, published posthumously in 1922 and edited by Robinson, this was repeated; but on page 80 was added: "Warner (1915) found that commercial nitrous oxide in Ohio often produced toxic symptoms."

operations, but as a preliminary to ether or chloroform anaesthesia, makes the adoption of a standard of purity for this substance highly desirable", the Section of Stomatology of the American Medical Association recommended, in 1909, the inclusion of liquid nitrous oxide with the U.S. Pharmacopoeia.* Meanwhile, it voted to describe nitrous oxide with New and Nonofficial Remedies until Pharmacopoeial recognition had been secured. Guidance as to how the standard of purity should be defined, however, was not forthcoming from either manufacturers or consumers. "It therefore became necessary to examine the product as it was found on the market" (Puckner, 1911). At that time nitrous oxide was commonly sold in America in cylinders containing 25 ounces of liquid (about 100 gallons of gas), and the contents of one such cylinder from each of the following firms were analyzed: (1) Johnson and Lund; (2) Ohio Chemical and Mfg. Co; (3) The Lennox Chemical Co.; and (4) S.S. White Dental Mfg. Co. Problems were encountered due to the solution of impurities in the liquid nitrous oxide. The greater part of the nitrogen was found to escape from the cylinders first, but oxygen and a small part of the nitrogen persisted as the cylinders were emptied. By passing 4 litres of gas from each cylinder through solutions of barium hydroxide, litmus, silver nitrate, potassium iodide and starch and Nessler's reagent, it was shown that the samples were free from acids, chlorine, the higher oxides of nitrogen, and ammonia. Carbon dioxide was found in one cylinder. The following results were quoted (Smith and Leman, 1911):

	1	2	3	4
	Per cent	Per cent	Per cent	Per cent
N_2O	95.4	93.4	95.8	96.1
O_2	0.0	1.4	1.1	0.1
N_2	4.6	5.2	3.1	3.5
CO_2	0.0	0.0	0.0	0.3

Baskerville (1912) reported further analyses of nitrous oxide manufactured in America. He found between 95.9 and 99.7 per cent nitrous oxide, the greatest contaminant being nitrogen. The water content was between 0.13 to 0.15 per cent. He suggested that "Nitrous oxide which is to be

* It was included in U.S.P. IX (1916).

used for anaesthesia should contain at least 95 per cent of N_2O and no solids, liquids, combustible organic material, chlorin, or other oxids of nitrogen. A small amount of carbon dioxid, according to the investigations of Gatch, can have no evil effects. If present, however, the percentage should be known."

Realization of danger in America.

Even then, however, some nitrous oxide used for anaesthesia was made in private plants. Haskins (1914), for example, investigated the impurities that may occur in nitrous oxide

at the suggestion of Doctor A. R. Warner, Superintendent of Lakeside Hospital. He had observed that "smoky" nitrous oxide gas was produced whenever the retort of the gas apparatus at the hospital was overheated. The visible vapor must necessarily be some impurity. The apparatus as improved by Doctor Warner removes all impurities, so that no ill effects of nitrous oxide administration have been observed for some time.

Haskins concluded that it was ammonia that was produced, and that this could be removed by bubbling the nitrous oxide through dilute sulphuric acid.

In the following year Warner (1915) disclosed the nature of the ill effects resulting from nitrous oxide administration, and gave a full account of the action taken to avoid and remove impurities.

At Lakeside Hospital, nitrous oxid gas has been used for anesthesia extensively for about eight years, and has been manufactured as a routine in the hospital for six years.

For the first four of these years, the gas we manufactured was not entirely satisfactory to any one, and at times not without harmful effects. This was overlooked at first, partly because, on the whole, we had as good results as others, and partly because it was then believed that a certain amount of cyanosis was necessarily present during nitrous oxid-oxygen anesthesia, and that bad after-effects were in a measure to be expected. As our anaesthetists developed more skill with this anaesthetic, they were able to demonstrate to us that the cyanosis, the irritation, and the symptoms of toxemia following the anesthesia were present to a greater or less extent in all or in several patients on the same day, and on other days there were no such symptoms at all: they convinced us that the gas made in the hospital contained a variable amount of some poison. Commercial gas, although producing at times the same symptoms of toxicity, seemed more uniform and distinctly less irritating. This difference was fairly constant, although our plant and methods of manufacture were the same as the commercial plants and methods known to us. On our worst day one patient of the gynecologic service died with all the symptoms of severe toxemia a few hours after a simple operation; one patient of the surgical service was severely poisoned, and three others suffered to a lesser extent.

The predominating symptom of the poisoning was a cyanosis that no amount of oxygen could dispel. The hemoglobin was evidently damaged. . . . The condition, with the exception of the color, resembled carbon monoxid poisoning, yet unfortunately no spectroscopic examinations of the blood of these patients were made.

. . . it became evident to all that nitrous oxid must be obtained in greater purity, or its use in the hospital abandoned . . .* The best consulting chemists obtainable were called to examine the plant and methods. . . . One of our trustees . . . offered to provide funds necessary to run an experimental plant . . ., and I undertook to solve . . . the two following problems:

1. To find a method for the manufacture of nitrous oxid of sufficient purity to be without poisonous effect.

2. To devise apparatus by which this can be done as a routine in hospitals under hospital conditions.

The entire plant was rebuilt several times . . . We found that nitric oxid, even when present in large amounts, was entirely removed from the nitrous oxid by confining in iron tanks or over water for a few hours. This explained the lesser irritation from commercial gas, which stands longer in the gasometers and is always shipped in iron cylinders. Commercial gas has always been free from nitric oxid, and our gas—sometimes used without standing long in the tanks—had not been. In these experiments we became convinced that the poisonous effects were, at times at least, not from nitric oxid, which has been the generally dreaded impurity. We learned, too, that the effect of the poison was cumulative, and that a long anaesthesia was the most delicate test available. In comparison with this, all anlayses and chemical tests were crude.

. . . a thorough washing with strong sulphuric acid was then added to the process of purification of the gas, for the purpose of removing all free basic radicals. On this day—now over a year ago—our gas became absolutely neutral in reaction, and the peculiar cyanosis and all other symptoms of toxicity disappeared from the operating rooms, never to appear again when acid-washed gas was used. We did, however, see it in varying degrees each time that the installation of new

---

* This would not have been entertained lightly because it was at this time and in this hospital that Crile (1911) was developing techniques based on the idea of anoci-association. In relation to the toxic manifestations encountered it is significant that these techniques would have heralded the use of nitrous oxide and oxygen for longer operations. Most operations, however, were still short. Crile (1911) indicated the durations of 20,448 anaesthetics administered at the Lakeside Hospital using the Teter anaesthetic apparatus. 12,886 anaesthetics lasted up to 5 minutes; 3,365, 5–15 minutes; 865, 15–30 minutes; 346, 30–60 minutes; 228, 1–2 hours; 22, 2–3 hours; and 2, 3–4 hours. The durations of 2,412 "personal cases" and 320 "colleagues at Lakeside" were not quoted, nor was it stated for how many of these anaesthetics nitrous oxide and oxygen was used. Of 10,787 surgical operations performed by Crile himself, however, 2,412 were performed under nitrous oxide and oxygen or nitrous oxide supplemented with ether. This was before the re-introduction of low-flow systems using carbon dioxide absorption, although Crile and his colleagues were experimenting with a closed system in 1916 (Jackson, 1955).

apparatus in the plant made it necessary to shut down and use for a few days commercial gas not scrubbed with acid. . . .

Confirming evidence came from independent sources. The Ohio Chemical Company of Cleveland noted our better results, and remodeled their plant. Three competent anesthetists, whom I have happened to meet, one from Boston, one from New York and one from Ithaca, volunteered information regarding the uniformly better results which they were having with the Ohio gas, all dating the better results from the date the company remodeled its plant and instituted the acid wash as part of the purification process. Later the Lennox Chemical Company remodeled its plant to include the acid wash. Since this date I have not heard of any evidence of toxicity or any bad results from the use of nitrous oxid in Cleveland or vicinity. These two plants manufacture all the gas sold in or about Cleveland.

The chemical work to identify the particular poison or poisons which have caused all the troubles has not been done. We know only that it is removed by the acid wash, and that it is found in the acid in the form of ammonium salts, which is consistent with the belief that it is one of the hydrazins or hydroxylamins. . . .

For the simple purpose of preventing commercial monopoly, application for patents . . . have been made. All patents issued will be held by the hospital to guarantee the unrestricted use of the apparatus and the methods covered by them.

To our mind the first problem has been solved. . . . We are not yet quite sure about the second problem. Lakeside can now manufacture nitrous oxide in sufficient purity to be absolutely safe in anesthesia as a routine, and safely, but the walls and the ceilings of our room still bear the marks made by pieces of bursted retorts,* and our colleagues have not forgotten the fumes which repeatedly filled the corridors "from the gas plant". It is never entirely safe to place a pot containing a nitrogenous and an oxidising substance over a fire . . .†

Baldwin (1916) published an article entitled "Nitrous oxide-oxygen, the most dangerous anesthetic" in which he wrote:

Practically all the anesthetists who have written on nitrous oxide-oxygen state most positively that death

---

* See also Brit. J. dent. Sci. (1905): "A great explosion of nitrous oxide gas took place in the surgery of Dr. J. W. Horner, Launceston, Tasmania . . . [He] barely escaped with his life, the surgery was wrecked . . . a piece of composition metal, part of the head of the retort was blown over the Bank of Australasia. . . . Dr. Horner . . . was suffering from severe pain in the back, but otherwise uninjured and quite collected . . . [he] had never heard an explosion like this before.

† These extracts speak for themselves. Warner's paper also gave data on the economics of the manufacture and the use of nitrous oxide, on piping it (it was piped from the basement to the operating theatres—see also Jackson, 1955), on metering the gas supplied to individual anaesthetic machines, on the pressure at which it should be delivered, and on the general benefits which accrued from the use of nitrous oxide and oxygen anaesthesia, supplemented if necessary with a little ether.

occurs *only* from asphyxia, and that if the anesthetist watches the color and pushes the oxygen death cannot occur. . . . In none of the cases detailed in this paper was death the result in any way whatever of asphyxia, but in all of them the death occurred without warning, in the midst of an apparently smooth anesthesia, and with the suddenness of an overdose of chloroform.

There is nothing to suggest that these deaths were the result of inhaling impurities with nitrous oxide, but writing so soon after Warner (1915) it is noteworthy that the possibility was not mentioned.

There was little further mention of the chemical aspects of nitrous oxide in the medical press until Baxter (1924) described its manufacture and chemical testing. Starting with the raw material he pointed out that because it was not always economically possible to get sufficiently pure nitrate, manufacturers should be equipped to purify the commercial grades commonly used for explosives. At that time much of the nitrate used for nitrous oxide manufacture was imported raw from Germany and then purified. He stipulated that a desirable nitrate should not contain more than 0.0015 per cent of chlorides (cf. I.C.I. Ltd. figures given in footnote on p. 129) and not more than 0.015 per cent sulphates, and that it should be free from organic impurities such as wood, etc. He made the point that however carefully the nitrates were selected, purified and heated, foreign gases were often generated, such as nitric acid, nitrogen peroxide, nitric oxide, or ammonium compounds such as hydrazins or hydroxylamins, all of which had to be completely removed. Many methods of purification were in vogue, but he stressed that

. . . the most important factor is, that there must be a safety factor created not only in the strength of the solutions used but also in the process of scrubbing which will effectively remove all impurities, and remove them under all conditions. In no other way can the users of nitrous oxide be protected. The purifying solution used should be of sufficient strength so that a 50 per cent safety factor is created. These solutions should be regularly sampled, titrated and built up to their full strength.

The nitrous oxide was dried using dehydrating chemicals such as calcium chloride, and compression, with cooling, was carried out in three stages.

Finally Baxter described the fifth and last stage of production as "of tremendous importance to all

concerned, namely, the analysis and certification of purity. Samples of gas should be secured throughout the day's run and analysed for various impurities such as chlorin, ammonia compounds, nitric oxid, and so forth." Methods of analysis were described, after commenting that "a much used quantitative test for nitric oxid will not respond to a five per cent mixture."*

Judging by their advertisements, American manufacturers of nitrous oxide were at that time acutely conscious of the customers' concern about purity. Lennox and Ohio, for example, illustrated a purifying tower, and added: "In addition, every

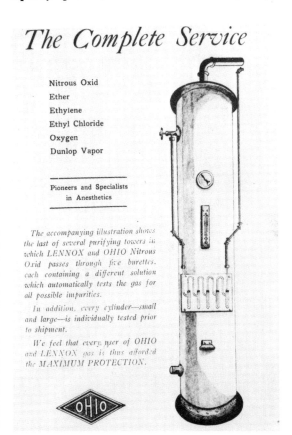

The Complete Service

Nitrous Oxid
Ether
Ethylene
Ethyl Chloride
Oxygen
Dunlop Vapor

———————
Pioneers and Specialists
in Anesthetics
———————

The accompanying illustration shows the last of several purifying towers in which LENNOX and OHIO Nitrous Oxid passes through five burettes, each containing a different solution which automatically tests the gas for all possible impurities.

In addition, every cylinder—small and large—is individually tested prior to shipment.

We feel that every user of OHIO and LENNOX gas is thus afforded the MAXIMUM PROTECTION.

Fig. 16

An American advertisement of 1924 placing great emphasis upon the purity of nitrous oxide and upon the individual testing of cylinders. (By kind permission of Ohio Chemical & Surgical Equipment Co.)

---

* See also Crowell (1925).

cylinder—small and large—is individually tested prior to shipment." The nature of the tests was not revealed (figs. 16, 17 and 18).

Some of Baxter's comments were reinforced the following year by a report of "An impure and dangerous sample of nitrous oxid gas" (Benson and Harding, 1925). This opened with the words:

IT IS OF GREAT IMPORTANCE that all necessary measures should be provided to insure the purity of chemicals used for anesthesia, and if the publication of this otherwise unimportant experiment helps, even in a small degree, in emphasising the necessity of a more adequate standardisation of nitrous oxide, we have accomplished our purpose.

They went on to describe the "examination of the gas in a small steel tank which we shall designate tank A, said to contain three pounds, 14½ ounces, and labelled 'Anhydrous Nitrous oxide'." They concluded that

From these results it is apparent that the nitrous oxid of Tank A was contaminated with nitric oxid and that it had a lethal effect on animals. No human mortality was reported from this sample. It is possible that the odor aroused suspicions before administration as an anesthetic. In any event we may conclude that dire results might follow human anesthesia with such a highly lethal gas.

It is the opinion of the writers that instances of the kind recited here should be reported, and that efforts should be made to obtain a thorough inspection and standardisation of all nitrous oxid used for anesthesia in surgery and dentistry.

Confidence in Your Anesthetic Gases

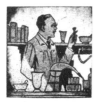

We furnish an analysis of our products

THE ANESTHETIST is continually dealing with life and death. For that reason he must have absolute confidence in the anesthetic gases he uses to put patients to sleep for various operative procedures.

Absolute confidence in nitrous oxide and oxygen for anesthesia can only be secured through constant analysis of these products, in addition to the most scientific methods of manufacture.

Clarke Nitrous Oxide is made from chemically pure Nitrate of Ammonia, distilled and refined in apparatus designed and constructed to produce a perfect product. It does not come in contact with metals which would affect its purity and reduce its efficiency; safeguarded by chemical tests at regular intervals during each day of manufacture, insuring uniform purity.

FIG. 17

This advertisement, together with those reproduced in figures 16 and 18, appeared in the same number of *Curr. Res. Anesth. Analg.* as Baxter's (1924) article on the manufacture and chemical testing of nitrous oxide gas.

S. S. WHITE
Non Freezing Nitrous Oxid
U. S. PATENT No. 1491740
and Oxygen

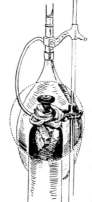

Necessity for hot towels, lamps and thermic devices to keep valve passages open, is eliminated by the use of S. S. White Nitrous Oxid. *It does not freeze*

THE LATEST and one of the most important steps in the advancement of gas anesthesia is the elimination of water vapor from Nitrous Oxid by a patented process.

From every aspect, Non-Freezing Nitrous Oxid is the best to use; it is safer in long continued administration, more efficient and economical in all administrations, and assures a continuous, even flow, at the volume ratio arranged for by the operator. Freezing of the water vapor in N_2O has been the cause of annoyance, anxiety and a source of actual danger necessitating the use of hot towels, lamps, and other heating devices to keep the valve passages free.

The freezing troubles are history when S. S. White Non-Freezing Nitrous Oxid is adopted as the anesthetic gas.

FIG. 18

In announcing the elimination of water vapour as the latest and one of the most important steps in the advancement of gas anaesthesia, S. S. White & Co. possibly intended to imply that the problem of purity had already been looked after. See also figures 16 and 17. (By kind permission of Messrs. S. S. White Company.)

Their experiments were carried out using guineapigs and mixtures of nitrous oxide and air or oxygen. One guineapig died after three exposures lasting 3, 2 and 25 minutes respectively, to the nitrous oxide mixed with "ample air to prevent asphyxia". A second guineapig was given a lower concentration for 30 minutes. "The animal revived, but with evidence of pulmonary irritation. The next day being Sunday, the animal was not observed, but on Monday it was found dead. . . . Autopsy revealed hyperemia of the lungs." A third guineapig was subjected to a mixture of the nitrous oxide and oxygen for 3 minutes, during which it

Exhibited dyspnea and salivation. It revived from the anesthetic, but the following day it was found dead in the cage. Autopsy disclosed an accumulation of serous fluid in both pleural cavities; considerable edema of both lungs; irregular congestion and hemorrhage; and muco-sanguinous tracheitis as well as bronchitis.

Another, anaesthetized with a similar mixture for 30 minutes, died one hour afterwards. "Immediate autopsy revealed extensive edema of the lungs combined with irregular congestion and hemorrhage."

In the same year Hoover (1925) reported an investigation of nitrous oxide by the Bureau of Chemistry.

Samples of Gas were not only tested for compliance with the U.S.P. requirements, but were subjected to further rigid examination for the presence of nitric oxid. It is particularly gratifying to the bureau that none of the samples examined contained enough impurities to warrant action under the Food and Drugs Act. While a few samples showed the presence of perceptible traces of nitric oxid, none contained harmful quantities. [The greatest concentration reported was 0.0008 per cent.]

Chaney (1933) drew attention to the fact that the presence of appreciable quantities of "inert gases" had been largely overlooked, and he suggested that these would increase the difficulties of inducing anaesthesia using nitrous oxide. He found that many cylinders of nitrous oxide, from different sources, contained 5–15 per cent of "inert gas" (nitrogen) in the gaseous phase of full cylinders. He did not report simultaneous tests for higher oxides of nitrogen. Clement (1945) also mentioned nitrogen as an impurity—"harmless, but decreases efficiency by dilution"—and he did not omit a warning about nitric oxide:

. . . [it] combines with hemoglobin like carbon monoxide, causing anoxia, or may form nitric acid in the tissues with resulting pulmonary edema. Nitric oxide may be suspected clinically by the presence of cyanosis which does not readily disappear with the administration of a high percentage of oxygen. A simple test for the detection of the higher oxides of nitrogen is to bubble gas through a starch iodide solution.

Recently (Hamelberg, Mahaffey and Bond, 1961) either nitric oxide or nitrogen dioxide was incriminated as the cause of the failure of nylon diaphragms of pressure regulating valves used with nitrous oxide cylinders in America, although there were no reports of any morbidity resulting from patients having breathed the gas.

Great Britain.

Warner (1915) performed a valuable service in reporting so fully the experience at Lakeside Hospital. Cleveland. He certainly stimulated at least two American firms to improve their methods of purification, and the remainder would have had to follow suit—unless their products had already reached the higher standard. That Warner's paper was not reported in the British medical press may have been because Hart and Minshall (1914), after analyzing cylinders of nitrous oxide manufactured in Great Britain, had concluded that

Considering the short interval of time that nitrous oxide is inhaled for anaesthesia and the large dilution of this by air or oxygen—administered during a longer period—for analgesia . . . the minute amounts of gaseous impurities found in the samples examined are, in general, too small to have any effect on the person.

Baldwin's article published the following year, with its dramatic title "Nitrous oxide-oxygen, the most dangerous anaesthetic", was noticed: but in the *Lancet* (1916) it was reported without comment, and in an editorial in the *British Journal of Dental Science* (1916) the opinion was expressed that "For the present we may reassure the public concerning the use of nitrous oxide and oxygen in producing anaesthesia during tooth extraction, provided the manipulation is conducted by those who possess sufficient knowledge and expert skill."

The findings of Hart and Minshall (1914) indicated that there had probably been an improvement in the purity of commercially prepared nitrous oxide since the days of Roberts (1884),

TABLE I

Hart and Minshall (1914): analysis of nitrous oxide cylinders in 1913 and 1914				Lehmann (1913) cited Hart and Minshall (1914): data on cats			
		Max. found	Min. found	Rapid death	Illness and danger $\frac{1}{2}$ to 1 hour	No serious illness $\frac{1}{2}$ to 1 hour	Slight symptoms after many hours
Dust	Grammes/100 c.c.	0.00015	nil				
Moisture	,,	0.00965	0.000121				
Carbon dioxide	Vols. per cent	0.3461	0.00398	30	6–8	4–6	2–3
Carbon monoxide	,,	0.00092	nil		0.2–0.3	0.3–0.1	0.02
Ammonia	,,	0.0045	0.00002		0.25–0.45	0.03	0.01
Nitric oxide	,,	0.0163	0.00013		0.005–0.007	0.0035	0.0018
Sulphur dioxide	,,	0.00004	nil		0.04–0.05	0.005	0.002–0.003
Hydrochloric acid	,,	0.00194	nil		0.15–0.2	0.005–0.01	0.001
Hydrogen sulphide	,,	0.00124	nil	0.1–0.2	0.05–0.07	0.02–0.03	0.01–0.015
Oxygen	,,	0.941	0.479				
Nitrogen	,,	4.710	2.555				

although only a few cylinders were sampled.* How the improvement came about is not clear. There was no published British counterpart of Warner's article to spell out the potential dangers of impurities to either producers or consumers.

Hart and Minshall, however, did not white-wash the nitrous oxide industry. They started their investigations in 1903 when "a cylinder of nitrous oxide was submitted to one of us for examination as to the presence of impurities, because of some apparent abnormal symptoms and possibly harmful effects during the anaesthetic administration of the gas." The impurities they reported were 0.0078 per cent carbon dioxide and 0.0264 per cent nitric oxide. The "possibly harmful effects" do not appear to have been published in 1903.

Reviewing the various methods of purification, they referred to this as

a matter of importance and attention, and its extent is restricted to and dependent on the limits of absorption, by and on the rate of gas passage through the absorbants, and on temperature. During the absorption, most of the impurities form definite stable compounds with the reagents used, nitric oxide being the exception.

In 1913, and again in 1914, Hart and Minshall examined gas "from a number of cylinders of the commercial product for anaesthetic use from various makers . . . the analyses being made,

except in the case of oxygen and nitrogen, on about 20 litres or 4.4 gallons, somewhere about the average quantity usually administered." They gave the results of analyses of five makes of gas, and the minimum and maximum quantities of the impurities found are given in table I.

In attempting to assess the significance of these findings they were handicapped by the fact that

Until recently, there were no published results as to the injurious effects of nitrous vapours, beyond the general fact that they were insidious in action, damage being done usually before the man is aware of the fact; it being generally stated that they can be inhaled at first without apparent inconvenience, but beyond a certain point they act suddenly and acutely, often with fatal results.

By 1913, however, Lehmann and his colleagues had at least defined levels of toxicity in cats, and some of the values quoted by Hart and Minshall, are given in table I beside the levels of impurities actually found. Hart and Minshall concluded that

. . . it would appear that nitric oxide is the impurity that calls for special attention. Since this impurity is generally removed by the passage of the gas throughout cold ferrous sulphate solution, with no formation of a definite stable compound, and from which solution the nitric oxide is easily liberated by rise in temperature, reduction of pressure, or by dilution, the remarks as to insufficiency of absorbent and rate of gas passage through it are of great importance in view of Lehmann's recent investigations stated above.

The purity of the gas can be maintained and the purification operation simplified by the use of raw materials of the best quality; in earlier years it was recognized that only the purest ammonium nitrate should be used; then followed, mainly for economic purposes, the use of ammonium sulphate and sodium nitrate, and in view of the varying quality of these materials on the commercial market, it is imperative that the question of their purity should be taken into consideration.

---

* They also implied that the use of nitrous oxide for dental anaesthesia might be on the wane: ". . . its importance in this direction is not so pronounced at the present time, due to the more extensive application of local anaesthesia, yet the production of this gas for dental purposes is still extensive."

Their recommendations were:

After careful considerations, both from the dental and the manufacturing points of view, and based on the analytical results obtained on and the difference found between the samples of 1913 and 1914, we propose the following recommendations as to the quality of commercial nitrous oxide for anaesthetic and analgesic use:—

Nitrous oxide, 98 per cent minimum; moisture, not to exceed 0.0002 grm. per 100 c.c.; carbon dioxide, not to exceed 0.05 per cent by volume; nitric oxide, not to exceed 0.001 per cent by volume; ammonia, not to exceed 0.001 per cent by volume. Hydrochloric acid, chlorine and its oxide, iodine, sulphur dioxide, sulphuric anhydride, hydrogen sulphide, carbon monoxide, nitrogen tri-, tetr- and pentoxides, cyanogen hydrocyanic acid, hydrogen phosphide, arsenide and antimonide, ozone, dust and all other impurities to be absent in the examination of 20 litres of gas.

The minimum concentration of 98 per cent nitrous oxide recommended by Hart and Minshall may be compared with the minimum concentration allowed by successive British Pharmacopoeias. When Nitrogenii Monoxidum was first included in the B.P. in 1932 (16 years after its first appearance in the U.S.P.) the entry stated that "When drawn from a cylinder in the upright position, it contains not less than 93 per cent nitrous oxide." In 1948 the minimum figure was raised to 95 per cent. It was not until 1953 (39 years after Hart and Minshall made their recommendations) that the figure was raised to 99 per cent, at which it still stands.*

That nitrous oxide featured in the British Pharmacopoeia as soon as it did was the result of the formation of a joint Anaesthetics Committee of the Medical Research Council and the Section of Anaesthetics of the Royal Society of Medicine, in 1924.

The formation of a joint committee of inquiry of this kind was first suggested by two factors: first, complaints as to abnormal effects of nitrous oxide in certain cases which from time to time reached the Anaesthetics Council, and secondly the fact that the "British Pharmacopoeia" does not include nitrous oxide and that therefore there were no official tests of purity by which this anaesthetic is to be judged in this country. [Blomfield, 1926.]

Hadfield (1935) confirmed that

With regard to nitrous oxide in particular, the [Pharmacopoeia] Commission drew largely from the information supplied by the Committee in laying down the official standards of purity. In fact it is almost true to say that the monograph on nitrous oxide in the present edition is due to the Committee.

*See *Brit. J. Anaesth* (1967), **39**, 445.

The abnormal effects of nitrous oxide do not appear to have been published in 1924. (Three advertisements for nitrous oxide of 1925 are shown in figures 19, 20 and 21.)

Hadfield (1926) defined the main stimulus for the formation of the Committee.

The complaint accompanied by the fullest clinical report, was that submitted by Dr. Ramsey Phillips; it was, in fact, the one largely responsible for the institution of the inquiry. . . .

Dr. Ramsey Phillips' Cases.—In October, 1924, Dr. Phillips anaesthetized six patients (four women and two men) with this particular gas for dental extractions. He reports:—

"The gas used had a strong smell like brown potash

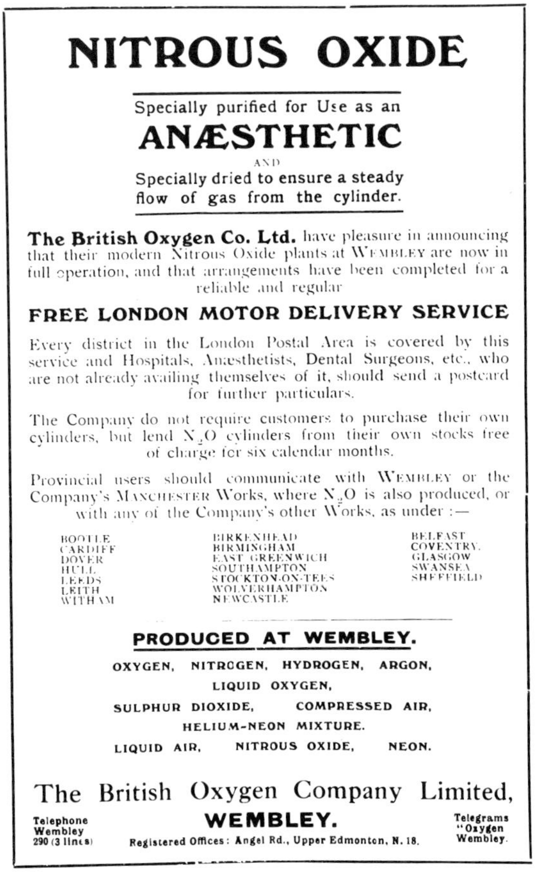

FIG. 19

An advertisement of the British Oxygen Co. Ltd. of 1925 announcing that their modern nitrous oxide plants at Wembley were in full operation producing nitrous oxide specially purified for use as an anaesthetic and specially dried to ensure a steady flow of gas from the cylinder. (By kind permission of the British Oxygen Company Ltd.)

or dirty wash-tub water. Clinically my complaint was that anaesthesia could not be produced without marked cyanosis; this led me to use the conjunctival reflex as a guide, a thing I never do in the ordinary way. This particular cyanosis was unusual. Lividity, white lips, grey colour of the skin, small to medium pupils, eye-balls looking directly forwards, and convulsions quite unlike the usual jactitation. In each case I gave large quantities of oxygen when this occurred, but the recovery was very slow. In some cases I had to reapply the gas with free supply of oxygen, as I had not allowed the operation to be commenced. Exactly the same thing occurred. There was no observable obstruction to the air-way in any of the cases. On recovery, all the patients felt very poorly, pulse small, irregular and soft. Nos. 1 and 2 gave rise to considerable anxiety at the time. No. 3 felt really ill when there should have been no cause for it. No. 4 also. No. 5 was not a dental case, but was having her neck stretched and manipulated for an alleged dislocation, and the con-vulsions were put down by the surgeon to his manipu-lations, who felt rather pleased, I think. No. 6 was badly knocked out, but she was a good subject for the gas. I heard afterwards that she had a severe cardiac

breakdown after it. I have not met with this before or since. My apparatus was in good working order, and in each case there was plenty of oxygen in the oxygen bag at the end of the case. The clinical picture was quite different from the cyanosis and jactitation common in cases where most of the air is washed out of the lungs and no oxygen is given. Again there was the strong smell of the gas, and the conjunctival reflex (taken well away from the cornea) was strongly present up to a point in some cases where I had to desist, and was unable to say that the patient would not feel the operation. No cough or sign of irritation in the air passages was present, and no nausea followed. I rather naturally dreaded to go to another gas case. I went to the makers and told them about it. While assuring me that the gas was good and normal, they showed me how to smell and taste it, and produced other gas which they acknowledged had no smell, while that which I had been using smelt strongly. I changed my stock of gas with the exception of the two bottles I sent you. While admitting that these difficulties may have been caused by myself, I felt it would be good to find out if the gas was good for human beings or not, since there are no regulations to control manufacture."

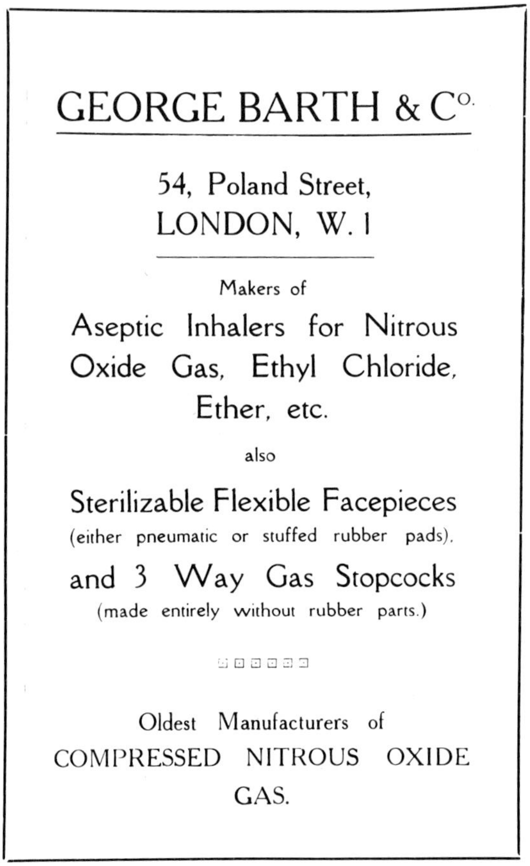

FIG. 20

This advertisement, together with those reproduced in figures 19 and 21, were bound with Hirsch (1925).

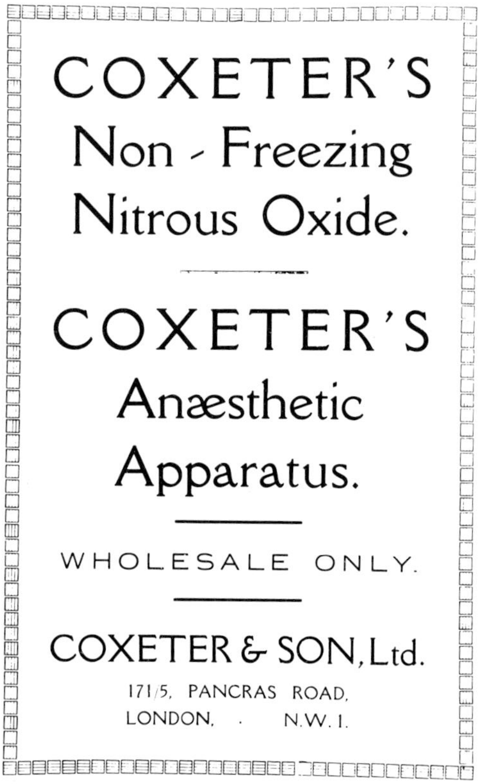

FIG. 21

Coxeter's advertisement for non-freezing nitrous oxide (cf. figure 18).

The unused gas was analyzed by Dr. King, chemist to the National Institute for Medical Research at Hampstead. He tested for halogens, reducing substances, acidic substances, carbon dioxide, nitric oxide (by bubbling for a long period through ferrous sulphate solution and looking for a "darkening" compared with a control), oxygen, carbon monoxide and nitrogen. The only impurities detected were "a small proportion of carbon dioxide and about 2 per cent of nitrogen" (King, 1926).

The absence of nitric oxide was confirmed by more sensitive tests. Quoting Hadfield (1926):

A few days later Dr. (now Sir Henry) Dale wrote to me as follows: "Since the last meeting, King and I have further examined the sample of nitrous oxide received from Ramsey Phillips. We passed the gas through a dilute solution of haemoglobin until all the oxygen was blown out and reduction complete. The spectrum was then that of reduced haemoglobin with only a single absorption band. This appears to me to exclude CO and NO beyond shadow of doubt, and much more decisively than any animal test could, or any ordinary chemical test. Pembrey agrees, but I am sending him the other cylinder of N_2O, so that he and Shipway may test it on some animals, if they think fit. King and I also tested the gas for nitrites, and, as a last shot, for cyanogen—both tests being completely negative."

Hadfield (1926) continued:

I think it was the negative result of this very thorough examination that made us realize the difficulty of the question under examination. We had all probably assumed that these irregular manifestations were due to the accidental presence of some obvious impurity such as halogen, nitric oxide or carbon monoxide. In this case, however, it seemed clear that all such substances were absent.

Despite the negative findings on analysis of the unused gas provided by Dr. Ramsey Phillips, his clinical descriptions suggest strongly that higher oxides of nitrogen were present. Dr. Ramsey Phillips was not reported as saying specifically that the clinical effects observed were all produced by gas from the same cylinder, but this is the natural assumption on first reading his account. He did, however, state that he changed his stock of gas except for two bottles. Sir Henry Dale also referred to two bottles. From the published evidence there is no guarantee that the nitrous oxide analyzed came from the same bottle as the nitrous oxide that produced the abnormal clinical signs and symptoms. It is also likely that the greater part of any nitric oxide present had already been blown off by the time that the gas was presented for analysis (see Austin, 1967).

Three further series of cases were reported. Cyanosis and difficulty in anaesthetizing the patients occurred in two of them, and the patients in the third showed convulsive movements during recovery. There was no mention of persistent cyanosis while breathing air or oxygen. Analysis of the gas remaining in the bottles used for the first two series revealed 5 per cent and 3.5 per cent nitrogen respectively, and the third a small quantity of carbon dioxide only. The concentration of nitrogen in the gas first released from the cylinders would have been higher, and dilution of nitrous oxide with nitrogen could have explained the clinical signs observed.

Messrs. Coxeter, supplied samples of gas which "although free from all ordinary impurities, did not in their opinion come up to standard and so was not issued. Dr. King confirmed the absence of these impurities but found that the gas contained 20 per cent of nitrogen and 3 per cent of oxygen."

An unnamed manufacturer provided details "of all complaints which had been received during the period of years in which he had been making nitrous oxide, and also with the results of detailed examination made in each case". There were five or six cases and "In most of them nothing was found at all, except sometimes a higher percentage than usual of nitrogen."

Dr. Maughan (1926) reported to the Committee:

Bad results obtained in anaesthetizing three children. . . . All three showed signs of collapse without cyanosis . . . in the remaining cases he gave half or three-quarters of the usual dose and obtained good anaesthesia followed by easy recovery. The remaining gas was returned to the makers and carefully examined by them—one of the partners himself inhaling it. He found it chemically quite pure, except that, as is so often the case, it contained nitrogen.

He amplified the account in the discussion of Hadfield's (1926) paper.

There was a definite and progressive failure of the circulation as from the tenth second. . . . He added that this was the first time in his experience of over forty years that three consecutive cases reacted to N_2O in the same abnormal manner. He felt it his duty in the circumstances to report the facts to the Section.

The absence of cyanosis may have meant that cyanosis did not appear to have been more marked than usual, and one is reminded that a constant finding of Greenbaum et al. (1967a, b), when administering nitric oxide or nitrogen dioxide to dogs, was an initial fall in arterial blood pressure. If nitric oxide had been present, most of it would have been blown off by the time that the remaining gas was analyzed.

That most of the nitrogen present as an impurity would be blown off early was pointed out to the Committee by Sir R. Robertson, but other impurities were not mentioned specifically in this connection. Hadfield (1926), however, did say:

I was discussing the matter with Mr. Trewby, whose skill and experience as a dental anaesthetist is well known. He assured me that we should never find much wrong with the cylinders of gas we examined, as it was always the gas delivered first that caused unpleasant symptoms. This was an interesting independent confirmation of what we had already learnt from Sir R. Robertson. I should like to add that Mr. Wellesley, of Messrs. Coxeter and Co., also drew our attention to this fact at the same time.

In reaching its final conclusions, the Committee of three anaesthetists and three Fellows of the Royal Society appeared to disregard the clinical evidence in favour of the analytical. It gave no indication as to what concentrations of the possible impurities might produce injurious effects in man, and it said little about the quantitative limits of the analytical methods used. Quoting from Hadfield (1926):

I think we are justified in concluding that the gas supplied to us anaesthetists by the three or four firms who make it in this country is a very pure product. We have never found any trace of such poisonous substances as the halogens, nitric oxide, nitric acid or carbon monoxide. . . . The only impurity which is at all frequently present is nitrogen . . . the possible source of much of this nitrogen [is] from the interaction of nitrous and nitric oxides. . . . The fact that the gas with which we are supplied is so pure speaks well for the methods adopted by the manufacturers.

But Hadfield went on to say:

In several cases we have been informed in confidence, of all the details of the process used, including sometimes secret "tips" of great utility. There is some variation in the methods, and some firms certainly appear to devote more attention to scrubbing than others, and possibly to control the whole plant in a more scientific manner. The end result appears, however, to be much the same. Again, in the testing of the finished product one firm differs from another in its methods and one may be more scientific than another. . . .

While thus, in the absence of any standard or official tests, it must be admitted that we have been well served in the past, it is not less obvious that such tests should be established and applied to each batch of nitrous oxide issued for use as an anaesthetic. I am possibly in error in speaking of batches of gas, as the process may be carried on as a continuous one. In this case standard tests should be applied to the product at certain fixed intervals.

That no such tests exist in England has already been stated. . . .

The Committee's work has shown that the impurity most frequently responsible for trouble is nitrogen, which on compression will tend to occur, in higher than general concentration, in the gas at the top of the cylinder. It is suggested that a sample of gas, taken with the cylinder upright, should contain at least 95 per cent N_2O.

The Committee's conclusions were not received altogether without reserve. In the discussion that followed, for example, Parkinson

. . . referred to Dr. Hadfield's account of the unsatisfactory anaesthesia obtained by Dr. Phillips in three consecutive cases from a single cylinder of gas. He expressed regret that the exhaustive chemical analysis of the residue of gas remaining in the cylinder should have revealed so little to account for the untoward symptoms . . . nitrogen . . . could hardly have accounted for the symptoms.

Boyle (1926), referring to the same series of cases, and the suggestion that most of the nitrogen would have been present in the gaseous phase, commented: "not only was the patient in the first case very ill after the administration, but other patients to whom gas had been given from the same cylinder were also affected. How could this be explained?" Then Dr. King spoke up and said that

. . . although all the previous cylinders of gas examined by him appeared to contain no impurities of note, within the last few days a cylinder of nitrous oxide had been received which undoubtedly contained higher oxides of nitrogen. The gas reduced permanganate and set free iodine from potassium iodide and starch. He also regarded as valueless the ferrous sulphate test for nitric oxide as an impurity in nitrous oxide.

Much of the information given by Hadfield (1926) was repeated by Blomfield (1926), who was chairman of the Committee, at a special session of the Section of Anaesthetics of the Royal Society of Medicine, with Canadian and American anaesthetists, five months later. Referring to the previous experiences at Lakeside Hospital (see Warner, 1915), which led to the installation of a complete plant for the manufacture of nitrous oxide in the hospital itself (this, in itself is a misleading statement), he said: "That plan has not yet been adopted in this country and it does not seem necessary. The general purity of the gas supplied by the makers in Great Britain appears to the Committee to redound highly to their credit." He made no mention of the fact that Dr. King had since come across a cylinder which contained some nitric oxide, and that he also expressed the opinion that he regarded the method of chemical analysis which was at first used for detecting nitric oxide, as valueless.

In the discussion that followed Blomfield's paper, Professor J. S. Haldane (1926) commented that nitrogen used to be an undesirable impurity in oxygen cylinders used in mines, and that this had now been reduced to less than $\frac{1}{2}$ per cent. He also believed that nitrogen was dissolved in nitrous oxide. Furthermore he remarked that

. . . there were serious casualties in coal mines from nitrous fumes, and he had carried out animal experiments dealing with the subject. The cyanosis was that which was associated with nitrites, and it was due to the presence of methaemoglobin in the blood. It was not dangerous unless it became extreme. What he would lay stress upon was the danger of bronchopneumonia of a fatal degree; the symptoms might not occur until twelve hours afterwards. This form of pneumonia was deadly.

Dr. F. H. McMechan (1926) added that

. . . there had recently occurred in the United States an interesting series of cases bearing on the purity of nitrous oxide. He was sure the finer tests would show the presence of nitric oxide. A chemist in the United States had discovered that nitrous oxide underwent decomposition in the fourth stage of compression in the cylinder on account of the temperature, which might be in the neighbourhood of 800° at that time. In order to eliminate any nitric oxide which might be formed at that point, the manufacturer had introduced Priestley's old method of reducing nitric oxide back to nitrous oxide by the presence of finely divided metal. Recently the container for this was thought to be cumbersome, and so the body of finely divided metal was cut down. Therefore the first batch of gas which went through, under the new conditions, gave identical results in the hands of four independent anaesthetists, namely, an absence of the cyanosis usually accompanying the drug until the thirty-fifth minute of anaesthesia. Most of the observers were using the same type of apparatus. The gas was then examined and found to contain minute traces of nitric oxide, though it would probably pass all Government standards. Oxygen did not relieve this lividity. He therefore hoped that the Committee, in its final report, would be very exigent about the elimination of nitric acid as an impurity. The standard of nitrous oxide purity in the United States was too low; 95 per cent purity was not compatible with the best type of nitrous anaesthesia; it should reach 98 or 99 per cent.

Mr. G. Wellesley (1926) then said

. . . he had taken a typical cylinder and worked down through every ounce. The first ounce contained an average of 8 per cent of nitrogen, the second ounce 6 per cent, the third ounce 4 per cent, the fourth 4 per cent, the sixth 3 per cent, the seventh 2 per cent, and the remainder 2 per cent, though the thirtieth gave only 1 per cent nitrogen. There was an average of 2 per cent throughout the cylinder. It would be easier to produce a purity of 98 per cent than 95 per cent.

It is curious that when nitrous oxide was first mentioned in the Pharmacopoeia, six years after Hadfield (1926) presented his report, as secretary of the Committee, the minimum acceptable concentration of nitrous oxide was given as 93 per cent instead of the Committee's recommended 95 per cent.

Hadfield (1935) later gave a retrospective report of eleven years work of the Joint Anaesthetics Committee. Dealing with nitrous oxide he made no mention of nitric oxide, although he did mention that a cylinder was found to be contaminated with traces of carbon monoxide, which were attributed to the presence of wood chips with the ammonium nitrate. He repeated that "The quality of the gas supplied by the various manufacturers had been found to be excellent." He also mentioned that further work had been done by Bennet (1930). I have not discovered what factors led to the upgrading of the purity of nitrous oxide allowed in the B.P., first in 1948, and then again in 1953.

IN RETROSPECT

Ever since Davy carried out his experiments on nitrous oxide in Bristol, there has been a general awareness of the desirability of inhaling the gas in a "pure" state. The degree of "purity" desirable has been less certain.

At first, producers of nitrous oxide lacked sensitive quantitative tests for impurities. They had to be content to select the best raw materials, to avoid overheating the ammonium nitrate, and to use various wash-bottles to remove such impurities as were liberated. The most sensitive tests were probably to smell the gas, and to observe patients when nitrous oxide was administered to them. As late as 1915, Warner was of the opinion that "a long anaesthetic was the most delicate test available. In comparison with this all analyses and chemical tests were crude." One is tempted to believe that this was still true in 1926 when Hadfield reported the conclusions of the Joint Anaesthetics Committee.

Recognition of the effects of nitrous oxide impurities was probably made more difficult in the early days when anaesthetics were brief, when cyanosis was the rule, and when the quantities inhaled were small. Warner (1915) and his colleagues were observing patients at a crucial period in the development of nitrous oxide anaesthesia. Oxygen was being administered with nitrous oxide for longer periods, but there was still a reluctance to associate the cyanosis observed with the presence of impurities, rather than with the administration of nitrous oxide itself. Using modern techniques, with muscle paralysis and controlled ventilation for long periods, the effects of low concentrations of impurities could be confused with postoperative complications of different aetiology, and the effects of high concentrations may be recognized too late. If, instead of giving dental anaesthetics in 1925, Dr. Ramsey Phillips had used the same nitrous oxide cylinder for anaesthetizing a curarized patient, it is possible that the Joint Anaesthetics Committee would have been more impressed by the clinical evidence than the analytical—but muscle relaxants had not then come into clinical use.

Before a satisfactory standard of purity can be established, the significant impurities must first be defined; adequate tests for their detection and quantitative analysis must then be found; the pharmacological and the pathological effects of known concentrations of the impurities should be determined in so far as this is practicable; and finally, due consideration should be given to what it is reasonable to expect from manufacturers. In Great Britain, the authors who at least attempted to consider all these factors, and who demonstrated the most balanced approach to the problem, were Hart and Minshall (1914). Their contribution appears to have been largely overlooked. They were about 40 years ahead of their time. One can only speculate as to what critical anaesthetists 40 years hence may think about the publications of today on the manufacture, storage and purity of nitrous oxide; but it may be salutary to compare them with those of the past.

Such evidence as is available from the literature suggests that the "purity" of nitrous oxide available for anaesthesia varied from time to time and from place to place. In the early days of nitrous oxide anaesthesia it is probable that the gas was often much diluted by nitrogen. This would have led to the same difficulties in the induction of anaesthesia as leaks around the mask, except that there would not have been the saving grace of oxygen in the diluent gas. There would have been the temptation to "push" the gas in order to get the patients anaesthetized. If any nitric oxide had also been present, there could have been the fatal combination of gross hypoxia and hypotension in the sitting patient. Whether the combination of nitrous oxide, nitrogen and nitric oxide has ever been the cause of death in the dental chair we shall probably never know, but the possibility needs to be considered. We should also be cautious in our assessment of accounts of early anaesthetics in the absence of evidence as to what gases were in fact administered. When, for example, Horace Wells failed in his attempt to give a public demonstration of nitrous oxide anaesthesia in 1844 (see Part V; Smith, 1966a), his misfortunes may have stemmed as much from the use of impure nitrous oxide—prepared and used in strange surroundings (or from an ill-fitting mask)—as from having removed the mask too soon (Wells, 1847), or from his patient having been "anaesthetic-resistant" (Macintosh and Pratt, 1940).*

---

* The following extract from the *British Journal of Dental Science* (1871b) gives an example of what can happen:

The following case has been forwarded to us for publication. We are in possession of proofs of its authenticity.

"Dear Doctor,—I went to the Dentist's in —— this morning to have my tooth extracted; they did not (three Dentists) give me enough gas, and I jumped up nearly mad, the operator cut out of the room and held the door, shouted for the servants. I stripped myself nearly naked to fight the lot, and I was some time before I was right again; they said they would not run the risk of being killed and having all their furniture broken, so my tooth is still in my head. It was a pantomime, but it has made me ill. I will tell you more when I see you. I shall be here for a week, and wish you were here to administer the gas and take out a tooth without *breaking* it."

The gentleman who forwarded the above relates another case in which he says:

"The patient in this instance drew a revolver from his pocket and fired at the operator, but fortunately missed him. I suppose there is no reason for the occurrence further than the mixture of air with the gas."

ACKNOWLEDGEMENTS

I am most grateful to Dr. O. P. Dinnick for drawing my attention to figures 16, 17 and 18, and to the Ohio Chemical & Surgical Equipment Co. and the S. S. White Company for permission to reproduce figures 16 and 18 respectively. The British Oxygen Company were also kind enough to allow reproduction of figure 19. I am indebted to Dr. E. A. Cooper for drawing my attention to Teleky (1948), to Dr. M. L. Kain for preventing the omission of Blomfield (1926), and to Mr. O. G. W. Stallybrass, librarian of the Royal Institution, Albermarle Street, for confirming the authorship of M.F. (1819) and drawing attention to Jeffreys (1960). In addition to providing information on the sources of ammonium nitrate used by Coxeter and Son when he was with that firm, Mr. W. Edmundson very kindly read through an early draft of this article. The prompt and full reply given by Mr. J. M. Peacock, of I.C.I. Ltd., to my queries about the purity of ammonium nitrate available in this country is also much appreciated.

REFERENCES

Austin, A. T. (1967). The chemistry of the higher oxides of nitrogen as related to manufacture, storage and adminstration of nitrous oxide. *Brit. J. Anaesth.*, **39**, 345.

Baldwin, J. F. (1916). Nitrous-oxide-oxygen, the most dangerous anaesthetic. *Med. Rec. (N.Y.)*, **90**, 176.

Barth, G., & Co. (1873). Correspondence. *Brit. J. dent. Sci.*, **16**, 140.

Baskerville, C. (1912). Chemistry of inhalation anaesthetics. *J. Amer. med. Ass.*, **59**, 1839.

Baxter, D. E. (1924). The manufacture and chemical testing of nitrous oxid gas. *Curr. Res. Anesth. Analg.*, **3**, 129.

Beddoes, T., and Watt, J. (1796). *Considerations on the Medicinal Use and on the Production of Factitious Airs*, 3rd ed. London: J. Johnson.

Bennet, A. N. C. (1930). Researches on nitrous oxide. *J. phys. Chem.*, **34**, 1137.

Benson, R. L., and Harding, E. P. W. (1925). An impure and dangerous sample of nitrous oxide gas. *Curr. Res. Anesth. Analg.*, **4**, 124.

Blomfield, J. (1926). Recent investigations concerning nitrous oxide, and the ignition points of some anaesthetic vapours. *Proc. roy. Soc. Med.*, **19**, 39.

Boyle, H. E. G. (1926). Discussion of Hadfield (1926). *Proc. roy. Soc. Med.*, **19**, 26.

—— (1934). Nitrous oxide: history and development. *Brit. med. J.*, **1**, 153.

Braine, C. (1870). Casual communication. *Trans. odont. Soc. N.S.*, **3**, 37.

Brande, W. T. (1827). Lectures on chemistry. XVII: On muriatic acid, hydriodic acid, and nitrous oxide. *Lancet*, **1**, 455.

Brit. J. dent. Sci. (1868a). Miscellanea. Barth's portable protoxide of nitrogen. **11**, 394.

—— (1868b). Miscellanea. Apparatus for the inhalation of nitrous oxide. **11**, 444.

—— (1868c). Nitrous oxide gas. **11**, 539.

—— (1869). Miscellanea. **12**, 206.

Brit. J. dent. Sci. (1870). Liquid gas. **13**, 145.

—— (1871a). Miscellanea. **14**, 36.

—— (1871b). Results of imperfect administration of nitrous oxide. **14**, 362.

—— (1871c). Miscellanea. Barth's liquid nitrous oxide bag. **14**, 589.

—— (1873). Death after the inhalation of nitrous oxide. **16**, 84.

—— (1905). Explosion of nitrous oxide gas, dentist's surgery wrecked. **48**, 332.

—— (1916). Editorial. **59**, 617.

Brit. med. J. (1868). Protoxide of nitrogen as an anaesthetic. **1**, 355.

—— (1870). Liquid nitrous oxide gas. **1**, 496.

Buxton, D. W. (1907). *Anaesthetics: Their Uses and Administration*. London: Lewis.

Chaney, A. L. (1933). The purity of nitrous oxid with especial reference to the nitrogen content. *Curr. Res. Anesth. Analg.*, **12**, 42.

Clement, F. W. (1945). *Nitrous Oxide-Oxygen Anaesthesia: McKesson-Clement Viewpoint and Technique*. London: Henry Kimpton.

Clover, J. T. (1868). Discussion. *Brit. J. dent. Sci.*, **11**, 212.

Cock, F. W. (1934). History of nitrous oxide anaesthesia. *Brit. med. J.*, **1**, 606.

Cohen, R. A. (1941). Some historical notes on dental anaesthesia with special reference to dentistry and nitrous oxide. *Dent. Gaz.*, **8**, 56.

Coleman, A. (1870a). Discussion. *Trans. odont. Soc. N.S.*, **2**, 216.

—— (1870b). Discussion. *Trans. odont. Soc. N.S.*, **2**, 244.

Colton, Q. C. (1868). Letter. *Brit. J. dent. Sci.*, **11**, 253.

Coxeter, J., & Son (1873). Correspondence. *Brit. J. dent. Sci.*, **16**, 195.

Crile, G. W. (1911). Nitrous oxide anesthesia and a note on anoci-association, a new principle in operative surgery. *Surg. Gynec. Obstet.*, **13**, 170.

Crowell, W. S. (1925). Chemistry and physics of "dry" nitrous oxid. *Curr. Res. Anesth. Analg.*, **4**, 241.

Davison, M. H. A. (1954). The first cylinder of gas. *Brit. J. Anaesth.*, **26**, 40.

Davy, H. (1799). Extract of a letter from Mr. H. Davy. *Nicholson's Journal*, **3**, 93.

—— (1800a). A letter from Mr. Davy, Superintendent of the Pneumatic Institution, to Mr. Nicholson, on the nitrous oxide, or gaseous oxide of azote, on certain factors relating to heat and light, and on the discovery of the decomposition of the carbonate and sulphite of ammoniac. *Nicholson's Journal*, **3**, 515.

—— (1800b). *Researches, Chemical and Philosophical; chiefly concerning nitrous oxide, or dephlogisticated nitrous air, and its respiration.* London: J. Johnson.

Duncum, B. M. (1947). *The Development of Inhalation Anaesthesia: with special reference to the years 1846–1900*. London: Oxford University Press.

Evans, T. W. (1868). Protoxide of nitrogen. *Brit. J. dent. Sci.*, **11**, 382.

Faraday, M. (1823). On the condensation of several gases into liquids. *Phil. Trans.*, **113**, 189.

—— (1845). On the liquification and solidification of bodies generally existing as gases. *Phil. Trans.*, **135**, 155.

Fox, C. J. (1868a). On the manufacture of nitrous oxide. *Brit. med. J.*, **2**, 201.

—— (1868b). On nitrous oxide. *Brit. J. dent. Sci.*, **11**, 519.

—— (1869). Coxeter's vessels for compressed gas. *Brit. J. dent. Sci.*, **12**, 441.

—— (1870a). Nitrous oxide gas as an anaesthetic in surgery, with Coxeter's liquid gas. *Lancet*, **1**, 515.

—— (1870b). Discussion. *Trans. odont. Soc. N.S.*, **2**, 216.

Greenbaum, R., Austin, A. T., Bay, J., Dixon-Lewis, G., Kain, M. L., Kelman, G. R., Nunn, J. F., Prys-Roberts, C., Shiel, F. A. O'M., and Toothill, C. (1967a). The effects of higher oxides of nitrogen during anaesthesia. *Brit. J. Anaesth.*, **39**, 87.

—— Bay, J., Hargreaves, M. D., Kain, M. L., Kelman, G. R., Nunn, J. F., Prys-Roberts, C., and Siebold, K. (1967b). Effects of higher oxides of nitrogen on the anaesthetized dog. *Brit. J. Anaesth.*, **39**, 393.

Hadfield, C. F. (1926). Nitrous oxide: its impurities and the establishment of tests suitable for official adoption. *Proc. roy. Soc. Med.*, **19**, 17.

—— (1935). The Joint Anaesthetics Committee. A retrospective of eleven years' work. *Proc. roy. Soc. Med.*, **28**, 1133.

Haldane, J. S. (1926). Discussion of Blomfield (1926). *Proc. roy. Soc. Med.*, **19**, 47.

Hamelberg, W., Mahaffey, J. S., and Bond, W. E. (1961). Nitrous oxide impurities. *Curr. Res. Anesth. Analg.*, **40**, 408.

Hart, W. B., and Minshall, F. W. (1914). The impurities in commercial nitrous oxide for dental use and their injurious effects by inhalation. *Brit. dent. J.*, **35**, 589.

Haskins, H. D. (1914). Impurities that may occur in nitrous oxide. *Cleveland med. J.*, **13**, 548.

Hewitt, F. W. (1893). *Anaesthetics and their Administration: a manual for medical and dental practitioners and students*, 1st ed. London: Charles Griffin.

—— (1907). *Anaesthetics and their Administration: a manual for medical and dental practitioners and students*, 3rd ed. London: Macmillan.

—— (1922). *Anaesthetics and their Administration: a manual for medical and dental practitioners and students*, 5th ed. (ed. Robinson, H.). London: Henry Froude and Hodder & Stoughton.

Hirsch, C. T. W. (1925). *A Chat on Anaesthetics*. London: John Bale, Sons & Danielsson.

Jackson, D. E. (1955). Anesthesia equipment from 1914 to 1954 and experiments relating to its development. *Anesthesiology*, **16**, 953.

Jeffreys, A. E. (1960). *Michael Faraday, a list of his lectures and published writings with a foreword by Sir Laurence Bragg*. London: Chapman & Hall on behalf of the Royal Institution.

Hoover, G. W. (1925). The quality of nitrous oxid manufactured in the United States. *J. Amer. med. Ass.*, **84**, 1472.

King, H. (1926). Discussion of Hadfield (1926). *Proc. roy. Soc. Med.*, **19**, 26.

Lancet (1916). Annotation. The danger of nitrous oxide and oxygen anaesthesia. **2**, 566.

—— (1920). Nitrous oxide gas for military hospitals. **1**, 349.

Lichtenstein, M. E., and Method, H. (1953). Edmund Andrews, M.D., a biographical sketch with historical notes concerning nitrous oxide-oxygen anaesthesia. *Northwest Univ. med. Sch. Quart. Bull.*, **27**, 337.

Macintosh, R., Mushin, W. W., and Epstein, H. G. (1958). *Physics for the Anaesthetist, including a section on explosions*, 2nd ed. Oxford: Blackwell.

Macintosh, R. R., and Pratt, F. B. (1940). *Essentials of General Anaesthesia with special reference to dentistry*. London: Blackwell.

McMechan, F. H. (1926). Discussion of Blomfield (1926). *Proc. roy. Soc. Med.*, **19**, 48.

Maughan, J. (1926). Discussion of Hadfield (1926). *Proc. roy. Soc. Med.*, **19**, 26.

M.F. (1819). Nitrous oxide. *Quart. J. Sci.*, **6**, 361.

Oscroft, E. (1934). History of nitrous oxide anaesthesia. *Brit. med. J.*, **1**, 516.

Parkinson,   (1926). Discussion of Hadfield (1926). *Proc. roy. Soc. Med.*, **19**, 25.

Pepys, W. H. (1802). Description of a new gas-holder. *Tilloch's Phil. Mag.*, **13**, 153.

Porter,   (1868). Mr. Porter's apparatus for making nitrous oxide gas. *Trans. odont. Soc. G.B.*, N.S., **1**, 29.

Puckner, W. A. (1911). Liquid nitrous oxide. Report of the Council on Pharmacy and Chemistry. *J. Amer. med. Ass.*, **57**, 576.

Ritson, J. L. (1871). Correspondence. *Brit. J. dent. Sci.*, **14**, 258.

Roberts, J. W. (1884). Anaesthetics and their administration. *Brit. J. dent. Sci.*, **27**, 1131.

Rottenstein, J. B. (1880). *Traité d'anesthésie chirurgicale contenant la description et les applications de la méthode anesthésique de M. Paul Bert*. Paris: Librairie Garmer Baillier.

Rymer, S. L. (1864). Remarks upon the use of nitrous oxide in dental operations. *Dent. Rev. N.S.*, **1**, 1.

Sculley, J. (1871). Dental *materia medica* and Therapeutics: nitrous oxide (not official). *Brit. J. dent. Sci.*, **14**, 272.

Shuter, G. P. (1912). The history of nitrous-oxide anaesthesia. *West Lond. med. J.*, **17**, 261.

Silk, J. F. (1888). *A Manual of Nitrous Oxide Anaesthesia*. London: Churchill.

Smith, W. D. A. (1965a). A history of nitrous oxide and oxygen anaesthesia. Part I: Joseph Priestley to Humphry Davy. *Brit. J. Anaesth.*, **37**, 790.

—— (1965b). A history of nitrous oxide and oxygen anaesthesia. Part II: Davy's researches in relation to inhalation anaesthesia. *Brit. J. Anaesth.*, **37**, 871.

Smith, W. D. A. (1966a). A history of nitrous oxide and oxygen anaesthesia. Part V: The crucial experiment, its eclipse, and its revival. *Brit. J. Anaesth.*, **38**, 143.

—— (1966b). A history of nitrous oxide and oxygen anaesthesia. Part VII: 1868—nitrous oxide anaesthesia takes root in Great Britain. *Brit. J. Anaesth.*, **38**, 551.

Smith, W. R., and Leman, E. D. (1911). The purity of nitrous oxide. *J. Amer. med. Ass.*, **57**, 577.

Snow, J. (1847). *On the Inhalation of the Vapour of Ether in Surgical Operations: containing a description of the various stages of etherization and a statement of the result of nearly eighty operations in which ether has been employed in St. George's and University College Hospitals.* London: John Churchill.

Sprague, A. W. (1864). Nitrous oxide as an anesthetic. *Boston med. sci. J.*, **71**, 169.

Stanley, F. (1842). Poisoning by the inhalation of impure nitrous oxide gas. *Lancet*, **1**, 395.

Sykes, W. S. (1960). *Essays on the First Hundred Years of Anaesthesia.* Edinburgh: Livingstone.

Teleky, L. (1948). *History of Factory and Mine Hygiene.* New York: Columbia University Press.

Thomas, F. R. (1870). *Manual of the Discovery, Manufacture, and Administration of Nitrous Oxide, or Laughing Gas, in its Relations to Dental or Minor Surgical Operations, and Particularly for the Extraction of Teeth.* Philadelphia: S. S. White.

Warner, A. R. (1915). Manufacture and administration of nitrous oxid for anesthesia: the experience of Lakeside Hospital. *J. Amer. med. Ass.*, **65**, 1973.

Wellesley, G. (1926). Discussion of Blomfield (1926). *Proc roy. Soc. Med.*, **19**, 48.

Wells, H. (1847). *A History of the Discovery of the Application of Nitrous Oxide Gas, Ether and other Vapours, to Surgical Operations.* Hartford: Gaylord Wells.

Willett, E. (1901). On a case of unusual symptoms following the administration of gas and oxygen. *Trans. Soc. Anaesth.*, **4**, 148.

Wylde, J. (c. 1872). *The Magic of Science: A Manual of Amusing and Scientific Experiments*, 3rd ed., London: Charles Griffin. (1st ed., 1861; 2nd ed., 1872.)

13

THE USE OF HEWITT'S "MIXTURE" AND THE DEVELOPMENT OF NASAL ADMINISTRATION

The development of the use of Hewitt's "mixture"
(of gas and oxygen)

Eleven years after beginning his studies on the use of oxygen (see Part IX; Smith, 1966), Hewitt (1897) decided to "place in the hands of the medical and dental professions (a) small treatise dealing more particularly with the practical aspects of the subject" and he published *The Administration of Nitrous Oxide and Oxygen for Dental Operations*. In the preface he wrote, quite uncompromisingly:

Safe and thoroughly efficient anaesthesia for dental operations is of such importance that it behoves every dental practitioner to carefully consider whether he should not abandon the prevalent but comparatively crude and unscientific method of producing insensibility from nitrous oxide, and avail himself of the new system.

Practical advice about the use of his apparatus indicates his appreciation of its limitations, and some of the difficulties in the manufacture of such devices.

All the valves are made of thin sheet india-rubber, and it is important that they should be in good order. Should they become inelastic from age, or should they in any way fail to act, as they are intended to act, with perfect accuracy, the apparatus will not produce good results. For example, an apparatus may let through much larger proportions of oxygen than usual if the nitrous oxide valve . . . should happen to adhere along part of its circumference, to the rim upon which it rests . . . trifling defects in the apparatus are liable to interfere with results. The connections must be tested, the bags inspected frequently; the stop cock taken to pieces occasionally—in fact, the anaesthetist must take a personal interest in his apparatus if he wishes to succeed with it.

Two years later Hewitt (1899) reported the investigation upon which much of his practical advice had been based. Using a gasometer of 20 gallons capacity (fig. 1), he used various known mixtures of nitrous oxide and air or oxygen in anaesthetizing 231 patients. With the aid of assistants, of whom one was Bellamy Gardner (fig. 2), he recorded each anaesthetic in detail, including notes on: (1) anoxaemic convulsions; (2) duskiness, lividity and cyanosis; (3) stertor; (4) retching movements; (5) phonation; (6) excitement and reflex movements; (7) after effects; (8) laboured or

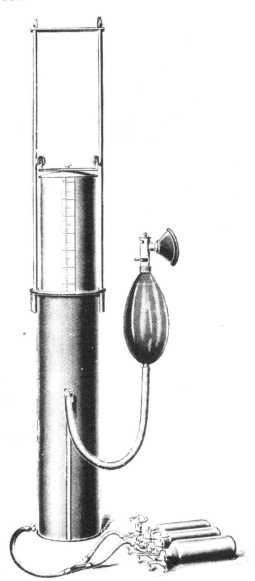

FIG. 1. The 20-gallon gasometer which Hewitt charged with various known mixtures of nitrous oxide and oxygen when seeking the optimum concentrations of oxygen for use during dental anaesthesia.

"catching" respiration; (9) unpleasant dreams; and (10) duration of anaesthesia after inhalation. He allocated "bad marks" to each of these side effects according to their importance and severity, for example, 20, 35 and 50 were allocated to slight, moderate and extreme anoxaemic convulsions; 10, 20 and 30 to change of colour; and 5, 15 and 40 to degrees of stertor. Anaesthetics lasting less than 20 seconds were allocated 20 marks; 25–29 seconds,

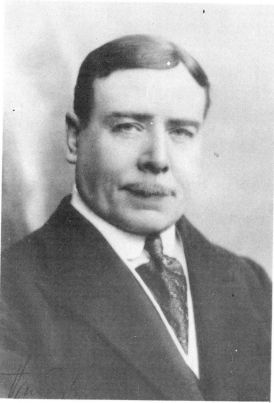

FIG. 2. Dr Harold Bellamy Gardner (1869–1943). "I would like to mention what a beautiful nasal gas Dr B. G. used to give. Good colour, quiet, it all looked so simple." (S. Coffin, 1968, personal communication.)

10 marks; and more than 30 seconds, no marks. In this way he was able to arrive at a figure for the "badness" of a given administration, which took into account all the above factors. A metronome was used for timing, its bell being adjusted to sound once every 3 seconds, and "metronome bells" were numbered down the lefthand margins of the record sheets so that notes could be timed accurately. He found that anoxaemic convulsions did not occur if he used more than 6 per cent oxygen or 25 per cent

air. He saw little or no alteration in colour if he used more than 9 per cent oxygen. Stertor was avoided by using more than 13 per cent oxygen. Reflex movements increased as the concentration of oxygen was increased above 7 per cent. Duration of anaesthesia was greatest when about 7 per cent oxygen was used, but the fewest "bad marks" were obtained with a concentration of 9 per cent oxygen, although he found "There is no one mixture of nitrous oxide with air or oxygen which will successfully anaesthetise every patient". He noted that

The more marked cyanosis is met with when very small percentages of air (3 to 6 per cent) or oxygen (under 3 per cent) are administered with nitrous oxide. With pure nitrous oxide cyanosis may not have time, as it were, to become pronounced, for the administration may be cut short by deep stertor.

He concluded that

In order to obtain the best form of anaesthesia, oxygen should be administered with nitrous oxide by means of a regulating apparatus, the percentage of the former gas being progressively increased from 2 per cent or 3 per cent at the commencement of the administration to 7, 8, 9 or 10 per cent according to the circumstances of the case. The longer the administration lasts, the greater may be the percentages of oxygen administered.

In discussion Dr John S. Haldane, "after complimenting the author", said:

. . . the paper raised the question, what was it that produced anaesthesia in nitrous oxide administration? Was it the want of oxygen or was it some definite specific action of the nitrous oxide gas? He thought that the paper proved that the anaesthesia was due to some specific action of the gas, since there was no lack of oxygen.

The slow acceptance of the virtues of using Hewitt's "mixture" is evident from a series of 6,657 anaesthetics administered at the London Hospital during the year 1897 (Hewitt, 1898). Of these, 1,362 were "straight" nitrous oxide anaesthetics, 282 used nitrous oxide as the induction agent before ether, and 240 were nitrous oxide and oxygen anaesthetics. In the same paper Hewitt described preliminary trials with the use of nitrous oxide and oxygen for surgical operations. The apparatus he used was similar to that devised for dental anaesthesia "except that the channels for the oxygen were double the size . . . and that the bags are about three times as large". While acknowledging that "it is quite possible, as our knowledge and experience increase, that further developments may render the use of nitrous oxide and oxygen more satisfactory for long operations than it is at present", and that "The two great recommendations of this plan of anaesthetising are that it is the safest at present known and that by its employment the often distressing after-effects of anaesthesia may usually be avoided", he reported that "I have used it in several surgical cases, but I cannot say that I have been satisfied with the results in many of them".

Bellamy Gardner (1899) reported more fully on the use of nitrous oxide and oxygen for surgical cases, but also with guarded enthusiasm. After initial trials he concluded

. . that 10 per cent of oxygen, the largest amount yielded by Dr Hewitt's apparatus, might be enough in dental cases and other short inhalations, but possibly a percentage of oxygen more nearly approaching that present in atmospheric air . . . would be required, after all the residual oxygen present in the patient's system at the moment of the first breath of the mixture, had been expired. . . . To obviate, as I thought, all symptoms of asphyxia in these anaesthesias with nitrous oxide gas, a percentage of 15 to 20 of oxygen should be available after the first few minutes of inhalation, and I therefore had the last three apertures in Dr Hewitt's regulating dial enlarged in diameter, so as to admit the necessary amount to the mixing chamber.

He also found that

Retching movements and sickness cannot be controlled by more gas and oxygen, as with other anaesthetics, this is a great drawback, and negatives the value of the mixture in boys and girls, about ten to fifteen years of age, who seem prone to sickness. . . . Profuse sweating is very common. . . . Florid, alcoholic, and muscular men are not such good subjects as the more ordinary type, nor can it be recommended for small children.

With regard to administering the mixture he made the particular point that "To obtain anything approaching accuracy in the percentage proportions of the mixture, the double gas bag of Dr Hewitt's apparatus must *hang free of the couch*. In conclusion he said

. . . from my experience of a thorough trial of the mixture in surgery, I must say that, though we have not discovered in this method an inhalation which can in any general sense supplant the use of ether or chloroform, we probably have one which has distinct advantages over gas or gas and ether for operations of minor and of very moderate severity.

In the discussion that followed, Dr Dudley Buxton commented that:

He had employed gas and oxygen for a good many years, both for surgical and dental work. He and Mr Gardner agreed in regard to it in many points, though perhaps Mr Gardner was more sanguine about the method than he was. . . . It had been demonstrated by not only Mr Gardner, but by others, that the anaesthetic was a very valuable mixture in its own place. The only danger was that it should be elevated as he feared it was, not by professional men, but by the public, into a position of absolute safety, absolute pleasantness, in fact into the position of an anaesthetic panacea . . . he thought they would agree

with Dr Silk and Mr Crouch in their wise remark that it was better to mark time for the present, and see how this matter was going to turn out.

In the same year Paterson (1899) also pleaded for a more extended use of nitrous oxide anaesthesia in general surgery, and "To prevent misunderstanding" he explained that "when I refer to the use of gas or nitrous oxide anaesthesia, I imply that the gas is given with suitable proportions of either air or oxygen". On seven occasions he had administered gas and oxygen for more than an hour.

Guy and Ross (1912) were unstinting in their praise of Hewitt's valuable series of experimental investigations, but they were critical of his method of administering the "mixture", on the grounds that it required complicated apparatus and considerable practice, and that the use of valves entailed the use of very large quantities of gases. As an alternative they adapted the method of Gatch (1910) (see Part XII). This entailed rebreathing gas and oxygen from a bag until the carbon dioxide level was considered to be as high as desirable, when the bag was emptied through an expiratory valve and then replenished. Their modification of the method was to allow for the injection of known increments of oxygen by means of a syringe bulb of 2-ounce capacity (fig. 3). For a dental anaesthetic the patient rebreathed nitrous oxide for 15–20 seconds when 4 ounces of oxygen were added by squeezing the bulb twice. Further known quantities of oxygen were supplied

. . . at such intervals as are indicated by the complexion, care being taken to steer between the two extremes of rosiness and cyanosis. Usually about four ounces of oxygen are required every 15 or 20 seconds, until from 6 to 10 ounces have been given in all; this will suffice for the 110 to 120 seconds required to induce anaesthesia for a dental case. . . . At the end of these two minutes the anaesthesia is quite deep enough for the extraction of two or three easy teeth, but if a deeper and more lasting anaesthesia is desired, from 1 to 3 cc of ethyl chloride (never more) is run in at the end of from twenty-five to forty seconds, and the mixture rebreathed for another thirty or more seconds, when a most beautiful anaesthesia lasting from 70 to 100 seconds, results.

Using this method, Guy and Ross reported 800 successful administrations over a period of five months. It is doubtful whether the concentration of oxygen in the bag ever exceeded 5 or 6 per cent, and it is perhaps not surprising that this method failed to supplant Hewitt's. It is worthy of notice, however, that two years previously work from the same centre (Guy, Goodall and Reid, 1910) had given particular attention to blood pressure during

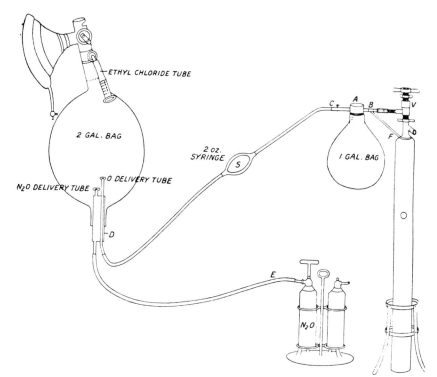

ETHYL CHLORIDE TUBE

2 GAL. BAG

2 OZ.
SYRINGE

S

1 GAL. BAG

N₂O DELIVERY TUBE   N₂O DELIVERY TUBE

D

E

N₂O

Fig. 3. The nitrous oxide and oxygen apparatus of Guy and Ross.

anaesthesia. It showed an awareness of the possible effects of posture and it compared the effects on blood pressure of: chloroform; ether; nitrous oxide with both rebreathing and non-rebreathing; nitrous oxide preceded by oxygen; nitrous oxide and ether given in sequence; ethyl chloride; nitrous oxide and ethyl chloride in sequence; and oxygen, nitrous oxide and ethyl chloride in sequence. Particular conclusions were

1. That there is no practical difference between the available anaesthesia brought about by nitrous oxide when rebreathing is allowed and that available when nitrous oxide is given with valves, but the effects of asphyxia are much more marked in the latter method.

2. The asphyxial element, present in the rebreathing method can be avoided by the previous inhalation of a gallon of oxygen, but the period of available anaesthesia is often shortened a few seconds.

The development of nasal administration of nitrous oxide.

At the end of the last century there was a revival of interest in prolonging unconsciousness during operations in the mouth when Coleman (1898a), Coxon (1898), Hilliard (1898, 1902) and McCardie (1899) presented papers on the subject. Alfred Coleman had by then retired so he relied upon the assistance of Dr Hewitt and Mr Paterson in trying

out his apparatus (fig. 4). This was a development of apparatus originally designed for the administration of chloroform through the nose. In his own words (at a meeting of the Society of Anaesthetists),

It consists of a nose-piece made to loosely cover the nose and fit accurately to its base, and which is connected with a very flat tube also adapted to fit accurately over the forehead. To the latter is attached a piece of stout rubber tubing having at its further extremity a very lightly constructed two-way stop-cock which is connected with the ordinary gas-bag, but between the two is placed a valve which opens towards the nose. The gas-bag is connected by a long tube to the gas-bottle. When using the apparatus it is well to instruct the patient to breath in at the nose and out at the mouth for a few times, and then to adapt the nose-piece, the same form of breathing being continued. An air-padded face-piece, rather larger than is ordinarily employed, and having only the outlet valve, is placed over the nose-piece and mouth and the gas turned on. When the patient is fully narcotised the face-piece is removed and the operation commenced, whilst sufficient gas is admitted into the bag to slightly distend it beyond its normal capacity.

Paterson had tried this out on fifteen patients, the average duration of anaesthesia being about $2\frac{1}{2}$ minutes and the longest anaesthetic 5 minutes.

Coxon (1898), at the same meeting, favoured playing a jet of gas into the mouth, using a curved tube which could also be employed as a tongue depressor. He found that the patient's mouth got following year, reported favourably on his own experience of Coxon's method of oral administration, to which he added the use of a nasal clamp. He noted that there was occasionally a feeling of faintness afterwards. Willett commented in the discussion that "it seemed to him that the gas and oxygen introduced by Dr Hewitt was so much superior to ordinary gas for dental cases that this new method of Mr McCardie's was not so important as it would have been if they had not had Dr Hewitt's method". Hilliard (1898) also presented a short paper on the use of a nasopharyngeal tube for the administration of nitrous oxide, which he elaborated in 1902 (fig. 5), but after that the idea seemed to peter out.

In passing, another method of prolonging nitrous oxide and oxygen anaesthesia may be mentioned, although its professed purpose was to make administration more comfortable for the patient, who was enabled to breathe the gas at atmospheric pressure,

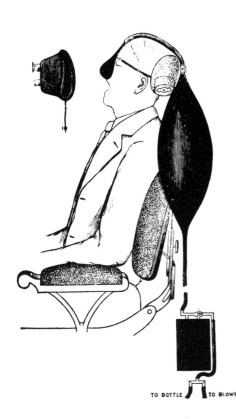

TO BOTTLE   TO BLOWER

FIG. 4. Coleman's apparatus. "In administering gas and ether and air through the same nose-piece I use much the same apparatus that I employed for many years at the Dental Hospital for giving gas and ether, but now, besides the gas bottle, I have connected with it a 'Fletcher's footblower'. I first give the patient nitrous oxide, and when rendered partially unconscious, divert the flow of gas through the ether, and when narcosis is fully established and the operation about to be commenced, turn off the gas and pump air by the foot bellows through the ether, and thus continue the anaesthesia by air and ether alone, effecting of course a very large saving of gas." (Coleman, 1898b; cf. Duncum, 1947.)

very cold, so he passed the gas through a copper coil immersed in hot water. Paterson (1898) had tried instead conveying nitrous oxide through a catheter inserted into the nose, but "He found hospital patients were very liable to bleed at the nose through the catheter being passed". Since then he had been lent Mr Coleman's apparatus and "All he could say was that from his short experience with it he could not commend it too highly in dental work . . . he thought that some modifications might be made with advantage". McCardie, in the

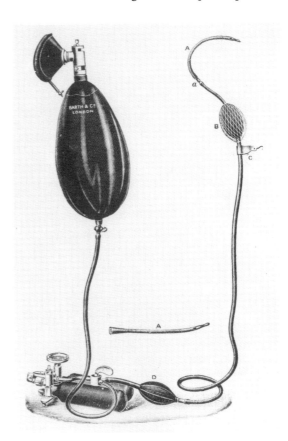

FIG. 5. Hilliard's apparatus for the nasopharyngeal administration of nitrous oxide.

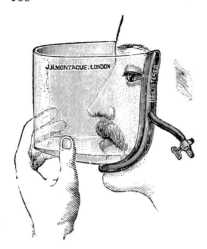

FIG. 6. Flux's open inhaler for use during dental surgical operations. Although Flux reported administrations lasting as long as 12 minutes, he did not indicate whether any of these were for dental cases. From the illustration it looks as if the inhaler would have been inconvenient for this purpose.

FIG. 7. Paterson's nosepiece, as modified by Kirkpatrick who incorporated an expiratory valve. The slotted cover over this valve could be rotated in order to put it out of action.

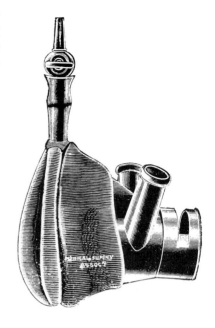

and to maintain free access of air. Flux (1899) introduced open inhalers (fig. 6) which could be applied to the face so that, with the face, the inhaler formed an open vessel into which nitrous oxide could be "poured" as required. He had used this method in 350 cases and for administrations lasting as long as 12 minutes.

Paterson (1899) took the next step in designing "a metal cover made to fit the nose accurately, with the aid of a rubber pad. . . . Two small metal tubes are let into the nose-piece, and to these are attached two rubber tubes which lead to an ordinary gas bag, a two way stop-cock intervening". After the patient had taken a few breaths of nitrous oxide, a celluloid cover, fitted with an expiratory valve, was placed over the mouth. This was removed after about 30 seconds, and, in his own words,

The patient is now taking in gas through the nose, and a limited amount of air through the mouth, and there is no difficulty in maintaining anaesthesia, indeed the stop-cock has often to be turned off occasionally in order to allow the patient to obtain more air than is admitted by the mouth.

Nine minutes and fifty-five seconds was the duration of the longest anaesthetic that he had given by this means. The only disadvantage that he reported was that he was unable to assist the operation as in giving the gas in the ordinary way.

Kirkpatrick (1902), however, found difficulty in getting patients to inspire by the nose and expire by the mouth and even using the mouth cover he experienced great difficulty in using Paterson's method. His solution was to fit an expiratory valve to the nosepiece so that the patient breathed entirely through the nose, keeping the mouth closed during the induction of anaesthesia (fig. 7). A Mason's gag was then used for opening the mouth (he checked the apposition of teeth beforehand, and if necessary inserted a small prop, just sufficient to keep the teeth apart). He also introduced a sponge into the back of the mouth so as to "occlude, or at all events limit, the air way from it". By fitting a movable cap over the expiratory valve he closed the valve when he wanted to increase the pressure in the gas bag and so "raise the gas pressure in the nasopharynx to such an extent that the soft palate was pushed forward against the tongue, so closing the mouth way from behind".

Throughout all these developments no one appears to have tried administering nitrous oxide and oxygen by the nasal route. One reason for this was probably that the administrators thought that the patients were getting enough air through the mouth and through leaks around the nosepiece. Another reason, explained by Bellamy Gardner (1907), was that it was not possible to use slight "plus pressure" on the bags of Hewitt's apparatus without altering the composition of the mixture delivered. Of this Hewitt was well aware (Smith, 1966; Part IX), and in an attempt to get over this difficulty, in the later models of his apparatus (Hewitt, 1897) he arranged for the two bags to share a common septum in the hope of keeping the two gases at the same pressure. Dr A. G. Levy (cited Gardner, 1907) went one

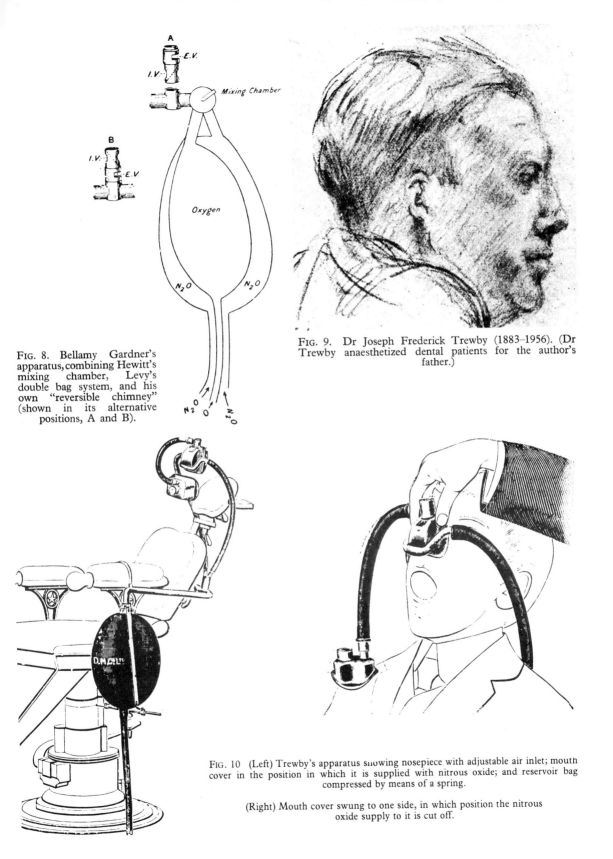

FIG. 8. Bellamy Gardner's apparatus, combining Hewitt's mixing chamber, Levy's double bag system, and his own "reversible chimney" (shown in its alternative positions, A and B).

FIG. 9. Dr Joseph Frederick Trewby (1883–1956). (Dr Trewby anaesthetized dental patients for the author's father.)

FIG. 10 (Left) Trewby's apparatus showing nosepiece with adjustable air inlet; mouth cover in the position in which it is supplied with nitrous oxide; and reservoir bag compressed by means of a spring.

(Right) Mouth cover swung to one side, in which position the nitrous oxide supply to it is cut off.

better than this by placing the oxygen bag inside the nitrous oxide bag, so that, provided the inner bag was not overdistended, the two gases were at approximately the same pressure. This development enabled Bellamy Gardner to introduce the technique of nasal administration of nitrous oxide and oxygen mixtures by combining the apparatuses of Hewitt and Paterson, incorporating the bag system of Levy (but enlarging the oxygen bag), and adding his own "reversible valve chimney" which permitted either rebreathing or non-rebreathing of gas and oxygen (fig. 8). His technique was to prop open the mouth, using a Hewitt's prop between the molar teeth, and administer 6 per cent oxygen with nitrous oxide through the nose; the patient was then allowed to rebreathe, a little nitrous oxide being run in to

replace that taken up; then the oxygen concentration was increased to 10 per cent after 1 minute and 15 per cent after $1\frac{1}{2}$ minutes. "Plus pressure" was used if the patient began to breathe through the mouth.

Frank Coleman (1908) (Alfred Coleman's son) introduced a sliding clamp to hold the twin tubes together, behind the patient's head (he had not begun to use oxygen).

Trewby (1909) (fig. 9) added a mouth cover, an air inlet on the nosepiece, and a means of supplying nitrous oxide at a steady even pressure a little above atmospheric pressure (fig. 10). The mouth cover was designed to make an efficient seal with the face while using a mouth prop. It was supplied by gas from the nosepiece, and a swivel connection on the nosepiece automatically cut off the gas supply to the mouth cover when this was swung out of the way. The adjustable air inlet on the nosepiece permitted air to be admitted instantly when required. The reservoir bag was compressed between two metal bands which were interconnected by means of a spring.

Coleman (1910) then observed that "no one form of inhaler is capable of satisfying the demands of every anaesthetist", and he presented an apparatus which "allows the induction of anaesthesia by the two chief methods at present employed" (fig. 11). This was followed by a "naso-oral inhaler" with

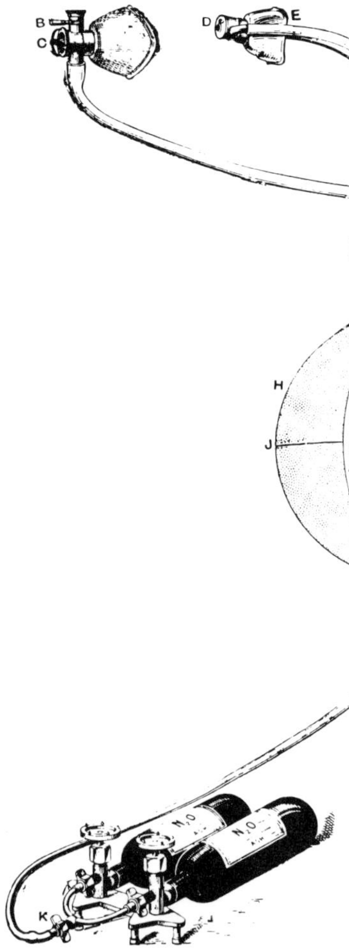

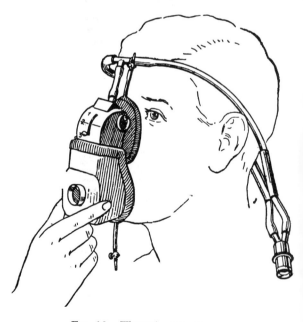

FIG. 11. Frank Coleman's apparatus providing for the use of either facemask or nosepiece.

FIG. 12. Warner's apparatus.

separate but communicating mouth- and nose-pieces, which has not survived (Warner, 1911) (fig. 12). This was really a development of Coleman's (1898) original design. There was, in fact, no real change in the design of apparatus for nasal administration until the invention of sophisticated anaesthetic machines and Goldman's (1936) introduction of a single wide-bore tube for connection to the nose-piece, in place of Paterson's twin tubes.

ACKNOWLEDGEMENTS

The photograph of Dr Bellamy Gardner was very kindly loaned by Mrs Kathleen Bellamy Gardner. I wish also to thank Mr Ronald B. Gardner for the loan of relevant documents, and Dr S. Coffin, who was Dr Bellamy Gardner's partner and who provided more information than I have been able to use in this article. The excellent likeness of Dr Joseph Frederick Trewby was drawn by his niece and it was very kindly loaned by his daughter, Mrs Diana Topham. The substance of this article has been extracted from the introductory chapter of a thesis approved for the degree of M.D. in the University of London.

REFERENCES

Coleman, A. (1898a). On a method of administering anaesthetics through the nose. Trans. Soc. Anaesth., 1, 117.
—— (1898b). Communication read in absentia. Trans. odont. Soc. G.B. (N.S. 30), 139.
Coleman, F. (1908). The Nasal Administration of Nitrous Oxide Gas. London: Claudius Ash.
—— (1910). A nasal inhaler for the continuous administration of nitrous oxide. Lancet, 2, 1840.
—— (1954). The history of nitrous oxide anaesthesia. Med. ill. (Lond.), 8, 419.
Coxon, S. A. (1898). The continuous administration of nitrous oxide. Trans. Soc Anaesth., 1, 123.
Duncum, B. (1947). The Development of Inhalation Anaesthesia, with special reference to the years 1846–1900, p. 490. London: Oxford University Press.
Flux, G. B. (1899). Administration of nitrous oxide gas by an open inhaler. Trans. Soc. Anaesth., 2, 140.
Gardner, B. (1899). Nitrous oxide gas and oxygen as an anaesthetic for surgical and dental operations. Trans. Soc. Anaesth., 2, 163.
Gardner, H. B. (1907). Prolonged Anaesthesia under Nitrous Oxide and Oxygen for Dental Operations. London: John Bale, Sons and Denielsson.
Gatch, W. D. (1910). Nitrous-oxide-oxygen anaesthesia by the method of rebreathing. J. Amer. med. Ass., 54, 775.
Goldman, V. (1936), cited Coleman (1954).
Guy, W., Goodall, A., and Reid, H. S. (1910). The blood-pressure in anaesthesia. Edinb. med. J. (N.S.), 4, 207.
—— Ross, J. S. (1912). Nitrous oxide and oxygen as an anaesthetic for dental and surgical purposes. Edinb. med. J. (N.S.), 9, 517.
Hewitt, F. W. (1897). The Administration of Nitrous Oxide and Oxygen for Dental Operations. London: Claudius Ash.
—— (1898). 6,657 administrations of anaesthetics conducted at the London Hospital during the year 1897. Lancet, 1, 483.
—— (1899). On the effects produced in the human subject by the administration of nitrous oxide and air and of nitrous oxide and oxygen. Med.-chir. Trans., 82, 163.
Hilliard, H. (1898). Nitrous oxide anaesthesia in dental practice. Lancet, 1, 655.
—— (1902). Further notes on the use of the nasopharyngeal tube for prolonged nitrous oxide anaesthesia. Lancet, 1, 1824.
Kirkpatrick, T. P. C. (1902). The prolongation of nitrous oxide anaesthesia for dental operations by Paterson's method. Med. Press, 125, 55.
McCardie, W. J. (1899). Meeting of the Society of Anaesthetists. On the prolongation of nitrous oxide anaesthesia in dental operations by means of a mouth-tube. Clin. J., 13, 379.
Paterson, H. J. (1898). Discussion. Trans. Soc. Anaesth., 1, 127.
—— (1899). The use of nitrous oxide gas in general and dental surgery. W. Lond. med. J., 4, 202.
Smith, W. D. A. (1966). A history of nitrous oxide and oxygen anaesthesia. Part IX: The introduction of nitrous oxide and oxygen anaesthesia. Brit. J. Anaesth., 38, 950.
—— (1972). A history of nitrous oxide and oxygen anaesthesia. Part XII: Developments in America and nitrous oxide anaesthesia between World Wars. Brit. J. Anaesth., 44 (in press).
Trewby, F. (1909). A combined ordinary and nasal apparatus for administering nitrous oxide. Brit. med. J., 2, 1805.
Warner, N. S. E. (1911). A new method for administering nitrous oxide, with or without oxygen, for prolonged dental operations. Lancet, 1, 371.

14

DEVELOPMENTS IN AMERICA AND NITROUS OXIDE ANAESTHESIA BETWEEN WORLD WARS

Developments in America.

In 1909, Teter wrote:

Thirteen thousand successful administrations of nitrous oxid and oxygen by one anesthetist covering a period of nine years for practically every kind of operation to its completion, under varying degrees of hazard, and varying in time from a few minutes to three hours, furnishes sufficient data, it seems to me, to establish to some degree, at least, the efficiency of nitrous oxid with oxygen as an anesthetic.

He went on to acknowledge that Hewitt had done more to bring this anaesthetic before the profession than any one man, and that his book was the best on the subject that had ever been published, but, he continued, "He, however, has not had the experience with this particular anaesthetic that some men in America have". Teter claimed to have used nitrous oxide with oxygen

. . . many times as an anesthetic throughout the following operations: laparotomies, consisting of hysterectomy, salpingectomy, oophorectomy, appendicectomy, cholecystectomy, choledochotomy, gastrectomy, gastroduodenostomy, ureterosigmoidostomy. Other operations, such as abdominal Caesarean section, prostatectomy, removal of large tumours and inflammatory adhesions, radical cure of hernia, varicocele, hydrocele and orchidectomy; amputations of breasts, amputations of extremities, and a large number of thoracentesis . . .

He continued:

In brain surgery nitrous oxid has been especially advised against, owing largely to the asphyxiation that is concomitant with the administration of nitrous oxid with air. . . . Nitrous oxid with varying proportions of oxygen, however, if skilfully given, is a different proposition. My experience in this line of work has been good, for I have not had a single case in which difficulties arose.

These claims contrast strikingly with the more cautious statements made in the United Kingdom. Teter, however, did acknowledge that he had learned that it was not always best to continue with nitrous oxide and oxygen under all circumstances "for it may be next to impossible to retain the desired depth of narcosis in certain cases". Since 1906, he had auscultated the chest continuously during anaesthesia. In order to overcome the rigidity which he found in about 10 per cent of cases in major surgery, he used injections of

morphine sulphate 7.5–15 mg and atropine 0.4–0.6 mg half an hour before the operation, but he warned against respiratory depression.

Teter also laid down specifications for the apparatus required and he designed his own. These included a spare cylinder for rapid change-over as each cylinder emptied; means of warming the gas; and large unobstructed channels from bag to inhaler, the gases being under a slight pressure. He thought that "A certain amount of cyanosis is not objectionable" and that "The most noticeable effect from extreme cyanosis is a severe headache, which will not subside in some cases for two to three hours". This cyanosis was of significance in relation to the contamination of nitrous oxide which occurred at Lakeside Hospital, Cleveland, where Teter worked (Smith, 1967, Part X).

As a result of the interest shown in Teter's (1909) article on nitrous oxide and oxygen, he felt it advisable, three years later, to follow with another (Teter, 1912)

. . . to make clear the requirements and limitations of this combination, in order to maintain its present popularity as approaching the principles of an ideal anaesthetic, and to avoid the sacrifice of life which may result in consequence of ignorance concerning the action of these peculiar gases.

He repeated the advisability of using premedication. He made it clear that anything from 80 to 95 per cent nitrous oxide might be necessary, the average patient requiring 88 per cent (although later he stated that the average amount of oxygen used was $16\frac{2}{3}$ per cent). He tried "to secure definite known percentages of nitrous oxid and oxygen put up in high-pressure cylinders. This was found to be impracticable for the reason that the percentages changed, as shown by daily tests". He pointed out:

Many accidents have been caused by the failure of the patients to receive the amount of oxygen indicated on the apparatus. It is impossible to control the percentages of the gases by having the controlling valves between the gas bags and the inhaler, on account of the impossibility of maintaining definite pressures in the bags. The only positive way is to have the gases at known pressures and the controlling valves between the gas bags and the gas supply.

He also favoured rebreathing nitrous oxide (see Gatch, 1910, below). He considered gas and oxygen to be contraindicated for children under 5 years of age, and in old people, and he did not consider it ideal for major surgery on patients possessing strong, vigorous constitutions or extremely nervous temperaments, or in those addicted to drugs or the excessive use of tobacco.

Gatch (1910) gave the "results of a trial of nitrous-oxid-oxygen anesthesia in the service of Professor Halsted at the Johns Hopkins Hospital". His object, at the outset, "was to develop a method of administering these gases so simple, cheap and effective as to make possible their more general use". It seemed to him "that the solution, in so far as cost and convenience are concerned, must be in using them over instead of wasting them after one inhalation". His results led him "to believe that within certain limits the method is not only harmless but beneficial". His apparatus did not allow accurate control of the composition of gas mixtures. A "valve box" on the facepiece provided for (1) non-rebreathing room air, (2) non-rebreathing gas "(with oxygen if desired)", (3) rebreathing into a bag of 6–8 litre capacity through a tube of 1 inch diameter and $2\frac{1}{2}$ feet long (capacity about 350 ml). Each of two nitrous oxide cylinders and one oxygen cylinder was connected, through its own narrow-bore tubing, to an L-shaped tube between the bag and the 1-inch diameter connecting tubing. An ether vaporizer was provided within the mask. The procedure was for the patient to non-rebreathe gas until he was slightly cyanotic. He then rebreathed into the bag and

At this moment a small puff of oxygen is admitted to the bag, just enough to restore the natural colour of the face. The patient now rebreathes a mixture of nitrous oxid and oxygen until the valve is moved back to its mid (non-rebreathing) position. He then exhales each breath into the air until the bag is empty. The anesthetizer then fills it with a fresh mixture of gases, which the patient again rebreathes. No attempt is made to measure the exact percentage of oxygen given. This we regard as unnecessary.

The patient rebreathed each bagful sixteen times. Gatch had used the method on about 700 patients for almost every abdominal and peripheral operation except craniotomy and operations on the female pelvic organs. The alleged advantages

appeared to be mainly theoretical and based upon his own interpretations of what was then known as the physiology of respiration and of "shock".

By the following year (Gatch, 1911) he had used this method for 2,500 gas-oxygen and gas-oxygen-ether anaesthesias. There were three deaths during or immediately after operations and one who never regained consciousness died 8 hours afterwards.

McKesson (1911) then brought out apparatus with a view to obtaining an easier and more accurate administration of nitrous oxide and oxygen. This incorporated a rebreathing bag, but check valves prevented expired gases from entering the two supply bags which, through valves, supplied a mixing chamber. The mixing chamber control had 20 graduations. The gases were warmed by an electric lamp. The rebreathing bag was also adjustable and calibrated for volume so that the amount of rebreathing could be controlled ("Fractional Rebreathing"). This could presumably have been adjusted so that only deadspace gas was rebreathed, in which case it would have functioned in a manner similar to the Magill breathing system (Kain and Nunn, 1967).

Peairs (1910) also devised apparatus with which nitrous oxide could be given pure or with oxygen in any proportion from 1 per cent to 15 per cent, but he did not give details of his mixing chamber. He wrote:

At the present time nitrous oxid and oxygen is the best anesthetic for short operations . . . but it is to its use in major surgery that I wish to draw attention. During the past two years I have administered the gas in a number of major surgical operations. My first experience was with a fixed mixture containing 2 per cent oxygen. This was satisfactory in some cases; in others it was not because the amount of oxygen could not be varied.

The concentration of oxygen administered to patients subsequently using his apparatus, was not stated. The longest administration was 1 hour 54 minutes.

Mandell (1911) preferred the Davis apparatus; it

. . . seemed less complicated that the Teter and was preferred to the "Gatch", only because the "Davis" has two bags, one for gas and one for oxygen, enabling the operator to stop gas instantly and give pure oxygen.

Early in 1912, Allen (1912) sounded a warning, drawing attention to the fact that the majority of the vast series of nitrous oxide and oxygen anaesthetics being reported were in fact for dentistry or minor surgical procedures—and not for major surgery. Quoting Crile, he provided the following table of 17,716 administrations by Teter of gas and oxygen without a death:

12,886	lasted less than	5 minutes
3,365	,,	5 to 15 ,,
865	,,	15 to 30 ,,
346	,,	30 to 60 ,,
228	,,	1 to 2 hours
22	,,	2 to 3 ,,
2	,,	3 to 4 ,,

He went on to say that anaesthetic deaths occurring during the use of nitrous oxide and oxygen in major surgery were not uncommon.

Skeel (1913), who also came from Cleveland, presented 1,120 anaesthetics, of which 731 were for laparotomies, with a view to discussing the selection of anaesthesia. He confessed that one of his motives was "a subconscious desire to stamp as altogether wrong the idea that there exists at the present time a universally safe anesthetic or one which under any and all circumstances meets every indication". He said that

Nitrous oxide and oxygen were selected for a great variety of reasons, first and foremost among which was the fact that a skilled and experienced nitrous oxide anesthetist was always available. In the absence of such an expert, nitrous oxide would have had a very limited field of application.

In this well-balanced but forthright paper, Skeel made plain the world of difference that lay between the use of nitrous oxide for dental operations and its use for major surgery, and he emphasized the potential danger of asphyxia. With frankness he asserted that

Exploitation by those personally interested is, I am sorry to say, another very potent reason for the popular belief in the safety of nitrous oxide. For this the exuberance and enthusiasm of some very prominent members of the profession are directly to blame, and I believe that could they have foreseen the results of their utterances they would have been more circumspect in what they said and wrote. Working under the most favourable circumstances with expert anesthetists they have not hesitated to proclaim the entire safety of nitrous oxide with the result that large numbers of medical men and dentists have equipped themselves with the necessary apparatus and after observing a half dozen administrations, have rushed home to announce the possibility of anesthesia without danger, discomfort during its use or uncomfortable after-effects.

In the discussion that followed, McKesson agreed that "There is more in the anesthetist than there is in the drug used". Humiston, also of Cleveland, confirmed,

In the hospital with which I am connected there have been cases recently of death following nitrous oxide and oxygen anesthesia. These deaths have not been published. One was a simple case of appendicitis, with a short operation. The patient expired at the close of the operation from nitrous oxide and oxygen given by a man who has had considerable experience.

Bainbridge, in support, said that

Many who attended (the discussion of anesthesia by the sections on Pharmacology and Physiology of the American Medical Association) and who listened attentively were appalled at the number of casualties presented by the honest statement of facts concerning the administration of nitrous oxide and the various inhalation anesthetics.

Meanwhile Boothby and Cotton (Boothby, 1912; Cotton and Boothby, 1912) had made worthwhile advances in the design of apparatus. In order to facilitate control of the flow of nitrous oxide and oxygen they used reducing valves to bring their pressures down from 700 and 200 Lb./sq.in. respectively, to 20 Lb./sq.in. (They cast special yokes for taking the cylinders so that they could be changed easily. Cut-out valves were incorporated. The nitrous oxide reducing valve was surrounded by an electric heating coil to prevent freezing.) Knowledge of the amount of each gas being used was

. . . obtained by passing the gases through water into a mixing chamber; the rate of the bubbling of the gas through the water gives a very accurate index of the percentages of the two gases as administered to the patient. In addition, this procedure adds a desirable degree of moisture to the gases.

An ether vaporizer was included and the gases were warmed. The action of the inspiratory valve could be controlled to allow some rebreathing. An electric motor and air pump were added so that the apparatus could be used for intratracheal insufflation. This system was fitted with a safety valve. In their description of the clinical use of this apparatus they were adamant that

To be safe, effective and suitable for major surgical work a nitrous oxide-oxygen anaesthesia must be so conducted that the patient is never in the least degree cyanotic; on the contrary the patient must always be pink. . . . In those cases that cannot be sufficiently relaxed for the purpose in hand by the use of nitrous oxide with a sufficient proportion of oxygen to prevent cyanosis, the anaesthesia should be deepened by the addition of as much ether vapour as may be needed.

The subsequent development of anaesthetic machines in America has been outlined by Miller (1941) and Jackson (1955). By 1915 they had standardized into the two main types: intermittent flow and steady flow. The use of the Rotameter for the latter type has been described by Foregger (1946, 1952) and by Mörch (1952).

Some of the stimulus to nitrous oxide and oxygen anaesthesia of those days came from Crile's interest in it in relation to his ideas on "anoci-association" (Crile, 1911). The details that he gave in his paper of 1911, however, referred more to nitrous oxide than to nitrous oxide and oxygen, although his anaesthetists were apparently using the latter. But he did give a few clues on their success. Apart from saying that "the anaesthetist must be an individual of the keenest perception of the precise condition of the patient at every moment, i.e., the anaesthetist must be a most delicate human recording apparatus", he mentioned that "The muscular rigidity may be overcome by switching on the ether in a Teter apparatus until relaxation is secured, after which nitrous oxide alone continues the relaxation". He also raised

a very important surgical point that relates to nitrous oxide anaesthesia—that is, rough surgery excites a greater involuntary reactive opposition of the patient to the surgeon than ether does. . . . Those who wish to do rough surgery will scarcely find nitrous oxide suitable for the purpose.

The use of premedicant drugs was mentioned by Teter (1909), but Crile added: "Combined with this method of anaesthesia there has also been developed a gentle technique and a more careful management of patients from the time of their entrance to the hospital until their discharge". And further, after commenting that "every surgeon can recall instances in which the combination of light anaesthesia and perhaps vigorous surgical procedure have elicited an unmistakable, perhaps even vigorous attempt at escape from the table", he described how:

If one combines a complete local anaesthesia with a general anaesthesia and avoids fear, then it matters not how poor the risk, nor how extensive the operation. . . . No one who has witnessed the astonishing immunity that is conferred upon the patient by this method could doubt the correctness of the premises.

Despite the claims of Teter, the apparatus and admonitions of Cotton and Boothby, and the approach and high example set by Crile, one cannot be too surprised at Baldwin publishing a paper in 1916 with the dramatic title "Nitrous oxide-oxygen, the most dangerous anesthetic" (Smith, 1967, Part X): although one may feel disappointment that McKesson (1920) should have introduced his "technic of secondary saturation" four years later—in his own words:

In a primary saturation only the actively circulating blood is saturated before oxygen must be administered. There remains in the muscles, and in all other tissues, consider-

able volumes of nitrogen and oxygen, which in the early minutes of narcosis enters the blood stream and dilutes the nitrous oxid which prevents a deeper anesthesia. In order to displace more of the non-anesthetic gases in the body with nitrous oxid, the technic to be described as secondary saturation has been devised. . . . The extraction specialists of years ago and today produced primary saturation and approached secondary saturation in many of their obstreperous patients before beginning to extract teeth. Had they required the relaxation needed in abdominal surgery and possessed the means for using oxygen which we now have, the technique for secondary saturation no doubt would have been developed by them, because they were not afraid of cyanosis, which is the stumbling block in the minds of ether or chloroform-trained anesthetists.

Nitrous oxide anaesthesia between the World Wars.

When nitrous oxide anaesthesia was first introduced it was used primarily for dental anaesthesia. Its use for minor surgery soon followed and there were a few reports of its use for operations such as amputation and mastectomy. Then during the early years of this century it began to be used more and more for major surgery. It was supplemented when necessary, usually with ether. With many of the large series of cases of nitrous oxide anaesthesia reported before the First World War it was not always clear what proportion of them referred to outpatient anaesthesia and what proportion to inpatient anaesthesia, but many of the problems were common to both, at least in kind, if not in degree.

The basic methods of outpatient anaesthesia changed little in the inter-war years. The anaesthesia machines used became, on the whole, more functional and accurate. New inhalation agents came to be used to supplement nitrous oxide and oxygen anaesthesia, and towards the end of the period intravenous induction agents were used. A particular advance in inpatient anaesthesia was the introduction of endotracheal intubation (Rowbotham and Magill, 1921; Magill, 1928), initially for plastic surgery. Some of the techniques before the First World War survived well into the post-Second World War era.

The best known anaesthetic machine in this country today is the so-called Boyle machine. This bears little relation to the "Nitrous Oxide-Oxygen-Ether Outfit" shown by Capt. H. E. G. Boyle, R.A.M.C.(T.) (fig. 1), at the Royal Society of Medicine in 1917 (Boyle, 1917a, 1919) (fig. 2). Boyle's first machine was in fact lent to him by Gwathmey (Boyle, 1917b, c). The "outfit" came in three sizes, and had two cylinders of nitrous oxide and two of oxygen. Each cylinder was provided with a fine adjustment valve and tap, and this was regarded as one of the main features of the machine. It was provided with a water sight feed and an ether bottle, together with rebreathing bag, facepiece and "ordinary three way valves". There was also a spirit lamp for warming the reducing valves of the nitrous oxide cylinders. An analysis of the developments in anaesthetic machines since that time could form a major study of its own.

In 1921, following a visit to Canada and America, Boyle gave a firsthand report of McKesson practising his own method:

He anaesthetized a young woman who was to have her knee opened. She had no preparation at all. McKesson began to get her under, and I noticed that her face was getting a curious gray colour, and that her breathing was becoming shallower, with a little prolonged expiration. Suddenly I heard a noise in the machine, and I realized Dr McKesson was giving oxygen under considerable pressure, so much so, that the patient's cheeks were blown out beneath the facepiece. Gradually she regained her colour, and he said "That is primary saturation". As soon as she became pink, he proceeded to saturate her a second time, and the same process was gone through. I must admit that the anaesthetic was very fine afterwards; he obtained good relaxation with it. I doubt whether we have

a machine in this country which would be capable of giving oxygen under the pressure he delivered it. I asked him subsequently whether this was a method one could teach students. He was perfectly candid about it; he said "No, it is a method for the expert, and for the expert only". He added, "You can do it perfectly well if you want to; I have done it for twelve years, and I believe in it".

McKesson (1926) described the method again on a visit to this country.

From a talk given by McCardie (1923), at the Royal Society of Medicine, it was apparent that even five years after the First World War the merits of the use of oxygen were far from generally recognized. McCardie used gas alone, at which Boyle expressed surprise in the discussion. Bellamy Gardner also expressed surprise that the benefits of nitrous oxide and oxygen were not more generally recognized for dental anaesthesia. Hughes, however, agreed that for most routine cases gas and air gave excellent results, especially by the nasal method. McCardie, in reply, said that he believed it was better for students to be taught to administer nitrous oxide alone because the signs of anaesthesia were so definite; it was used in practice by both

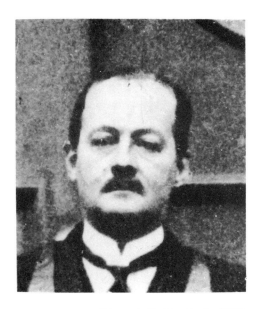

FIG. 1. Henry Edmund Gaskin Boyle (1875–1941) (Hadfield, 1950).

FIG. 2. The original Boyle's anaesthetic machine, described by Boyle as an "outfit".

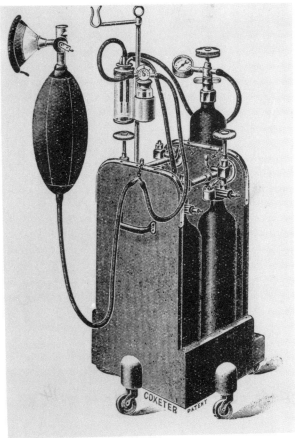

doctor and dentist, and the necessary apparatus was simple. By properly regulated admission of air nearly as good a result could be attained as by the addition of oxygen.

At the next discussion on dental anaesthesia at the Royal Society of Medicine (Gardner and Spain, 1927) both the main speakers advocated the use of gas and oxygen for the majority of cases, and there was no serious argument from the floor. The use of ethyl chloride appeared to be gaining popularity at that time and Magill said that more stress might have been laid on the value of endotracheal anaesthesia in long and difficult dental operations. Then in a further discussion in 1944, the use of cyclopropane (Pinson, 1944; Gillies, 1944), thiopentone (Roberts, 1944), nitrous oxide and oxygen anaesthesia (Marston, 1944) and trichloroethylene (Galley, 1944) were described. Public discussion of "straight gas" or "gas and air" appeared to have disappeared, but Marston (1944) described the initial administration of pure nitrous oxide until the onset of slight cyanosis, twitchings of the palpebral muscles, absence of the conjunctival reflex and automatic respiration. Marston then suggested: "In the average case, if the gases are being delivered at a pressure between 5 and 10 mm Hg, then 5% O_2, gradually increased to 7% and then, if necessary, to 10%, will suffice".

We will probably never know how many patients died needlessly from anoxia in the years before the First World War. In the light of published papers we should not be surprised that Courville (1939) was able to report in some detail on a series of deaths during anaesthesia, due to anoxia, in the inter-war years. Few of his cases, however, can be placed under the heading of "outpatient" anaesthesia. Usually we can survive brief anoxic assaults, but we may never know at what cost in intellectual capacity.

ACKNOWLEDGEMENTS

I am indebted to Dr T. B. Boulton for figure 1. The substance of this article has been abstracted from the introductory chapter of a thesis approved for the degree of M.D. in the University of London. This research has received support from the Wellcome Trust.

REFERENCES

Allen, F. (1912). Nitrous oxid and oxygen anesthesia in major surgery. *J. Amer. med. Ass.*, **58**, 395.

Baldwin, J. F. (1916). Nitrous oxide-oxygen, the most dangerous anesthetic. *Med. Rec.*, **90**, 176.

Boothby, W. M. (1912). Nitrous oxide-oxygen anesthesia with a description of a new apparatus. *Boston med. surg. J.*, **166**, 86.

Boyle, H. E. G. (1917a). Nitrous oxide-oxygen-ether outfit. *Proc. roy. Soc. Med.*, **11**, 30.

—— (1917b). The use of nitrous oxide and oxygen with rebreathing in military surgery. *Lancet*, **2**, 667.

—— (1917c). The use of nitrous oxide and oxygen with rebreathing in military surgery. *Brit. med. J.*, **2**, 653.

—— (1919). Nitrous oxide-oxygen-ether outfit. *Lancet*, **1**, 226.

—— (1921). Report on visit as official representative of the Section of Anaesthetics to the first meeting of the Canadian Society of Anaesthetists at Niagara, and to the Meeting of the American Society of Anesthetists at Boston, in June, 1921. *Proc. roy. Soc. Med.*, **15**, 1.

Cotton, F. J., and Boothby, W. M. (1912). Nitrous oxide-oxygen-ether anesthesia: notes on administration; a perfected apparatus. *Surg. Gynec. Obstet.*, **15**, 281.

Courville, C. B. (1939). *Untoward Effects of Nitrous Oxide Anesthesia with particular reference to Residual Neurologic and Psychiatric Manifestations.* Mountain View, California: Pacific Press Publishing Association.

Crile, G. W. (1911). Nitrous oxide anaesthesia and a note on anoci-association, a new principle in operative surgery. *Surg. Gynec. Obstet.*, **13**, 170.

Foregger, R. (1946). The Rotameter in anesthesia. *Anesthesiology*, **7**, 549.

—— (1952). Early use of Rotameter in anaesthesia. *Brit. J. Anaesth.*, **24**, 187.

Galley, A. H. (1944). Discussion on anaesthesia in the dental chair. *Proc. roy. Soc. Med.*, **38**, 236.

Gardner, H. B., and Spain, I. S. (1927). Discussion on anaesthetics in dental operations. *Proc. roy. Soc. Med.*, **20**, 1297.

Gatch, W. D. (1910). Nitrous-oxid-oxygen anesthesia by the method of rebreathing. *J. Amer. med. Ass.*, **54**, 775.

—— (1911). The use of rebreathing in the administration of anesthetics. *J. Amer. med. Ass.*, **57**, 1593.

Gillies, J. (1944). Discussion on anaesthesia in the dental chair. *Proc. roy. Soc. Med.*, **38**, 235.

Hadfield, C. F. (1950). Eminent anaesthetists. No. 4: H. Edmund G. Boyle. *Brit. J. Anaesth.*, **22**, 107.

Jackson, D. E. (1955). Anesthesia equipment from 1914 to 1954 and experiments leading to its development. *Anesthesiology*, **16**, 953.

Kain, M. L., and Nunn, J. F. (1967). Fresh gas flow and rebreathing in the Magill circuit with spontaneous respiration. *Proc. roy. Soc. Med.*, **60**, 749.

McCardie, W. J. (1923). General anaesthesia in dental surgery. *Proc. roy. Soc. Med.*, **16**, 11.

McKesson, E. I. (1911). Nitrous oxid-oxygen anesthesia with a description of a new apparatus. *Surg. Gynec. Obstet.*, **13**, 456.

—— (1920). Advances in pure nitrous oxid-oxygen anesthesia: with considerations of cyanosis, the signs of anesthesia and a description of the technic of secondary saturation. *Anesth. Suppl. Amer. J. Surg.*, **34**, 98.

—— (1926). Gas-and-oxygen anaesthesia in abdominal surgery; and "secondary saturation". *Proc. roy. Soc. Med.*, **19**, 57.

Magill, I. W. (1928). Endotracheal anaesthesia. *Proc. roy. Soc. Med.*, **22**, 83.

Mandell, A. H. (1911). Nitrous oxid and oxygen anesthesia. *Boston med. surg. J.*, **165**, 592.

Marston, A. D. (1944). Discussion on anaesthesia in the dental chair. *Proc. roy. Soc. Med.*, **38**, 233.

Miller, A. H. (1941). Technical development of gas anesthesia. *Anesthesiology*, **2**, 398.

Mörch, E. T. (1952). Rotameters in anaesthesia. *Brit. J. Anaesth.*, **24**, 196.

Peairs, R. P. (1910). Nitrous oxid and oxygen in major surgery. *J. Amer. med. Ass.*, **54**, 1422.

Pinson, K. B. (1944). Discussion on anaesthesia in the dental chair. *Proc. roy. Soc. Med.*, **38**, 231.

Roberts, F. W. (1944). Discussion on anaesthesia in the dental chair. *Proc. roy. Soc. Med.*, **38**, 232.

Rowbotham, E. S., and Magill, I. (1921). Anaesthetics in the plastic surgery of the face and jaws. *Proc. roy. Soc. Med.*, **14**, 17.

Skeel, R. E. (1913). The selection of the anesthetic for abdominal and pelvic surgery. *Amer. J. Obstet. Dis. Wom.*, **67**, 102.

Smith, W. D. A. (1967). A history of nitrous oxide and oxygen anaesthesia. Part X: The early manufacture, storage and purity of nitrous oxide. *Brit. J. Anaesth.*, **39**, 351.

Teter, C. K. (1909). Thirteen thousand administrations of nitrous oxid with oxygen as an anesthetic. *J. Amer. med. Ass.*, **53**, 448.

—— (1912). The limitations of nitrous oxid with oxygen as a general anesthetic. *J. Amer. med. Ass.*, **59**, 1849.

15

NITROUS OXIDE ANAESTHESIA FOR AMBULATORY PATIENTS*

The object of this paper is to review some anaesthetic techniques, clinical observations and theoretical points which were considered while seeking a satisfactory method for the administration of nitrous oxide to ambulatory patients. Most of the personal observations described were made during anaesthetics which were administered in the casualty department of the Royal South Hants Hospital. For these a Boyle anaesthetic machine was used. Oxygen, nitrous oxide and cyclopropane were available for use in a Magill semiclosed system. Latterly the standard vaporizer bottle for trichloroethylene was replaced by a bottle calibrated by I.C.I. for halothane administration. For dental anaesthesia, an old Walton machine was used with a thick-walled reservoir bag in circuit. The nasal masks were fitted with Coxeter expiratory valves. A vaporizer calibrated for halothane administration was not available. All the anaesthetics administered in the casualty department were recorded in a notebook in as much detail as circumstances permitted, a stopwatch being used to observe times. Latterly a home-made apparatus was used to keep continuous record of respiration during anaesthesia. The pressure changes occurring in the anaesthetic circuit adjacent to the reservoir bag were transmitted to a thin rubber diaphragm. This was connected to a simple ink writer. The recording paper was propelled by clockwork which also actuated a one-minute time marker. An additional marker was used to indicate the times of incidents recorded in the notebook. Deflections of the pen were non-linear with respect to pressure change and full scale deflection was produced by a pressure of about 10 mm Hg under static conditions.

*Based on a paper read before the South-West Metropolitan and Wessex Regional Society of Anaesthetists, on May 30. 1959.

In all the records obtained full deflection nearly always occurred during expiration but the overshoot due to the inertia of the system was not known. When using this apparatus induction of anaesthesia was preceded by inhalations of 100 per cent oxygen while securing an airtight seal between mask and face. The simultaneous administration and recording of anaesthesia in the dental outpatient department was not practicable.

A common technique of nitrous oxide administration and its modification following experience with pigmented patients.

The author was trained to induce anaesthesia in the casualty department with 100 per cent nitrous oxide until the onset of "regular respiration" and then to use a mixture of nitrous oxide and oxygen. The emphasis was more upon the maintenance of anaesthesia using nitrous oxide than upon the maintenance of adequate oxygenation. Experience of anaesthetizing pigmented patients in Jamaica led to a modification of this technique. It was found difficult to assess cyanosis through pigmented skin. Furthermore, many Jamaicans were so anaemic that concentrations of reduced haemoglobin sufficient to exhibit cyanosis were barely possible without dangerous hypoxia. There was also the possibility of precipitating a sickle cell crisis (Golding, 1956). To allow for these conditions, and to avoid excessive hypoxia, induction was started with 6 breaths of 100 per cent nitrous oxide and continued with 2 litres of oxygen and not more than 10 litres of nitrous oxide per minute. If anaesthesia was still inadequate, trichloroethylene was introduced as a supplement.

The dangers of hypoxia.

The dangers of hypoxia during anaesthesia have been emphasized. Bedford (1955) observed that in a group of 1,193 patients over the age of

50 years who had had operations, 120 showed some degree of mental deterioration, while 29 had become demented. Discussing hypoxia as a possible cause, he mentioned the occasional catastrophic effects of anoxia during nitrous oxide anaesthesia, which had been vigorously emphasized by Courville (1955) and by Bourne, J. G. (1952). Bourne stressed the inevitable hypoxia associated with brief nitrous oxide anaesthetics and quoted Macintosh as having knowledge of five deaths, within as many months, due to the effects of such hypoxia upon the myocardium. Bourne, J. G. (1957) has also remarked upon the hazard of fainting in the dental chair. Bourne, W. (1936) has shown that hypoxia may produce reversible yet undesirable damage, such as that suggested by the impairment of hepatic function produced by nitrous oxide with cyanosis

The partial pressures of oxygen in anaesthetic mixtures compared with those in air at various altitudes.

Hypoxia occurring during nitrous oxide anaes-

thesia may be put into perspective by relating given mixtures of nitrous oxide and oxygen, inhaled at sea level, with the altitudes at which atmospheric air would contain the same partial pressures of oxygen. For example, the mixture of 2 litres of oxygen with 10 litres of nitrous oxide per minute, described above for the maintenance of anaesthesia, allows for a minimum inspired oxygen concentration of 16.7 per cent. The partial pressure of this corresponds with that in air at 6,000 feet.

The relationships between anaesthetic mixtures at sea level, partial pressures of oxygen and altitude are indicated in figure 1. This has been derived from tables (Dittmer and Grebe, 1958). It can be seen that in a mixture of 10 litres of nitrous oxide with 1 litre of oxygen (or 9 per cent oxygen), the partial pressure of oxygen is the same as that in air at an altitude of 22,500 feet. At this height above sea level even the fittest of acclimatized mountaineers become dyspnoeic upon the slightest exertion. A patient inspiring such

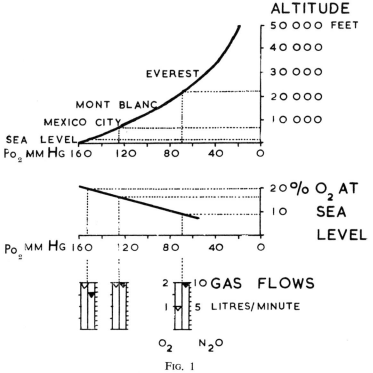

FIG. 1

Altitudes at which the partial pressure of inspired oxygen would be the same as that of given nitrous oxide and oxygen mixtures at sea level.

a mixture during anaesthesia would also be subjected to the resistances of an anaesthetic circuit, in particular to that of the expiratory valve. To what height would it be reasonable suddenly to project a patient with whom one has made only the briefest acquaintance, within whom may lurk unsuspected disease, and whose physiological powers of adaptation may be limited?

The induction of "amnalgesia" using 100 per cent nitrous oxide.

With the object of avoiding the hazards of hypoxia, Tom (1956) applied what Klock (1951, 1955) had earlier described as "amnalgesia" to anaesthesia for dental extractions. In Tom's technique induction is commenced using a few breaths of 100 per cent nitrous oxide and is then continued with 15 per cent oxygen. The state of "amnalgesia" is produced after about 40 breaths, and is often preceded by a hesitation in breathing. (Tom claimed to correct this by verbal encouragement to "keep blowing.") Breathing then becomes free and regular and after a few more breaths the patient is ready. Dental extraction is accompanied by some movement and occasionally by phonation. This technique is similar to that described above and used by the author for anaesthesia in the casualty department, except that Tom did not describe the use of supplementary agents, such as trichloroethylene. In practice the technique may permit more hypoxia than might be expected to occur during the maintenance of anaesthesia with 15 per cent oxygen, since the calibration of apparatus used in dental departments may be grossly inaccurate (Bourne, 1960).

The induction of anaesthesia using 100 per cent nitrous oxide following pre-oxygenation.

Whereas Tom sought to avoid dangerous hypoxia by administering not less than 15 per cent oxygen during the maintenance of anaesthesia, Mostert (1958) claimed to achieve safety by using pre-oxygenation. He affirmed that 85 to 90 per cent nitrous oxide was required to produce anaesthesia and that 20.93 per cent oxygen could not be allowed for short anaesthetics. He therefore advocated pre-oxygenation for 2 minutes in order to replace 98 per cent of the nitrogen in the lungs by oxygen and so provide a reserve of oxygen to cover the period of nitrous oxide

induction. Following pre-oxygenation 100 per cent nitrous oxide was given for 1 minute at a flow rate greater than the patient's assumed minute volume. This was stated to provide adequate anaesthesia within the next half-minute. Breath-holding was said to be rare. For 15 to 30 seconds, while the surgeon started, 10 to 15 per cent oxygen was administered. This was followed by 20 per cent oxygen. Supplementary agents were added if the operation lasted for more than 2 to 3 minutes.

Considering the many differences between patients, the set time of 1 minute for 100 per cent nitrous oxide inhalation seemed too rigid. An alternative suggested itself in the administration of 100 per cent nitrous oxide for as long as the patient would respond, by nodding, to the anaesthetist counting aloud each breath taken (see "Loss of consciousness, amnesia and analgesia" below). This was tried once.

Case history.

The patient was a tall active female of 67 years, requiring reduction of a Colles fracture. She nodded in response to the counting aloud of 25 breaths during induction, but at this stage cyanosis was detected. It was realized afterwards that those 25 breaths had taken nearly 2 minutes. Gas flows were then altered to 6 litres of nitrous oxide and two litres of oxygen per minute. There was a short period of apnoea but cyanosis soon disappeared as respiration resumed. Respiration then became obstructed and an airway was inserted. The conditions for operation were excellent. The management of anaesthesia could have been much safer.

The latent period between the inhalation and the action of an anaesthetic agent.

One obvious factor overlooked in the above reasoning was the delay between the inhalation of a gas, its transport in solution and its effective action upon the central nervous system. To investigate this, 15 patients, of average age 38 years, were asked to signal, by raising a hand, the very first onset of subjective change after inhaling a single deep breath of nitrous oxide. The delays ranged from 15 to 55 seconds and averaged 32 seconds. These figures may be compared with the figure of 35 seconds given by Wylie (1953) as the time taken for 75 per cent nitrous oxide with oxygen to become fully effective when used in midwifery; and with the 12 to 15 seconds given by Guedel (1953) as the time of passage of blood from the lungs to the brain. The author experienced a delay of 20 seconds between taking a single breath of nitrous oxide and noting any subjective effects. This was consistent with the half-dozen breaths actually counted before appreciating any change during a nitrous oxide induction (see below). No subjective effects followed the inhalation of a single deep breath of 100 per cent nitrogen.

A comparison of induction techniques using nitrous oxide without and with pre-oxygenation.

Apart from the knowledge of the composition of gases inhaled by the patient, the only clinical guide to alveolar oxygen tension in a normal patient is peripheral cyanosis. If it be accepted that cyanosis is indicative of excessive hypoxia, then there is no clinical warning of its approach during a nitrous oxide induction. Since measurement of breath-by-breath alveolar composition is not practicable during anaesthesia in outpatient departments, an attempt has been made to calculate approximate values that might be expected

to occur during the induction of a hypothetical patient by each of two techniques. The results are shown in figure 2. Allowance has been made for the dilution of 3,000 ml of functional residual air with an effective tidal volume of 300 ml at a respiratory rate of 15 per minute; for the solution and transport away from the alveoli during each respiratory cycle of 20 ml of oxygen plus the volume of nitrous oxide calculated to be soluble in one-fifteenth of a cardiac output of 5,000 ml per minute, at the calculated prevailing partial pressure (blood/gas partition coefficient was taken as 0.47); and for the replacement of these dissolved gases by carbon dioxide and dead-space gas from the previous expiration. The figures chosen and calculated may have a very doubtful relationship with the true state of affairs existing in any given patient, but they should give some idea of the relative orders and patterns of change in alveolar composition when the techniques of Tom and Mostert are used. The results suggest that there is a greater margin of safety after pre-

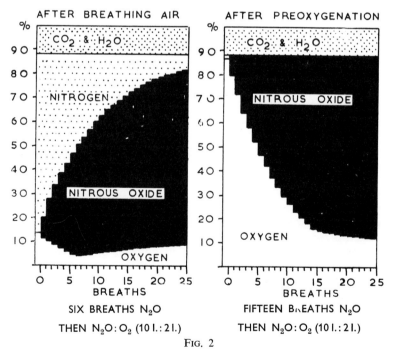

FIG. 2

See text. Calculated breath-by-breath alveolar gas concentrations during induction of nitrous oxide anaesthesia, in a hypothetical patient, by two techniques.

oxygenation. When induction is started with six breaths of 100 per cent nitrous oxide without pre-oxygenation hypoxia may contribute to loss of consciousness, especially in those patients with whom contact is quickly lost (see "Loss of consciousness, amnesia and analgesia" below). The justification for this short period of hypoxia is open to question.

Loss of consciousness, amnesia and analgesia.

The author has personally experienced an induction by Tom's technique for a dental extraction.

From the start the author counted each breath to himself. A subjective change was noted at the 6th or 7th breath. At the 12th breath the anaesthetist was heard to say, "He seems to be taking it all right". At the 13th breath there was cerebration to the extent of realizing that 13 was an "unlucky number", of calculating that twice 13 was 26 and of wondering whether breaths could be counted up to that number. In retrospect there was no memory of counting beyond 13. Upon recovery there was an awareness of an indistinct figure who clarified into the anaesthetist. The author was soon feeling fully awake, standing up and asking how long it had taken. Before this, however, he had apparently asked the anaesthetist, "Who are you?" Of this there is no memory. He had then made an exclamation which cannot be remembered with certainty. Was the author still unconscious at this time and talking like someone talking in his sleep, or was he subsequently just amnesic?

Following this experience, breath counting was used to find out when patients lost consciousness during induction of nitrous oxide anaesthesia. Each breath taken by the patient was counted aloud by the anaesthetist and the patient was asked to nod slightly in response. Upon recovery enquiry was made of the last count heard. Figure 3 shows the results arranged from above downwards in order of the number of nods observed. Each horizontal stick represents an anaesthetic. Its length indicates the number of nods observed by the anaesthetist and the black portion indicates the number of nods remembered by the patient. There was much variation. On average just over half the nods were remembered. Counts were not always definite. Some patients stopped nodding early but resumed on command. Nodding sometimes became unrelated to counting. Some patients began shaking their heads instead of nodding and occasionally nodding became so exaggerated as to require restraint. The last number remembered was not always definite, a

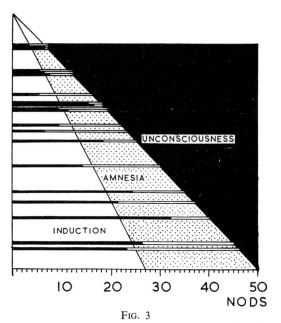

FIG. 3

See text. Number of nods made by 20 patients in response to the anaesthetist counting aloud each breath taken during induction of nitrous oxide anaesthesia.

lower figure often being given soon after return to consciousness than could be given later. That patients were in fact responding to the spoken voice and not nodding automatically with respiration was sometimes checked by asking them to shake the head instead of nod. Compliance with this request was variable and noncompliance was of uncertain significance, as shown by the following example.

Case history.

An engineer of 44 years nodded 25 times. The later nods looked automatic. He did not comply with the request to shake his head. Other observers considered that he had responded satisfactorily to only 21 or 22 counts. In fact he not only remembered counts up to the 25th, thereby demonstrating negligible amnesia, but he also remembered being asked to shake his head. He could not explain why he had not done so.

Any hesitation in breathing that occurred was always noted after the last nod. It seems unlikely that exhortations to "keep blowing" would have made any difference.

If this experiment were to be repeated with the lower partial pressures of nitrous oxide commonly used in abdominal and thoracic surgery, it might be found that we are more often "amnalgetists" than anaesthetists. Indeed, Gray (1954) and Rosen

(1959) have made relevant observations. Gray described a level of narcosis at which subjects obey commands yet afterwards assert that they have been unconscious. He also found that onset of analgesia was close in time to loss of consciousness. Rosen was able to establish contact, in some instances, with patients stabilized on being given nitrous oxide and oxygen mixtures containing up to 73 per cent nitrous oxide. Almost half the patients with whom good contact was made had total amnesia.

The late onset of analgesia referred to by Gray had been suspected from observation of those patients in the casualty department who had preoperative pain. Relief from pain during induction of anaesthesia was denied by headshaking even when attempts were made to ameliorate the pain by suggestion. Although Chapman, Arrowood and Beecher (1943) concluded that 20 per cent nitrous oxide with oxygen had an analgesic potency equivalent to morphine 16 mg against pain produced by radiant heat and ischaemia, this effect took 10 minutes to reach maximum. "Gas" and hypoxia, however, are still combined in midwifery in the use of self-administered gas and air.

The use of supplementary agents.

The indications for the use of particular gas mixtures and supplementary anaesthetic agents vary with the anaesthetist. An examination of the casualty operations register at the Royal South Hants Hospital was made to ascertain how frequently nitrous oxide and oxygen mixtures were in fact administered with and without supplementary agents. Over a 17-month period 45 per cent of 1,259 nitrous oxide anaesthetics were administered without the use of supplementary agents. A more detailed analysis was made of a group of 131 personally administered anaesthetics, 48 per cent of which were not supplemented. Anaesthetics were given twice as often for bone and joint surgery as for scissions and sutures, but supplementation of nitrous oxide was required twice as frequently for the latter as for the former. This was presumably related to the intensity and duration of the surgical stimuli, and perhaps also to ease of restraint. The greatest incidence of bone and joint surgery was in the early and later years of life. The early years involved males more than females and the later years females more than

males. Those patients who were over the age of 50 years were more easily anaesthetized by nitrous oxide and oxygen alone than those below this age. The incidence of scissions and sutures declined steadily with increasing age.

Walsh (1958) described the use of halothane as a supplement to nitrous oxide anaesthesia for dental extractions. Subsequently he introduced it to the casualty department of the Royal South Hants Hospital. Previously trichloroethylene had been the most favoured supplementary agent. A technique tried by the author latterly was to induce anaesthesia with 8 litres of nitrous oxide and 2 litres of oxygen per minute with 0.15 to 0.3 per cent halothane. The halothane administration was then stopped, maintained or increased according to the reaction of the patient to surgical stimulation. The cost of using halothane in the casualty department was about two shillings per anaesthetic. Impressions from brief experience with this technique suggest that induction is not unpleasant and that it takes about 5 minutes. Loss of consciousness appears to be rapid after allowing for the delay between first inhalation and effective action. Restraint may be needed in the early stages but relaxation soon follows. There may be some movement upon surgical stimulation. Return to consciousness is a little slower than after nitrous oxide and oxygen anaesthesia. The time at which recovery is complete is difficult to assess but it appears to be much later. The ears remain flushed and nystagamus may be observed even after the patient has risen from the table and professed to be fully recovered.

The following case report provides a warning about the use of this particular technique for patients in the dental chair.

Case history.

A tall, fit, tough welder in his early twenties attended for dental extraction with a note to the effect that it was not possible to anaesthetize him with nitrous oxide. The halothane technique was tried using an uncalibrated vaporizer. The anaesthetic appeared to be entirely satisfactory. The patient recovered consciousness quickly, smiled and expressed surprise and pleasure at the ease with which the operation had been carried out. Shortly afterwards he slumped in the dental chair and lost consciousness. He was pink. His superficial temporal pulse was still palpable but rather slow and of low tension. He was placed in a horizontal position, whereupon he repeated the performance of waking up, smiling, talking, sitting up and slumping. After being kept horizontal for a period there was no further trouble.

CONCLUSION

An ideal anaesthetic for an ambulatory patient should please the patient, the surgeon and the anaesthetist. It should have a high margin of safety and recovery should be complete and immediate. These requirements would seem to be most nearly met when the least hypoxic nitrous oxide and oxygen techniques prove adequate without supplementation using more potent drugs, but this requires more patience than when hypoxic methods are used. If supplementary agents are needed they should be used sparingly.

SUMMARY

Some techniques for inducing and maintaining nitrous oxide anaesthesia are reviewed with particular reference to the oxygen content of inspired and of alveolar gases. A method of recording observations during such anaesthesia is mentioned. The use of supplementary anaesthetic agents is considered.

Attention is drawn to the variable latent period between the inhalation of an anaesthetic agent and the onset of subjective effects.

A breath-counting technique for assessing the time of loss of consciousness and of amnesia is described and reference is made to the circumstances of analgesia, amnesia and loss of consciousness.

The register of anaesthetics administered in a particular casualty department is examined with particular regard to the use of supplementary agents in relation to the type of surgery performed and the age and sex of the patients.

ACKNOWLEDGMENTS

The author wishes to thank Dr. R. P. W. Shackleton for his encouragement and permission to publish this paper. He is also particularly appreciative of the patient co-operation of Sister D. S. Wilkes and her staff and of the succession of casualty officers in the casualty department of the Royal South Hants Hospital from 1957 to 1959.

REFERENCES

Bedford, P. D. (1955). Adverse cerebral effects of anaesthesia in old people. *Lancet*, **2**, 259.

Bourne, J. G. (1952). Cyclopropane anaesthesia for dental extraction and other surgery in outpatients. *Lancet*, **2**, 705.

—— (1957). Fainting and cerebral damage. *Lancet*, **2**, 499.

—— (1960). *Nitrous Oxide in Dentistry: Its Danger and alternatives*, appendix F. London: Lloyd-Luke (Medical Books).

Bourne, W. (1936). Anaesthetics and liver function. *Amer. J. Surg.*, **34**, 486.

Chapman, W. P., Arrowood, J. G., and Beecher, H. K. (1943). The analgetic effects of low concentrations of nitrous oxide compared in man with morphine sulphate. *J. Clin. Invest.*, **1**, 871.

Courville, C. B. (1955). Narcosis and cerebral anoxia. *Anesth. and Analges.*, **34**, 61.

Dittmer, D. S., and Grebe, R. M. (1958). *Handbook of Respiration*, p. 2. Philadelphia and London: W. B. Saunders Company.

Golding, J. S. R. (1956). Bone changes in sickle cell anaemia. *Ann. roy. Coll. Surg.*, **19**, 296.

Gray, T. C. (1954). Disintegration of the nervous system. *Ann. roy. Coll. Surg.*, **15**, 402.

Guedel, A. E. (1953). *Inhalation Anaesthesia*, 2nd ed., p. 5. New York: Macmillan.

Klock, J. H. (1951). "Amnalgesia": a technique of supplemental anaesthesia in oral surgery. *Anesth. and Analges.*, **30**, 151.

—— (1955). New concept of nitrous oxide anaesthesia. *Curr. Res. Anesth.*, **34**, 379.

Mostert, J. W. (1958). Nitrous oxide anaesthesia without harm. *Brit. med. J.*, **1**, 502.

Rosen, J. (1959). Hearing tests during anaesthesia with nitrous oxide and relaxants. *Acta Anaesth. Scand.*, **3**, 1.

Tom, A. (1956). An innovation in technique for dental gas. *Brit. med. J.*, **1**, 1085.

Walsh, R. S. (1958). Halothane as an adjuvant to nitrous oxide in outpatient dental anaesthesia. *Brit. J. Anaesth.*, **30**, 578.

Wylie, W. D. (1953). *The Practical Management of Pain in Labour*, p. 73. London: Lloyd-Luke (Medical Books).

INDEX*

*f denotes a figure and n a footnote.